Mosby's Color Atlas and Text of

Gastroenterology and Liver Disease

Commissioning Editor: Laurence Hunter
Project Development: Fiona Conn
Project Management: Frances Affleck
Design Direction: Judith Wright
Page Layout: Alan Palfreyman

Mosby's Color Atlas and Text of

Gastroenterology and Liver Disease

Dr Richard J. Aspinall BSc MBChB MRCP
Lecturer in Medicine,
Gastroenterology Unit
Hammersmith Hospital
London
UK

Dr Simon D. Taylor-Robinson MD MRCP FRCP
Senior Lecturer and Consultant Physician
Division of Medicine
Imperial College School of Medicine
St Mary's Hospital and Hammersmith Hospital
London
UK

Illustrated by Joanna Cameron MMAA RMIP

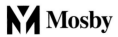 Mosby

EDINBURGH LONDON NEW YORK OXFORD PHILADELPHIA ST LOUIS SYDNEY TORONTO 2002

MOSBY
An affiliate of Elsevier Science Limited

© Mosby International Limited 2002

First published 2002
Reprinted 2003

ISBN 0 723 43103 5

British Library Cataloguing in Publication Data
A catalogue record for this book is available from the British Library

Library of Congress Cataloging in Publication Data
A catalog record for this book is available from the Library of Congress

Note
Medical knowledge is constantly changing. As new information becomes
available, changes in treatment, procedures, equipment and the use of
drugs become necessary. The authors and the publishers have, as far as it is
possible, taken care to ensure that the information given in this text is
accurate and up-to-date. However, readers are strongly advised to confirm
that the information, especially with regard to drug usage, complies with
the latest legislation and standards of practice.

ELSEVIER
SCIENCE

your source for books,
journals and multimedia
in the health sciences

www.elsevierhealth.com

The
publisher's
policy is to use
**paper manufactured
from sustainable forests**

Printed in China

Contents

Foreword

There are plenty of textbooks and some atlases of gastroenterology, but fewer of hepatology. In this new enterprise, you have the two together on both subjects. The coverage is comprehensive and should attract the specialist registrar studying for accreditation and the consultant needing re-accreditation. *Mosby's Color Atlas and Text of Gastroenterology and Liver Disease* covers medical, surgical, radiological and pathological aspects in a very accessible format. I have no doubt that this book will successfully fill a gap in the market and prove popular with undergraduate and postgraduate alike.

Professor Howard Thomas
Imperial College School of Medicine,
London

Preface

This book was born out of a need to combine both clinical material and relevant anatomical, embryological and basic science material with the more visual aspects of gastroenterology and liver disease that today's doctors in training require. Constantly developing technology dictates that new diagnostic media are coming into clinical usage all the time. We have attempted to provide the reader of this book with insight into new diagnostic techniques and have provided information on those that are still research tools at present, but may well become commonplace in this new century.

The chapters have been arranged with an embryological format into foregut, midgut and hindgut, with separate chapters on the liver, the pancreas, the systemic manifestations of gastrointestinal disease, and the gastrointestinal manifestations of systemic disease. Each chapter starts with the relevant anatomical and embryological information in the appropriate area of the gastrointestinal tract and then a problem-based approach to diagnosis has been adopted. Therefore, we have discussed the common symptoms afflicting patients presenting in the typical gastrointestinal clinic or emergency department. We have then suggested appropriate pathways of investigation and documented rarer 'special case' investigations, before detailing individual diseases and their management.

Each chapter is accompanied by endoscopic, histological, radiological and diagrammatic information which may act as an *aide-mémoire*, or else as a useful means to diagnosis for newcomers to the field.

We hope that the book will be accessible not only to gastroenterology and hepatology doctors in training, but also to those who may need a readily available reference point without resorting to a larger text. We also believe that our *Color Atlas and Text* will be useful to specialist nurses, radiologists and pathologists who wish to read further in this area, and of course, to enquiring medical students.

We are particularly grateful to Professor Howard Thomas for providing the Foreword to this book and to all those who contributed clinical material and artwork.

Richard Aspinall
Simon Taylor-Robinson

Acknowledgements

In the preparation of this book, we have received invaluable help from numerous individuals at the hospitals of the Imperial College School of Medicine and the University of London. We particularly wish to thank the following:

Hammersmith Hospital
Dr Massimo Pignatelli (Department of Histopathology); Dr Tony Chu (Dermatology); Mr John Spencer and Dr Mohammed Aslam (Surgery); Dr David Swirsky (Haematology); Professor Graeme Bydder, Dr Nandita de Souza, Dr Jane Cox, Dr Alastair Hall and Adreanna Williams (MRI Unit); Dr Martin Blomley, Dr James Jackson, Dr Chris Harvey, Dr Walter Curati, Dr Claire Cousins and Kim Williams (Radiology); Jenny Butler-Barnes and Nayna Patel (Ultrasound); Professor Mike Peters and Daphne Glass (Nuclear Medicine); Professor Philip Hawkins (Immunological Medicine); Dr Gary Frost and Dr Louise Thomas (Clinical Nutrition); Dr Jason Wilson (Anaesthesia); Zeinab Nadiadi, Dr Neil Jackson and Dr John Martin (Gastroenterology); Martina Dineen, Heena Khagram, Teresa Darowska and Ciesta de Raux (Endoscopy Unit); Margarete Haywood (Medicine).

St Mary's Hospital
Dr Rob Goldin and Dr Marjorie Walker (Histopathology); Dr Mike de Jode, Dr Gabrielle Lamb, Sarah Hockley-Refson, Alison Gwynne-Davis, Joanne Kelly, Dr Wladyslaw Gedroyc (iMR Unit); Dr Janice Main, Mary Crossey, Susan Jackson and Teresita Roguin (Medicine).

Charing Cross Hospital
Dr Andrew Thillainayagam and Dr Marta Carpani de Kaski (Gastroenterology).

St Bartholomew's Hospital
Dr Alison McLean (Radiology).

We wish to express our admiration for the patience and encouragement of our publishers, Mosby, and in particular, Fiona Conn, Maria Stewart, Gina Almond, Claire Hooper, Laurence Hunter and Richard Furn.

Richard J. Aspinall
Simon Taylor-Robinson

chapter 1

The Foregut

STRUCTURE AND FUNCTION

EMBRYOLOGY AND ANATOMY

In embryological terms, the digestive tract is divided into three parts: the *foregut*, comprising the oesophagus, stomach and the proximal part of the duodenum; the *midgut*, from the distal half of the duodenum to the distal third of the colon; and the *hindgut*, which forms the remainder of the colon and rectum (**Fig. 1.1**).

The oesophagus

The oesophagus connects the pharynx to the stomach and is approximately 25 cm in length. Its lower end is approximately 40 cm from the incisor teeth, a useful measurement to remember when performing an endoscopy. At the upper end, the contractions of the cricopharyngeus muscle form the upper oesophageal sphincter. The body of the oesophagus has two muscle layers – an inner circular layer and an outer longitudinal layer, which contract and relax during peristalsis. The upper third of the oesophagus is composed of striated muscle; the lower third consists of smooth muscle, and in the middle third there is an overlapping region of both muscle types. Between the muscle layers there is a myenteric plexus which coordinates swallowing and peristaltic activity. There is a rich autonomic nerve supply and the vagus provides both parasympathetic and motor fibres. The mucosal lining is made up of stratified squamous epithelium, but this changes to columnar epithelium at or near the gastro-oesophageal junction. Unlike at the pharyngeal end, the lower oesophageal sphincter (LOS) is not formed from a distinct muscle, but is a physiological entity with high resting muscle tone at the distal end of the oesophagus in order to prevent or minimise gastro-oesophageal reflux. However, anatomical studies have defined a muscular component.

Congenital abnormalities of the oesophagus include oesophageal atresia (**Fig. 1.2**) and oesophageal stenosis.

The stomach

Anatomically, the stomach can be divided into the fundus, the corpus or body, and the antrum. The short gastric vessels supply the majority of the fundus with blood, while the gastroepiploics supply the rest of the stomach (**Fig. 1.3(a)**). The lymphatic drainage generally follows the blood supply, draining to regional lymph nodes in the greater and lesser omentum. There are three layers of smooth muscle in the stomach wall: an inner oblique layer, an outer longitudinal layer and a circular layer between them (**Fig. 1.3(b)**). The stomach is innervated with a myenteric plexus which includes a profuse autonomic supply, including parasympathetic fibres from the vagus nerve. The mucosal lining of the stomach forms thick folds or rugae. It has a honeycombed appearance and contains

The digestive tract

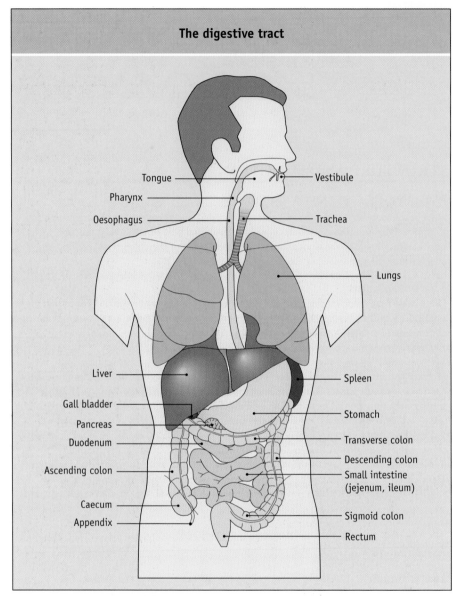

Tongue

Pharynx

Oesophagus

Vestibule

Trachea

Lungs

Liver

Gall bladder

Pancreas

Duodenum

Ascending colon

Caecum

Appendix

Spleen

Stomach

Transverse colon

Descending colon

Small intestine
(jejunum, ileum)

Sigmoid colon

Rectum

Fig. 1.1 *The digestive tract.*

specialised glands (**Fig. 1.4**). The gastro-oesophageal sphincter is at the top of the stomach, with the pyloric sphincter at the lower end, formed from a thickening of the circular muscle coat.

The commonest developmental abnormality is congenital hypertrophic pyloric stenosis, where there is considerable narrowing of the pyloric canal owing to hypertrophy of the circular smooth muscle.

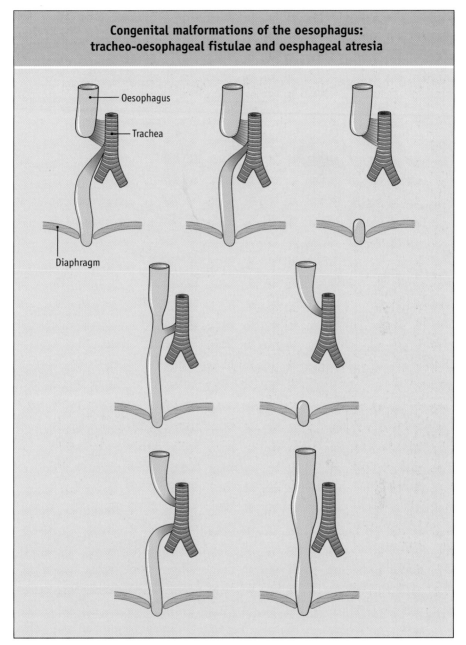

Congenital malformations of the oesophagus: tracheo-oesophageal fistulae and oesphageal atresia

Oesophagus

Trachea

Diaphragm

Fig. 1.2 *Congenital malformations of the oesophagus. Oesophageal atresia occurs in a number of different forms, but most commonly with an associated tracheo-oesophageal fistula.*

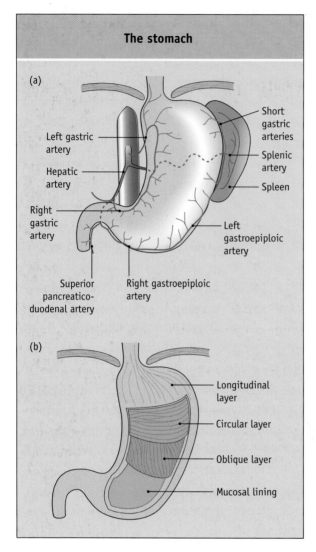

Fig. 1.3 *The stomach: anatomical aspects. (a) The arterial blood supply. Ischaemia of the stomach is rare owing to its profuse blood supply from numerous sources. (b) The muscular layers of the stomach wall.*

The duodenum

The duodenum is formed from the distal part of the foregut and the proximal midgut, the embryonic liver and pancreas developing from 'entodermic buds' or outgrowths of the gut lining from the embryonic duodenum. When fully formed, the duodenum has a C shape, with the pancreas situated in its concavity (**Fig. 1.5**). The biliary and pancreatic ducts empty into the second part of the duodenum at the ampulla of Vater.

PHYSIOLOGY

The oesophagus

The upper oesophageal sphincter relaxes and then the muscle in the body of the oesophagus contracts involuntarily in a wave of peristalsis, following the voluntary

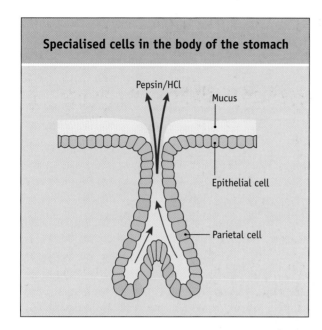

Specialised cells in the body of the stomach

Pepsin/HCl

Mucus

Epithelial cell

Parietal cell

Fig. 1.4 *Specialised cells in the body of the stomach. The various cells within the gastric glands have specific functions. Parietal (oxyntic) cells secrete hydrochloric acid and intrinsic factor. The cells above and between the parietal cells are a mixture of mucus-secreting cells, enterochromaffin cells and chief cells. Pepsinogen, the precursor of the enzyme pepsin, is produced by the chief cells.*

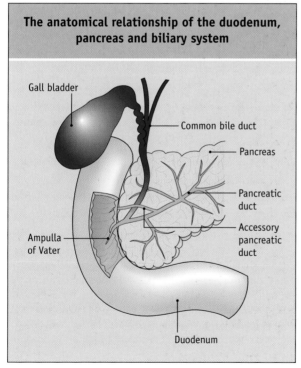

The anatomical relationship of the duodenum, pancreas and biliary system

Gall bladder

Common bile duct

Pancreas

Pancreatic duct

Accessory pancreatic duct

Ampulla of Vater

Duodenum

Fig. 1.5 *The anatomical relationship of the duodenum, pancreas and biliary system.*

The functions of the stomach	
Motor function	Reservoir for food 'storage' to regulate digestion downstream Mixing of food with gastric secretions Controlled release of food into small bowel
Luminal secretion	Hydrochloric acid Pepsin(ogen) Mucus Bicarbonate Intrinsic factor Water
Endocrine secretion	Gastrin Somatostatin

Fig. 1.6 *The functions of the stomach.*

initiation of swallowing. The contractions propel food boluses down the oesophagus. The LOS, normally an area of high resting muscular tone, relaxes to allow the passage of the bolus into the stomach.

The stomach

The stomach has a number of functions (**Fig. 1.6**). The body of the stomach contains oxyntic mucosa, richly supplied with gastric glands containing parietal cells which secrete both hydrochloric acid and intrinsic factor. Some of these glands are also present in the fundus. They also contain mucus-secreting cells and pepsinogen-secreting chief cells. This protease precursor is converted to the active enzyme, pepsin, in the stomach lumen in the presence of hydrochloric acid. The contributory neural, hormonal and paracrine factors influencing the secretion of gastric acid are shown in **Fig. 1.7**. Parietal cells bear receptors for acetylcholine (muscarinic), gastrin and histamine, all of which can stimulate gastric acid secretion. The gastric body contains significant numbers of enterochromaffin (ECL) cells, which secrete histamine to act in a paracrine manner on parietal cells. The ECL cells release histamine when stimulated by acetylcholine or gastrin.

The antrum contains G cells which secrete gastrin (in response to the presence of food in the lumen as well as neural and neuronal release of GRP – gastrin releasing peptide) and cells which produce mucus.

The duodenum

The duodenal mucosa contains Brunner's glands; these secrete an alkaline mucus which neutralises the acidic gastric contents. Bile and pancreatic juices in the duodenum also perform a similar function. The neural and hormonal mechanisms governing the digestion of proteins, carbohydrates and fats are summarised in chapter 2.

Pancreatic proteases are secreted in inactive form and only activated in the duodenum and small intestine by the presence of enterokinase, an endopeptidase produced by small intestinal villi.

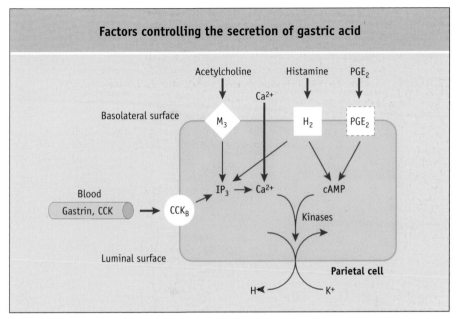

Fig. 1.7 *Factors controlling the secretion of gastric acid from the oxyntic parietal cell. Each of the major secretagogues has its own membrane-bound receptor. Gastrin stimulates acid secretion via receptors that are also sensitive to cholecystokinin (CCK) with which it shares some homology. Acetylcholine (acting via M_3 muscarinic receptors) and histamine (via H_2 receptors), like gastrin, are able to elevate intracellular calcium levels by generating inositol trisphosphate (IP_3). Histamine additionally causes an increase in cyclic adenosine monophosphate (cAMP) levels, which can be opposed by mucosal prostaglandin E_2 (PGE_2). Elevated levels of these second messengers lead to a kinase-dependent activation of the apical hydrogen/potassium ATPase pump resulting in the net secretion of acid into the lumen.*

SYMPTOMS AND SIGNS

Difficulty in swallowing

Dysphagia or difficulty in swallowing is a worrying symptom which merits further investigation because it is invariably caused by organic disease. A proper history should be taken (**Fig. 1.8**) from the patient and this should establish whether there is actually an inability or impairment of deglutition (suggesting dysmotility of the cricopharyngeus muscle) or whether the patient feels retrosternal holdup of food at any point after swallowing has taken place (suggesting an oesophageal stricture).

A long history of heartburn is more likely to point to a benign peptic stricture, but the *de novo* development of dysphagia to solids in the absence of reflux symptoms may indicate a more sinister underlying cause. Regurgitation of solids or liquids may suggest achalasia or perhaps a pharyngeal pouch. Patients with functional dysphagia or '*globus hystericus*' can generally be discerned since they usually complain of a constant sensation of a 'lump in the throat'.

The differential diagnosis of dysphagia	
Peptic oesophageal stricture	Usually gradual onset Preceding reflux symptoms Solids > liquids (at least initially)
Achalasia/oesophageal spasm	Usually sudden onset May be intermittent Difficulty in belching in achalasia +/− Reflux symptoms in spasm Solids = liquids
Globus syndrome	Intermittent symptoms Discomfort unrelated to meals 'Lumps in throat'
Oesophageal malignancy	Weight loss common Gradual onset May not have reflux symptoms Solids > liquids Often painful
Pharyngeal/oesophageal pouch	May have regurgitation

Fig. 1.8 *The differential diagnosis of dysphagia.*

Odynophagia and oesophageal spasm

A proper history is very helpful in discriminating the cause of oesophageal pain. Odynophagia is a severe, intense pain on swallowing and is often a feature of conditions which ulcerate the oesophagus such as cytomegalovirus or *Herpes simplex* oesophagitis.

Oesophageal spasm can mimic cardiac pain almost entirely, even to the point of seeming to be induced by exercise (since acid reflux may be precipitated, which then causes the spasm). This is therefore a diagnostic dilemma and most patients generally go along the route of cardiological investigation before they are referred to the gastroenterologist.

Simple heartburn as a result of gastro-oesophageal reflux may be distinguished from other causes of oesophageal pain as it is usually made worse by bending or lying flat.

Regurgitation

Accurate history-taking can be helpful. Individuals with pharyngeal pouches often complain of dysphagia when the pouch is full and can regurgitate food in an undigested form at variable intervals, even days after the original meal. Regurgitation is a feature of achalasia. A column of food may be present in the oesophagus which puts the patient at risk of aspiration. Patients may complain of 'asthma' as a presenting symptom or dysphagia to both solids and liquids.

Dyspepsia and reflux

The most frequent presenting complaint is of 'indigestion', by which most patients mean epigastric discomfort and heartburn, often accompanied by belching. Individuals are commonly overweight and have their symptoms exacerbated on bending over or at night when they lie flat, particularly when they have eaten heavily. Significant gastro-oesophageal

Causes of nausea and vomiting	
Gastrointestinal	Gastric outlet obstruction Intestinal obstruction Pancreatitis Gastritis – viral, alcohol, biliary Toxins – e.g. staphylococcal Diabetic gastroparesis Peptic ulceration Acute hepatitis Appendicitis Cholecystitis
Neurological	Migraine Meningitis Raised intracranial pressure Motion sickness Labyrinthitis Psychogenic vomiting
Metabolic	Diabetic ketoacidosis Uraemia Hypercalcaemia Addison's disease
Drugs	Alcohol Opiate analgesics Cytotoxic agents Colchicine Digoxin Erythromycin Many others
Miscellaneous	Pregnancy Irradiation Renal colic Myocardial infarction

Fig. 1.9 *Causes of nausea and vomiting.*

reflux can result in oesophagitis and patients may complain of increased heartburn with spicy or acidic foods. Causes of dyspepsia/'indigestion' symptoms include:

- Non-ulcer dyspepsia
- Irritable bowel syndrome
- Peptic ulcer disease
- Gastro-oesophageal reflux disease (GORD)
- Gastric cancer
- Pancreatitis
- Gallstone disease
- Oesophageal dysmotility
- Ischaemic heart disease

Nausea and vomiting

The history usually provides clues to the cause (**Fig. 1.9**). With an acute onset of vomiting in a previously well patient, a detailed food history, including whether there are other afflicted individuals, is important. An alcohol and drug history should not be forgotten. Underlying metabolic causes such as Addison's disease may have a more insidious onset, while patients with diabetes often have recurrent episodes which may be related to an underlying autonomic neuropathy. Neurological causes for vomiting such as raised intracranial pressure may present without nausea.

Epigastric pain

Classically patients with duodenal ulceration give a history of epigastric pain which wakes them at night (hunger pains) and is relieved by drinking milk. Symptoms are typically recurrent, lasting for a few weeks at a time. Unfortunately, the symptoms of benign or malignant gastric ulceration and gastritis are not distinguishable on historical grounds. In both there is classically epigastric pain which is exacerbated by eating. However, the only definite way to discern gastric from duodenal disease is with further endoscopic or radiological investigation.

A sensation of abdominal distension generally points towards functional disorders (irritable bowel or non-ulcer dyspepsia), particularly in younger patients. Epigastric pain may also be experienced by those who have symptoms caused by gallstones (see chapter 4). These patients often have a nebulous intolerance of fatty foods. However, it is a mistake to ascribe epigastric pain simply to gallstones if there is a convenient radiological diagnosis, because around 10–15% of the adult population in the western world have cholelithiasis anyway.

Pancreatitis (see chapter 5) may also present with epigastric pain, but this usually radiates through to the back, a symptom which may also be present with a posterior duodenal ulcer. A serum amylase test should always be requested in acute abdominal pain and wherever the clinical suspicion of pancreatitis is high (for example, in alcohol abusers). In cases of chronic pancreatitis, however, the serum amylase level may not necessarily be raised.

Haematemesis and melaena

A significant bleed from oesophageal, gastric or duodenal pathology (see **Fig. 1.46**) is usually unequivocal. Patients may present with *haematemesis*, which may involve altered (so-called 'coffee grounds') or fresh red blood; with *melaena* (black, tarry stool with a characteristic smell); or with *hypotensive shock* without external evidence of bleeding. Bleeding from oesophageal varices is usually brisk and should always be considered in those patients with a history of alcohol abuse and/or stigmata of chronic liver disease (see chapter 4).

Sometimes it is not clear whether an upper gastrointestinal bleed has taken place. Confounding factors which mimic haematemesis include haemoptysis and swallowed blood from nose bleeds. Persistent retching may lead to small amounts of blood-stained vomit, while vomit from any cause can contain 'coffee grounds'. Patients who are taking oral iron or bismuth preparations may have dark stools which can be confused with melaena.

INVESTIGATIONS

DIAGNOSTIC RADIOLOGY

An initial barium swallow is generally advisable in patients complaining of dysphagia, since the site and nature of the lesion can be defined prior to endoscopy (**Fig. 1.10**). This limits the risk of inadvertent endoscopic perforation, including intubation of an unsuspected pharyngeal or oesophageal pouch.

The barium meal remains a good diagnostic test for patients with dyspepsia (**Fig. 1.11**), but is performed less often where good endoscopic facilities exist. The two investigations are used for different indications, rather than being mutually exclusive. A barium meal will effectively demonstrate abnormal motility or anatomical variations (such as hiatus hernia or duodenal diverticulae), while endoscopy is preferred when fine mucosal detail is sought (if the patient is thought to be bleeding, for example).

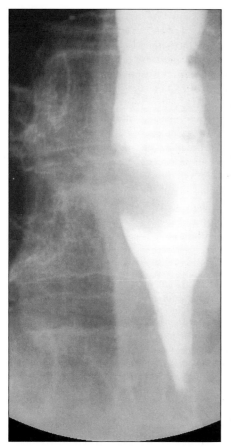

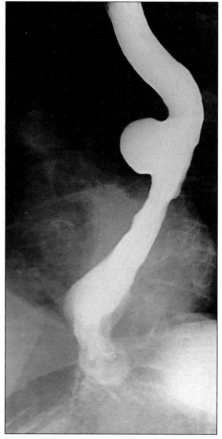

Fig. 1.10 *Barium swallow in a patient with oesphageal cancer. An oesophageal carcinoma is visible as a polypoid filling defect extending into the lumen.*

Fig. 1.11 *Hiatus hernia on barium study. A sliding hiatus hernia together with reflux of barium into the oesophagus. The patient also has a mid-oesophageal diverticulum.*

Ultrasound

An ultrasound of the liver, gall bladder and pancreas is invaluable where cholelithiasis or pancreatitis is suspected as the cause of epigastric pain (see chapters 4 and 5).

ENDOSCOPY

The advent of flexible fibreoptic (and later video chip) endoscopy (**Fig. 1.12**) was a major turning point in clinical gastroenterology, allowing the relatively easy visualisation of the foregut and the performance of numerous diagnostic and therapeutic procedures.

Complication rates for diagnostic upper gastrointestinal endoscopy are very low, with significant events occurring in less than 1 in 1000 cases and a mortality of below 1 in 10 000. They are most likely to occur in emergency situations, with acutely ill patients and the elderly. Oversedation, respiratory difficulties (particularly aspiration of gastric contents), perforation or cardiac dysrhythmia may occur. It is vital that patients are closely monitored (**Fig. 1.13**) and that there is appropriate care of the airway and sufficient nursing support during both the procedure and the subsequent recovery period.

Oesophagogastroduodenoscopy (OGD) is superior to barium meal in the investigation of dyspeptic patients, where it can be performed safely and effectively, since it offers the opportunity to obtain specimens for histological, cytological and microbiological analysis. This is in addition to determining *Helicobacter pylori* status from rapid urease testing of biopsy material from the antrum and/or the body of the stomach (see **Fig. 1.19**). Therapeutic manoeuvres can be performed including oesophageal dilatation (see **Fig. 1.24**); oesophageal variceal sclerotherapy and band ligation (**Fig. 1.14**); injection, laser or heat ablation of bleeding gastric and duodenal ulcers or other bleeding lesions such as haemorrhagic telangiectasia (**Fig. 1.15**); and removal of both foreign bodies (**Fig. 1.16**) and lesions such as gastric polyps (see **Fig. 1.60**).

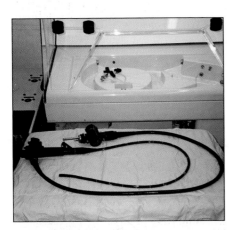

Fig. 1.12 *A typical upper gastrointestinal video endoscope, disconnected from its supporting machinery. The control head (with steering wheels) is on the left. The metallic plug marks the end of the 'umbilical cord' that connects the scope to the supporting light source and suction apparatus. The narrower shaft of the scope itself (centre) has white markings that indicate the length of instrument in centimetres. In the background is a dedicated machine for cleaning and disinfecting the endoscope.*

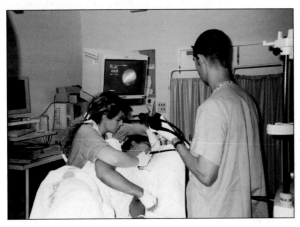

Fig. 1.13 *Upper gastrointestinal endoscopy. The endoscopist is able to view the images conveniently on a mounted video screen, holding the shaft of the scope in the right hand and the control head of the instrument in the left. The nurse helps to maintain the sedated patient's airway and reduce the possibility of aspiration by regular pharyngeal suction. Supplementary oxygen is given by a nasal cannula and pulse oximetry is monitored.*

Endoscopic criteria for evidence of recent bleeding from gastric and duodenal ulcers are summarised on page 32.

Endoscopic ultrasound and endoscopic magnetic resonance imaging (MRI)

These cross-sectional imaging techniques are currently being developed to scrutinise mural lesions in the oesophagus and stomach. Endoscopic ultrasonography allows the depth of

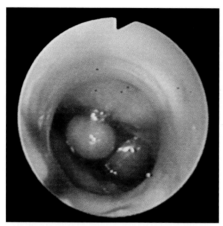

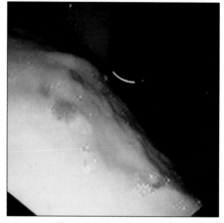

Fig. 1.14 *Endoscopic band ligation of oesophageal varices. The base of the oesophageal varix in the foreground has been constricted using a rubber band. A similarly treated varix lies in the background. After ligation the varices thrombose and degenerate.*

Fig. 1.15 *Gastric telangiectasia in a patient with Osler–Weber–Rendu disease. The gastric fundus and cardia are seen using a 'J' manoeuvre where the endoscope (top) looks back on itself. This vascular lesion would be suitable for heater-probe treatment.*

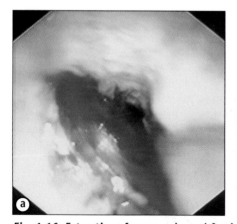

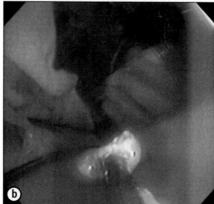

Fig. 1.16 *Extraction of an oesophageal foreign body. This female patient with Alzheimer's disease presented with dysphagia and haematemesis. (a) The foreign body in the oesophagus. (b) The foreign body is extracted using endoscopic grasping forceps. The object was revealed to be a swallowed pendant.*

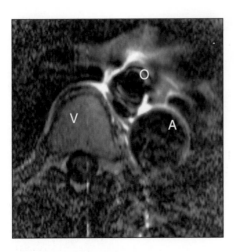

Fig. 1.17 *Upper gastrointestinal endoscopic magnetic resonance image. Obtained using an endoscopic probe, this image shows the mucosa, muscular wall and external relations of the oesophagus (O = oesophagus; V = vertebra; A = aorta).*

invasive tumours to be assessed, but the operative technique is not easy to acquire and is subject to a considerable learning curve. An example of endoscopic ultrasound is shown on page 27 (**Fig. 1.36**).

MRI endoscopy remains largely experimental at present. Patients undergo an endoscopic examination within the bore of an MR magnet, with a radiofrequency coil built into the tip of a specially designed, non-magnetic endoscope. The aim is to produce high-quality images of the mucosa and submucosa. This may be useful in conditions such as Barrett's oesophagus, where patients are regularly screened for the development of an invasive carcinoma (**Fig. 1.17**).

OESOPHAGEAL MANOMETRY AND PH MONITORING

Oesophageal spasm can present like angina, but may be diagnosed on manometry (**Fig. 1.18(a) and (b)**). This is usually available in specialised centres. For the most part, therapeutic trials of antireflux treatments and antispasmodics such as nifedipine are carried out on an empirical basis in patients who have a normal resting and exercise ECG tracing.

Ambulatory intra-oesophageal pH monitoring (**Fig. 1.18(c) and (d)**) is also a specialised investigation which is probably best reserved for those patients who have atypical symptoms and signs or who do not respond well to standard antireflux treatment. A pH electrode 5 cm above the lower oesophageal sphincter is connected to a portable microprocessor that records the episodes of oesophageal pH below a set limit (usually a pH of 4). The data can be used to seek a correlation between acid reflux and symptoms, as well as judging the efficacy of therapeutic regimens. The test is seldom required for the majority of patients with reflux disease.

UREASE TESTS

The organism *Helicobacter pylori* has the ability to split urea and this property can be utilised in a number of diagnostic tests. In addition to being detectable at endoscopy on rapid urease testing (**Fig. 1.19**), microbiological culture or histological analysis of endoscopic biopsy specimens (see **Fig. 1.21**), *non-invasive* tests are available which make use of the ability of the organism to split either ^{13}C- or ^{14}C- labelled urea into ammonia and the labelled carbon dioxide, which is absorbed and exhaled (**Fig. 1.20**). *H. pylori* status can also be ascertained serologically using an antibody test, but this does not necessarily distinguish between an active infection and a recently eradicated one.

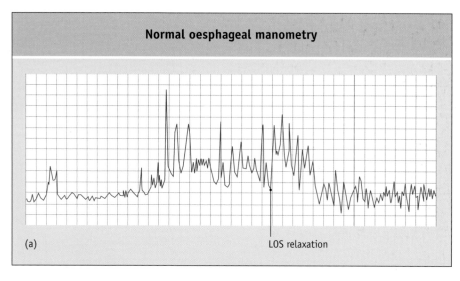

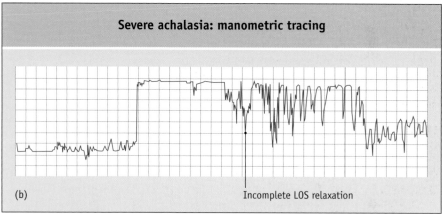

Fig. 1.18 *Oesophageal manometry and pH monitoring. (a) Normal oesophageal manometry. This tracing, taken at the level of the lower oesophageal sphincter (LOS), shows a normal resting tone, regular contractions and a relaxation response following deglutition. (b) Severe achalasia. The tracing shows high pressure at the LOS, disordered motor contractions and a failure to relax after swallowing.*

OTHER DIAGNOSTIC TESTS FOR *HELICOBACTER PYLORI*

There are several other methods available for the diagnosis of *H. pylori*. The organism may be observed on histological examination of gastric biopsies from the antrum (**Fig. 1.21**) and also the corpus, particularly in patients on long-term acid suppressant drugs. However, colonisation of the stomach may be patchy and this method can therefore be subject to sampling error.

The use of the polymerase chain reaction (PCR) allows specific DNA sequences from the *H. pylori* genome to be amplified. The bacteria do not need to be viable when the test is performed and samples can be taken from mucosal biopsies, gastric juice or even faeces.

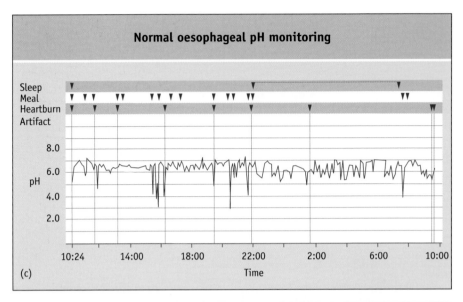

(c)

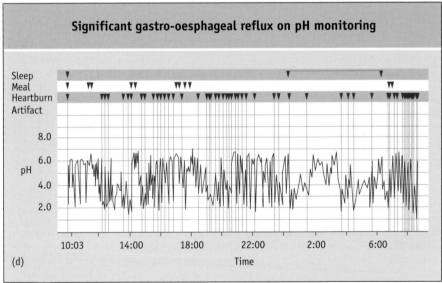

(d)

Fig. 1.18 *(Cont.) (c) Normal oesophageal pH monitoring. A pH monitoring probe is positioned 5 cm above the lower oesophageal sphincter. The marks on the top of the graph record periods of symptoms, sleep and meal times over the 24-hour period. Significant acid reflux is defined by a drop in pH below 4. This normal trace demonstrates that a few episodes of mild reflux do occur, but these do not coincide with the patient's symptoms of heartburn. (d) Significant gastro-oesophageal reflux. This tracing demonstrates severe episodes of acid reflux, many of which are prolonged (> 5 minutes); the oesophageal pH is below 4 for about 25% of the total recording time. The reflux is at its worst in the postprandial periods and there is good correlation with the symptoms of heartburn.*

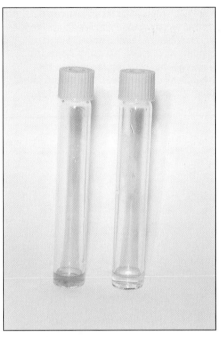

Fig. 1.19 *Gastric biopsy rapid urease test for* Helicobacter pylori. *Endoscopic antral biopsy specimens are placed in a medium containing urea. If* H. pylori *is present, its urease activity splits the urea into ammonia and carbon dioxide with a consequent rise in pH that can be detected using a pH-sensitive dye in the medium (pink sample). Depending on the brand of test, the reaction may be visible in just a few minutes or several hours.*

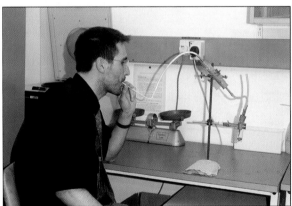

Fig. 1.20 *Urease breath test for* Helicobacter pylori. *The individual fasts overnight and then provides a baseline breath sample. A known quantity of radiolabelled (^{13}C or ^{14}C) urea is drunk and if* H. pylori *is present, its urease enzyme liberates the radioactive ligand as CO_2. The patient's exhaled breath is passed first through a chamber containing anhydrous calcium chloride, which absorbs water, so as to make the final counting process more accurate. It is then bubbled through the blue solution, which contains phenolphthalein and a carbon dioxide-trapping agent such as hyamine. Once the hyamine is saturated, the increased pH renders the solution colourless and the exhaled radiolabelled CO_2 is calculated by liquid scintillation counting.*

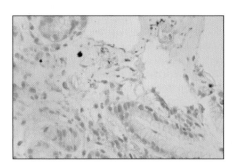

Fig. 1.21 Helicobacter pylori *gastritis. An antral biopsy specimen showing evidence of gastritis, with mucosal* H. pylori *organisms present. By using a specific Helicobacter-staining technique, the organisms can be identified as the small, dark 'S' shapes on the mucosal surface.*

Relative attributes of different tests for *Helicobacter pylori*

	Sensitivity	Specificity	Rapidity	Cost
Serology	+++	++	++	++
^{13}C urease breath test	+++	+++	+++	+
Biopsy urease tests	++	+++	+++	+++
Biopsy Gram stain smear	+	++	+++	+++
Biopsy histology	+++	++	+	+
Biopsy for bacterial culture	+++	+++	+	+
Biopsy with polymerase chain reaction test	+++	+++	++	+

+ = reasonable, ++ = good, +++ = excellent

Fig. 1.22 *Relative attributes of different tests for* Helicobacter pylori.

Microbiological culture is still probably the gold standard diagnostic method. It is particularly important in determining sensitivity or resistance to antibiotic therapy. The prevalence of metronidazole resistance, for example, can vary widely in different communities.

A comparison of the different diagnostic tests is shown in **Fig. 1.22**.

DIFFERENTIAL DIAGNOSIS

DISEASES OF THE OESOPHAGUS
Oesophageal web
These fibrous structures may be seen on barium swallow in the upper oesophagus and postcricoid webs can be associated with iron deficiency anaemia, koilonychia, angular stomatitis and glossitis (Paterson–Brown–Kelly or Plummer–Vinson syndrome). The condition is underdiagnosed endoscopically, probably because the webs are easily broken with the endoscope or negotiated before adequate vision of the oesophageal lumen has been obtained.

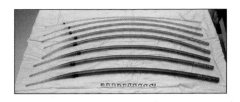

Fig. 1.23 *Savary–Guilliard oesophageal bougies. These soft, tapering plastic wands are used to dilate oesophageal strictures. The lubricated bougie is passed over a guide-wire across the stricture, ideally under X-ray fluoroscopic control. The size of bougie used is gradually increased.*

Benign and malignant oesophageal stricture

Oesophageal stricturing may be benign in aetiology and secondary to gastro-oesophageal reflux, often in association with a hiatus hernia, while the oesophageal dysmotility in systemic sclerosis may lead to reflux and subsequent stricturing. Deliberate or accidental swallowing of strongly acidic or alkaline substances may cause a similar problem, but usually the stricture is sited higher up in the oesophagus.

Malignant strictures can occur at any level in the oesophagus and are usually caused by squamous carcinomas. However, there is an increasing incidence of adenocarcinoma of the oesophagus, which is related to the premalignant lesion, Barrett's oesophagus. At endoscopy, all strictures should be brushed for cytological analysis and biopsies taken. Dilatation can either be performed using metal rods with olive-shaped dilators of varying sizes or gently tapering plastic rods known as 'bougies' (**Fig. 1.23**); alternatively the procedure may be performed under direct vision at endoscopy using oesophageal balloons (**Fig. 1.24**).

Oesophagitis

Peptic oesophagitis. This is the commonest cause of oesophagitis, due to reflux of gastric acid or more rarely to biliary reflux through an incompetent LOS. Patients tend to complain of heartburn, worsened by lying flat or bending forwards. Belching and epigastric discomfort are other symptoms. The presence of a hiatus hernia, where the gastro-oesophageal junction is intrathoracic (**Fig. 1.25**), tends to exacerbate the problem. The endoscopic and barium swallow appearances of a hiatus hernia are shown in **Figs 1.26** and **1.11** (see pp. 26, 11) respectively.

Other factors that may worsen reflux include the consumption of foods that relax the LOS, such as coffee, chocolate, tea, raw onions, cucumber and marmalades which contain lots of citrus peel. Spicy or acid foods may irritate established areas of oesophagitis directly on ingestion, while carbonated drinks exacerbate reflux. GORD may also be more marked when there is increased intra-abdominal pressure, such as in pregnancy or in the obese. This acid reflux can lead to varying degrees of oesophagitis (**Fig. 1.27**), although patients can be strongly symptomatic even in the absence of endoscopic evidence of inflammation. In severe or prolonged cases, peptic oesophagitis may result in mucosal ulceration (**Fig. 1.28**) or stricture formation (**Fig. 1.29**). Another long-term sequel is Barrett's oesophagus (see below).

Patients with oesophageal reflux should be given specific advice on weight reduction if overweight, eating smaller meals at more frequent intervals and not eating immediately prior to going to bed, together with avoidance of foods which may exacerbate the problem. Other lifestyle modifications include reducing alcohol intake, stopping smoking and sleeping at a slight incline in the 'head-up' position to prevent nocturnal acid reflux. This may be effected by placing a builder's brick or heavy book under the legs of the bed.

Simple antacids may provide symptomatic relief, but acid suppression is usually required with H_2 antagonists or with proton pump inhibitors (PPIs) if symptoms are more

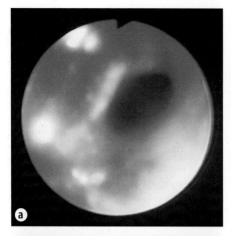

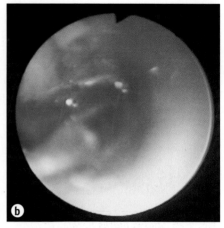

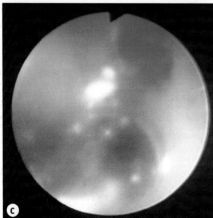

Fig. 1.24 *Endoscopic balloon dilatation of an oesophageal stricture. (a) This patient has a benign peptic stricture of the oesophagus. (b) A balloon is threaded down the endoscope and placed across the stricture. (c) It is then inflated under direct vision. This technique does not usually require fluoroscopic monitoring.*

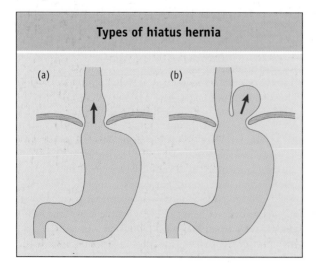

Types of hiatus hernia

(a)   (b)

Fig. 1.25 *Types of hiatus hernia. (a) Sliding. (b) Paraoesophageal.*

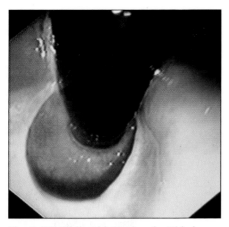

Fig. 1.26 *Sliding hiatus hernia. This is a 'J' view, with the endoscope looking back on itself towards the gastro-oesophageal junction, which can be seen to lie within a hiatus hernia.*

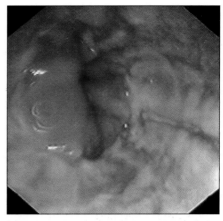

Fig. 1.27 *Reflux oesophagitis. Endoscopic view showing linear streaks of oesophagitis in two patients with gastro-oesophageal reflux disease.*

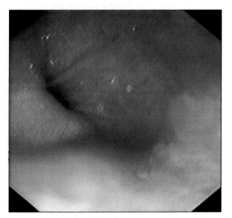

Fig. 1.28 *Chronic oesphagitis with ulceration. Two small oesophageal ulcers are visible in this endoscopic view.*

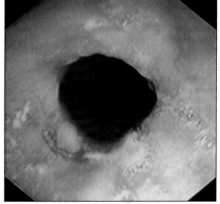

Fig. 1.29 *Peptic stricture of the oesophagus. This patient had a long history of heartburn and developed dysphagia. There is an obvious stricture of the oesophagus with some associated inflammation. Endoscopic balloon dilatation relieved the difficulty in swallowing. The appearance of this peptic stricture should be contrasted with the malignant lesion shown in Fig. 1.38.*

severe. Patients who have persistent symptoms or who relapse after a course of acid suppression should undergo endoscopy to assess the extent and severity of the oesophagitis (**Fig. 1.27**) and any of its sequelae, to establish the presence of a hiatus hernia and to rule out other pathology in the upper gastrointestinal tract. PPI treatment is in widespread use, but prokinetic agents may be effective in increasing LOS pressure and promoting gastric emptying.

In persistent, severe GORD with significant hiatus hernia, there are surgical alternatives such as formal or laparoscopic fundoplication. These operations reduce the hiatus hernia by creating an intra-abdominal segment of oesophagus, which then has a portion of the gastric fundus wrapped around it.

Oesophageal infections. Ulceration and oesophagitis are frequently found in immunosuppressed patients, particularly transplant recipients and individuals with the acquired immune deficiency syndrome (AIDS). These conditions can result from opportunistic fungal and viral infections, the most common being *Candida albicans*, cytomegalovirus (CMV) and *Herpes simplex* virus (HSV).

Candidal oesophagitis is often an asymptomatic finding in the diabetic, the immunosuppressed or those receiving long-term antibiotics. Many of these patients will have oral candidiasis, but its absence does not exclude significant oesophageal involvement. A ragged mucosal appearance is seen on barium swallow and there are characteristic cheesy-looking plaques at endoscopy (**Fig. 1.30**).

In patients with AIDS, candidiasis often presents with dysphagia and is sufficiently common for many experts to recommend a course of systemic antifungal treatment (usually 1 week of oral fluconazole) for symptomatic patients; endoscopy is reserved for those who fail to respond.

Odynophagia, rather than dysphagia, usually implies oesophageal ulceration. In the immunocompromised patient this may be caused by CMV or HSV infection. CMV is particularly common. It is estimated that some 50% of adults in the USA are seropositive for CMV, with the consequent risk of reactivation under conditions of immune deficiency (approximately 80% of CMV-seropositive bone marrow transplant recipients reactivate their infections).

There may be vesicles or frank oesophageal ulceration at endoscopy with oral or perioral herpetic lesions noted at intubation. The endoscopist should take care to wear protective clothing including goggles, since viral particles are transmissible across mucosal surfaces. Plaques of oesophageal candidiasis should be removed with the endoscope to allow inspection of any underlying viral ulcers. The diagnosis is clinched on brush cytology (where intranuclear inclusion bodies are seen), viral culture techniques or histological biopsy of the ulcer itself.

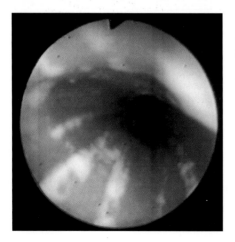

Fig. 1.30 *Oesophageal candidiasis. White plaques of oesophageal candidiasis in a patient on immunosuppressive treatment.*

Treatment includes acid suppression, antiviral drugs (aciclovir or famciclovir for HSV; ganciclovir or foscarnet for CMV) and, in transplant patients, reducing or altering the immunosuppressive regimens.

Idiopathic oesophageal ulceration (IOU) is the second commonest cause, after CMV, of ulceration in AIDS patients. It seems to be a form of aphthous ulceration, which may respond to oral corticosteroids or thalidomide.

Rare causes of oesophagitis. Other infections such as syphilis and tuberculosis are rare but recognised causes of oesophagitis and ulceration. Crohn's disease can affect any part of the gastrointestinal tract from mouth to anus and may occasionally affect the oesophagus. Radiotherapy for bronchial carcinoma or intrathoracic lymphoma can result in a radiation-induced oesophagitis.

Certain drugs, such as iron preparations, potassium salts, non-steroidal anti-inflammatory agents (NSAIDs) and beta-blockers, can cause a chemical oesophagitis through local contact, particularly in the elderly who may find difficulty in swallowing tablets.

Systemic conditions such as Behçet's disease and skin conditions such as pemphigoid and pemphigus may occasionally cause inflammation and ulceration in the oesophagus.

Barrett's oesophagus

This condition, characterised by oesophageal columnar metaplasia, probably occurs as a consequence of long-term GORD. Indeed, Barrett's oesophagus can be found in 10–20% of GORD cases.

The change from normal squamous oesophageal mucosa to the more acid-resistant columnar epithelium of a gastric or intestinal type is initially brought about by recurrent peptic oesophagitis and ulceration. Barrett's oesophagus is an endoscopic diagnosis (**Fig. 1.31**), confirmed by histology (**Fig. 1.32**), where islands of darker pink columnar

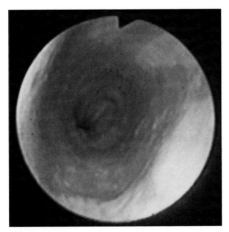

Fig. 1.31 *Barrett's oesophagus. Characteristic endoscopic appearance of Barrett's oesophagus, showing red, velvety mucosa extending up into the oesophagus. Such an area should be biopsied and cytological brushings taken to exclude dysplasia.*

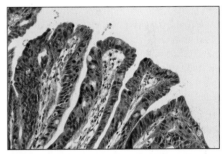

Fig. 1.32 *Histological appearance of Barrett's oesophagus. This oesophageal biopsy specimen shows an area of villiform intestinal metaplasia, together with evidence of severely dysplastic changes.*

mucosa may be seen at the lower end of the oesophagus, surrounded by lighter pink squamous mucosa. This usually occurs as an accompaniment to peptic oesophagitis, but the metaplastic change may be confluent and result in migration of the squamo-columnar junction up the oesophagus.

This is not simply an endoscopic curiosity, since the condition has a premalignant potential. There is an increased risk of adenocarcinoma of the oesophagus of at least 30 times, particularly with intestinal metaplasia. The annual incidence of oesophageal cancer in patients with Barrett's oesophagus is 0.8%.

Patients with Barrett's oesophagus should receive appropriate acid suppression for GORD and undergo regular surveillance endoscopies with multiple biopsies to rule out any early malignant change. On balance, this should be performed every 12–18 months, but there should be increased vigilance if dysplastic change is seen. However, the exact monitoring and treatment of patients with oesophageal dysplasia remains controversial. Many authorities would rebiopsy in each of the four quadrants of the oesophagus at 1 cm intervals along the length of the Barrett's segment within 1 month. If severe dysplastic change is seen on biopsy, then the patient is at significant risk of developing oesophageal adenocarcinoma. Indeed, in cases of severe dysplasia, there is an estimated 30% chance that the patient may already have coexisting malignant change. Because of these risks, many gastroenterologists recommend that patients with severe dysplasia should be referred for oesophageal resection, particularly younger and fitter individuals. As many patients with Barrett's oesophagus are elderly or have other medical comorbidity, an alternative approach is to use endoscopic mucosal ablative techniques, such as laser photodynamic therapy.

Oesophageal cancer

Most oesophageal cancers are squamous and this remains a tumour with a very poor prognosis, since patients usually present when the disease is at an advanced stage. Dysphagia is a late sign (see **Fig. 1.10**).

Epidemiology. There is a marked geographical variation in incidence, being most common along the southern shores of the Caspian Sea, in Iran and in certain areas of China and southern Africa (**Fig. 1.33**).

Alcohol, tobacco, fungal contamination of the food supply and diets rich in nitrites and nitrosamines have been causally implicated. There may be a genetic predisposition like that in familial conditions such as tylosis. Achalasia of the cardia and caustic strictures have both been associated with oesophageal tumours, but the rising incidence of adenocarcinoma of the oesophagus has been linked to Barrett's oesophagus. Factors associated with oesophageal cancer include:

Squamous carcinoma
- Tobacco smoking
- Alcohol excess
- Dietary deficiencies – vitamins A and C, riboflavin, molybdenum
- Caustic stricture
- Tylosis
- Plummer–Vinson syndrome
- History of squamous head and neck cancer
- Long-standing achalasia
- Mouldy food

Adenocarcinoma
- Chronic gastro-oesophageal reflux
- Barrett's oesophagus
- Tobacco smoking

Diagnosis. Tumours may be demonstrated by barium swallow (**Fig. 1.34**) but the specific diagnosis is obtained by using endoscopic biopsy (**Fig. 1.35**) or brush cytology.

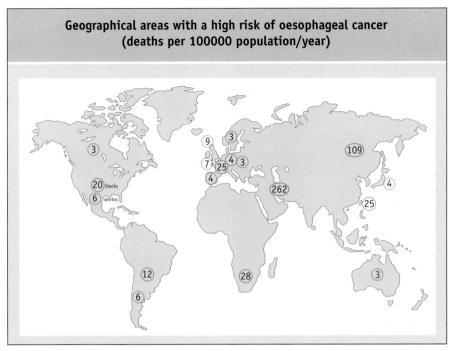

**Geographical areas with a high risk of oesophageal cancer
(deaths per 100000 population/year)**

Fig. 1.33 *Geographical areas with a high risk of oesophageal cancer. Incidence rates are expressed as the number of deaths per 100 000 population per year.*

Management. Definitive oesophageal resection provides a better chance of cure than radiotherapy. However, this operation is not without its complications and combined treatment with radiotherapy and/or chemotherapy with agents such as bleomycin, doxorubicin and cisplatin have sometimes been used as adjuvant treatment. Tumour staging procedures such as spiral computed tomography (CT) of the chest, hepatic ultrasound, endoscopy and (increasingly) endoscopic ultrasound (**Fig. 1.36**) are used to determine whether the tumour is resectable. Unfortunately, some 50% of oesophageal cancers are unresectable at the time of presentation and so the therapeutic aim is to achieve palliation by relieving dysphagia with the minimum morbidity and allowing the patient to continue on as normal a diet as possible. The main palliative options are summarised in **Fig. 1.37**.

Oesophageal strictures (**Fig. 1.38**) may be dilated endoscopically and oesophageal stents can be inserted by this route. Laser photocoagulation of exophytic tumours using Nd YAG (neodymium yttrium aluminium garnet) can provide similar palliative results to endoscopic intubation although the laser is perhaps best reserved for polypoid lesions. Recanalisation of the lumen is almost always achieved, but experience and care are needed to avoid complications such as oesophageal perforation.

Luminal patency can be maintained with oesophageal stents, although traditionally plastic stents have been prone to problems with migration (particularly if the stricture is located close to the cardia) and blockage with either food debris or tumour. Newer self-expanding metallic stents (SEMS) are being used more widely. Covered metallic stents reduce the incidence of tumour ingrowth; those with a conical shape are claimed to suffer less from migration and may be more suitable for lesions at the lower end of the oesophagus.

25

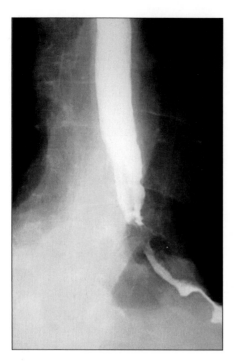

Fig. 1.34 *Malignant oesophageal stricture on barium swallow. This stenosing, ulcerated stricture in the lower oesophagus is due to an adenocarcinoma. Its appearance contrasts with the polypoid lesion shown in Fig 1.10.*

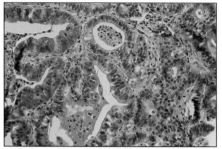

Fig. 1.35 *Adenocarcinoma of the oesophagus. This histopathology specimen shows a moderately differentiated adenocarcinoma of the oesophagus.*

In additional to these 'mechanical' treatments, palliation can be furthered by adding radiotherapy (either intracavitary or external beam) for cases of squamous carcinoma and chemotherapy for those with adenocarcinoma. Chemotherapy regimens vary, but the combination of epirubicin, cisplatin and 5-fluorouracil has been shown to produce a therapeutic response in more than two-thirds of patients.

Other tumours in the oesophagus include leiomyomas, lymphomas and Kaposi's sarcomas.

Achalasia of the oesophagus

Achalasia is characterised by an aperistaltic segment in the body of the oesophagus and failure of the LOS to relax in the normal way after swallowing. These motility defects can be picked up on oesophageal manometry and are due, among other denervation abnormalities, to an absence or reduction in ganglion cells within the myenteric plexus.

The disease can present at any age, but rarely does so in childhood. The cause is unknown. In Latin America, infection with *Trypanosoma cruzi* may cause a similar appearance in patients with Chagas' disease.

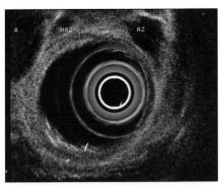 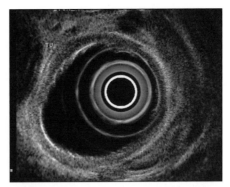

Fig. 1.36 *Endoscopic ultrasound of oesophageal malignancy. (a and b) Views of an oesophageal adenocarcinoma taken at distances of 26 and 27 cm respectively from the incisor teeth. The ultrasound probe is clearly visible in the centre of each radial image; the surrounding structures are the aorta (A), hemiazygos vein (HAZ), spine (SP), azygos vein (AZ) and the tumour itself (TU), with mucosal irregularity particularly obvious in (b). The adenocarcinoma is seen to extend no further than the muscularis propria, indicating a T2 lesion which is potentially resectable. As part of the same examination, a thorough search is made for any surrounding lymphadenopathy. Endoscopic ultrasound has an accuracy of around 90% in the staging of oesophageal tumours.*

Palliation for oesophageal carcinoma	
Palliative surgery	Resection or bypass procedures May be limited by comorbidity
Chemotherapy	Retard tumour growth
Radiotherapy	May be combined with endoscopic therapies below (to prolong intervals between treatments)
Endoscopic laser therapy	Best used for polypoid tumours Repeated treatments usually required ~ monthly Recanalisation achieved in > 90% cases Significant improvement in dysphagia in > 70% Complications (e.g. perforation) in < 6% Procedural mortality 1–2%
Plastic stents	Used less commonly now Migration and blockage frequently occur Dysphagia relief usually only moderate
Self-expanding metallic stents	Can be covered/uncovered/conical/cylindrical Symptom relief better than plastic devices Lower complication rate (~ 20%) but tumour ingrowth and stent migration can still occur

Fig. 1.37 *Palliation for oesophageal carcinoma.*

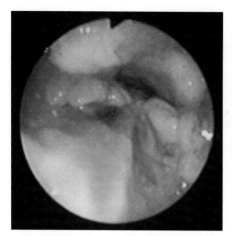

Fig. 1.38 *Malignant stricture of the oesophagus. Gross mucosal irregularity and stricturing in a patient with an adenocarcinoma.*

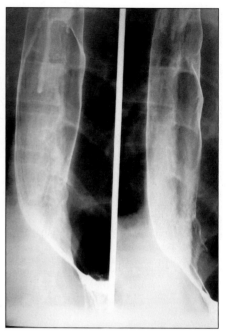

Fig. 1.39 *Achalasia. Barium swallow showing characteristic sharp narrowing of the lower oesophagus with holdup of barium. The proximal oesophagus is distended as a result.*

The most obvious feature of the condition at barium swallow (**Fig. 1.39**) is dilatation of the oesophagus, which may be filled with a column of food debris and fluid that can be the cause of recurrent aspiration pneumonia.

Management is aimed at reducing LOS pressures. Occasionally drug therapy is effective with nitrates or nifedipine, but usually serial endoscopic oesophageal balloon dilatation is required. Some patients may need surgical myotomy (Heller's operation) if endoscopic treatment is ineffective. Recently, the use of botulinum toxin has been explored, given by endoscopic intrasphincteric injection.

Schatzki ring

This is an annular fibromuscular condensation in the lower end of the oesophagus, which is often seen on barium swallow as an incidental finding (**Fig. 1.40**), but may be a cause of dysphagia to solids. Endoscopic dilatation may stretch the Schatzki ring, but usually nothing needs to be done apart from advising the patient to chew food properly before swallowing.

Oesophageal diverticula

These pouches can pose potential hazards for the unwary endoscopist.

The Zenker's diverticulum or pharyngeal pouch is the commonest type (**Fig. 1.41**), occurring in the defect between the inferior constrictor muscle and the cricopharyngeus muscle in older patients. Food tends to accumulate in the diverticulum as it enlarges, with intermittent regurgitation of its contents. Patients may complain of being 'chesty' because of recurrent nocturnal aspiration. Surgical excision is the standard treatment.

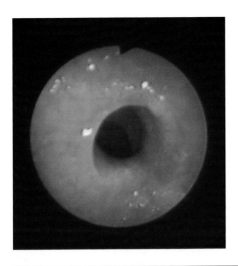

Fig. 1.40 *Schatzki oesophageal ring. Endoscopic view showing the characteristic appearance of a Schatzki fibrous ring encroaching on the oesophageal lumen.*

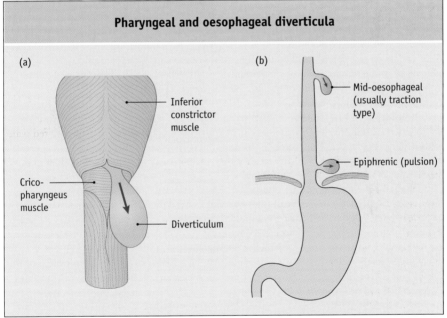

Fig. 1.41 *Pharyngeal and oesophageal diverticula. (a) Posterior view of pharynx. The pharyngeal pouch is usually a posteromedial pulsion diverticulum. (b) Pouches lower down in the oesophagus may result from traction (usually caused by tethering from adjacent inflammation) or pulsion (usually due to dysmotility). An oesophageal diverticulum is also shown in Fig. 1.11.*

Other diverticula may be 'epiphrenic', consequent to motility disorders at the lower end of the oesophagus, or occur in the mid-oesophagus, secondary to oesophageal tethering in conditions where there is mediastinal inflammation such as tuberculous mediastinal lymphadenitis.

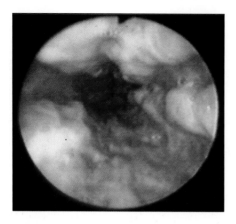

Fig. 1.42 *Oesophagoscopy showing four large columns of varices.*

Oesophageal varices

Portal hypertension may be *prehepatic*, secondary to portal vein or splenic vein thrombosis; *intrahepatic*, secondary to chronic liver disease; or *post-hepatic*, following conditions such as hepatic vein thrombosis (Budd–Chiari syndrome). The aetiology of portal hypertension is discussed in greater detail in chapter 4. Regardless of the cause, elevated portal pressures may result in the development of a collateral circulation between the systemic and portal systems, including, most commonly, oesophageal varices (**Fig. 1.42**).

On barium swallow, worm-like filling defects may be seen at the lower end of the oesophagus (**Fig. 1.43**), while at endoscopy the varices may appear as bluish or white submucosal dilatations. Stigmata of recent bleeding include the cherry red spot or red wale (ridge) signs (**Fig. 1.44**). The treatment of portal hypertension is also outlined in chapter 4.

Oesophageal spasm

Diffuse spasm is characterised by intermittent chest pain and sometimes dysphagia. Barium swallow or manometry may reveal non-peristaltic contractions. Some patients may experience peristaltic hyperactivity, manifested clinically by chest pain which may be severe enough to mimic angina with increased amplitude and duration of contractions observed on manometry – the so-called 'nutcracker oesophagus'.

Diffuse spasm and nutcracker oesophagus may be relieved by glyceryl trinitrate, but the use of long-acting nitrates has been disappointing owing to side-effects such as headaches. Calcium channel antagonists such as nifedipine have been advocated, but they rarely provide sustained relief.

Many patients' symptoms are exacerbated by stress and antidepressants are effective treatment in some individuals. Acid suppression is useful in cases where symptoms are clearly provoked by gastro-oesophageal reflux (oesophageal pH monitoring may be helpful in deciding this).

Pneumatic dilatation or surgical myotomy should only be reserved for very severe unrelenting symptoms.

Mallory–Weiss syndrome

This syndrome is the consequence of forced vomiting or retching, which causes longitudinal mucosal tearing at the gastro-oesophageal junction. It is a common cause of acute upper gastrointestinal bleeding and classically occurs after an alcoholic binge.

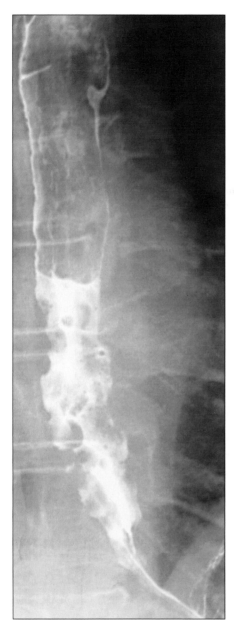

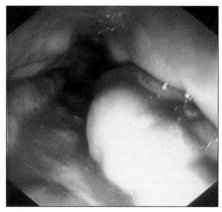

Fig. 1.43 *Oesophageal varices visible on barium swallow.*

Fig. 1.44 *Large oesophageal varices with signs of recent haemorrhage.*

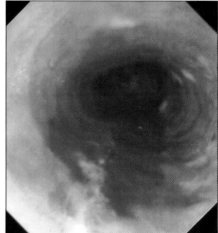

Fig. 1.45 *Mallory–Weiss tear. Endoscopic view of a young man admitted with haematemesis following an alcoholic binge. A linear tear in the mucosa is shown at about 6 o'clock.*

However, at endoscopy (**Fig. 1.45**) it is a common incidental finding in other conditions which cause vomiting or haematemesis.

Bleeding from Mallory–Weiss tears is usually only mild and transitory; hence management is largely conservative. Very rarely, massive bleeding may result, requiring surgical repair.

DISEASES OF THE STOMACH

Gastric bleeding

Causes of bleeding from the upper gastrointestinal tract are shown in **Fig. 1.46**; the diagnostic approach is the same for bleeding from anywhere in the foregut. A management algorithm is shown in **Fig. 1.47**. Endoscopic signs of recent haemorrhage are as follows:

Ulcers
- Visible vessel with spurting arterial bleeding
- Non-bleeding visible vessel
- Overlying fresh clot
- Blue or red pigmented macules in ulcer floor

Varices
- Visible ooze
- Fresh clot
- Cherry red spots*
- Red wales (ridges)*
- Size of varices*

Data from the North Italian Endoscopy Club studies revealed that these factors, together with the Child's grade of severity of cirrhosis, could accurately predict potential variceal haemorrhage. The size of oesophageal varix can be graded as: Grade I (small varices that flatten with air insufflation), Grade II (do not flatten, but occupy less than 50% of the oesophageal diameter) and Grade III (large varices that individually meet the midpoint of the lumen and may collectively occlude the view).

Patients who have had a haematemesis or melaena within the last 48 hours should be admitted to hospital for assessment. Haemodynamic stability should be assessed (including signs of poor peripheral perfusion, anaemia, tachycardia, hypotension or a postural drop in blood pressure). Adequate, large-bore venous access should be secured and blood cross-matched. Patients with significant hypotension or evidence of on-going haemorrhage should have a central venous line inserted, particularly those who are elderly or who have concomitant cardiac, renal or hepatic disease.

The causes of haematemesis and melaena	
Common causes	Duodenal ulceration
	Gastric ulceration
	Oesophageal ulceration
	Portal hypertension – oesophageal varices, gastric varices, portal gastropathy, duodenal varices
	Gastritis and gastric erosions
	Duodenitis
	Oesophagitis
	Oesophageal tear (Mallory–Weiss)
Uncommon causes	Malignancy of oesophagus or stomach
	Dieulafoy lesion
	Benign tumours – e.g. gastric leiomyoma
Rare causes	Foreign body
	Telangiectasia
	Angiodysplasia
	Amyloidosis
	Pseudoxanthoma elasticum
	Ehlers–Danlos syndrome
	Haemobilia
	Bleeding from pancreatic lesion

Fig. 1.46 *The causes of haematemesis and melaena.*

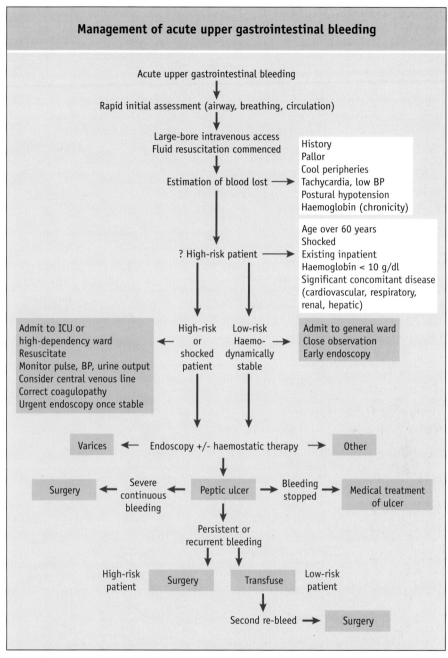

Management of acute upper gastrointestinal bleeding

Acute upper gastrointestinal bleeding

Rapid initial assessment (airway, breathing, circulation)

Large-bore intravenous access
Fluid resuscitation commenced

History
Pallor
Cool peripheries
Estimation of blood lost ⟶ Tachycardia, low BP
Postural hypotension
Haemoglobin (chronicity)

Age over 60 years
Shocked
? High-risk patient ⟶ Existing inpatient
Haemoglobin < 10 g/dl
Significant concomitant disease
(cardiovascular, respiratory,
renal, hepatic)

| Admit to ICU or high-dependency ward Resuscitate Monitor pulse, BP, urine output Consider central venous line Correct coagulopathy Urgent endoscopy once stable | ← | High-risk or shocked patient | Low-risk Haemo-dynamically stable | → | Admit to general ward Close observation Early endoscopy |

Varices ← Endoscopy +/- haemostatic therapy ⟶ Other

Surgery ← Severe continuous bleeding ← Peptic ulcer ⟶ Bleeding stopped ⟶ Medical treatment of ulcer

Persistent or recurrent bleeding

High-risk patient   Surgery   Transfuse   Low-risk patient

Second re-bleed ⟶ Surgery

Fig. 1.47 *Management of acute upper gastrointestinal bleeding. Patients should ideally be managed in collaboration with the surgical team. The three main indications for surgical intervention are massive continued bleeding, the loss of more than 8 units of blood and episodes of rebleeding (once in those over the age of 60 years and twice in those younger). The specific management of bleeding varices is discussed in chapter 4.*

Upper gastrointestinal endoscopy should be sought as soon as possible, although in many cases this can be deferred to within the next 24 hours. However, earlier intervention is usually required where bleeding oesophageal varices are suspected (such as those patients with clinical stigmata of chronic liver disease or a history of previous oesophageal varices), in patients who have had a significant bleed requiring a 4-unit blood transfusion or more, or where recurrent bleeding has taken place. The elderly have a considerable mortality from rebleeding and so emergency endoscopy should always be offered in order to staunch any bleeding lesion acutely.

Upper gastrointestinal endoscopy has a high diagnostic yield and most published studies have shown that the source of bleeding can be identified in around 90% of patients with acute haemorrhage. Endoscopy also allows therapeutic interventions aimed at achieving haemostasis. Actively bleeding lesions can be injected with adrenaline, alcohol or a sclerosant such as ethanolamine. Alternative endoscopic therapeutic strategies are outlined in **Fig. 1.48**.

Sometimes the cause of bleeding is not immediately obvious at endoscopy. If the endoscopy is entirely negative in a patient with 'melaena', a colonoscopy should be performed to exclude a proximal colonic source. If this is unrevealing, radionuclide red cell scans or visceral angiography may help to localise the bleeding lesion. However, the lesion has to be bleeding fairly briskly for these tests to be positive (usually greater than 0.5 ml per minute), although even in the absence of active bleeding an angiogram may demonstrate an area of abnormal circulation. Many centres now have access to small-bowel enteroscopy. In some cases of obscure bleeding, an 'on-table' enteroscopy, performed at laparotomy, is the final resort.

Endoscopic treatment of bleeding lesions		
Ulcers	**Injection therapy**	Adrenaline
		Alcohol
		Sclerosants
		Thrombin
	Thermal methods	Heater probe
		Electrocoagulation
		Argon beamer
		Neodymium YAG laser
	Other techniques	Microwave coagulation
		Cyanoacrylate glue
Varices*	**Injection therapy**	Sclerosants
		(polidocanol; ethanolamine oleate;
		sodium tetradecyl sulphate; alcohol)
		Thrombin*
		Glue*
	Band ligation	

In general, gastric varices are much less responsive to endoscopic treatment than oesophageal varices. The use of adhesives or thrombin may be more effective for gastric varices, but better results may be seen with treatment modalities aimed at lowering the portal pressure, such as octreotide, somatostatin, vasopressin or transjugular intrahepatic portasystemic stent shunts (TIPSS).

Fig. 1.48 *Endoscopic treatment of bleeding lesions.*

Gastritis

Gastritis is a frequent endoscopic finding in patients with dyspepsia or epigastric pain (although the single commonest finding in these patients is actually a normal endoscopy). Inflammation of the lining of the stomach can be due to a wide range of insults, including infection, autoimmunity, drugs and alcohol. Infection with *Helicobacter pylori* is an important cause of gastritis and a number of other foregut disorders.

Helicobacter pylori. Spiral organisms were first found in the mammalian stomach around a hundred years ago and at the turn of the century such bacteria were noted in biopsies of human gastric carcinomas. Little attention was paid to these findings until 1982, when Marshall and colleagues grew a *Campylobacter*-like organism from the stomach of a patient with peptic ulcer disease. The organism was initially named *Campylobacter pyloridis*, but this was subsequently changed to *Helicobacter pylori* on account of its spiral shape *in vivo* and lack of genomic similarities with 'true' campylobacters.

This microaerophilic Gram-negative bacterium is a common cause of chronic gastritis and peptic ulceration. The organism infects gastric-type mucosa (and therefore may also be found where there is gastric metaplasia in the oesophagus or duodenum). In most western countries, its prevalence is highest in the older age groups, with about 60% of 60-year-olds being infected compared with about 10% of children. This higher prevalence with increasing age is thought to be at least partly a 'cohort effect', suggestive of higher rates of infection in past decades.

The exact mode of transmission is still not fully clear, but the worldwide geographical and sociological patterns of *H. pylori* infections suggest a faeco-oral or possibly oro-oral route. Rates of infection are higher with poor socio-economic conditions, overcrowding and lack of sanitation.

H. pylori selectively colonises gastric epithelium, particularly the antrum, and can infect such epithelium at sites other than in the stomach, such as a Meckel's diverticulum, duodenal metaplasia or Barrett's epithelium in the oesophagus.

Chronic infection of the gastric antrum can lead to enhanced gastrin production and consequently increased secretion of gastric acid. The bacterium itself produces large amounts of the enzyme urease. PPI drugs may inhibit urease and can lead to false-negative results on diagnostic urease tests (see pp 14, 15, 17, 18). In the corpus, chronic infection may progress to atrophic gastritis.

Genetic analysis has revealed that strains of *H. pylori* are actually very diverse. Certain polymorphisms of the bacterial gene encoding a vacuolating cytotoxin ('vacA') or the presence of the cytotoxin-association gene ('cagA') appear to be more closely associated with peptic ulceration. Intense research is currently under way into different aspects of the *H. pylori* genome and how these may be linked to particularly pathogenic strains of the bacterium.

Apart from gastritis, the organism is causally associated with duodenal and gastric ulceration (in > 90% and 70% of cases, respectively) and the development of MALT (mucosa-associated lymphoid tissue) lymphomas, and has been implicated in the genesis of gastric adenocarcinoma. Exactly which patients develop these diseases is likely to be determined by the presence of 'toxigenic' strains of bacteria (see above) together with host factors influencing the immune response. Research is continuing into the roles of genes that encode blood group antigens (which may affect bacterial adhesion to the mucosa) and human leucocyte antigen (HLA) status.

The treatment of *H. pylori* infection is dealt with in the section on duodenal ulceration. The full range of conditions associated with this organism are as follows:

Common
- Chronic gastritis
- Duodenal ulceration
- Gastric ulceration
- Non-ulcer dyspepsia (controversial)

Less common
- Gastric adenocarcinoma
- Gastric lymphoma

?Unproven
- Ischaemic heart disease (controversial)

Aetiology of gastritis. Gastritis may be the result of a number of different pathological processes. Histological and endoscopic classifications of gastritis are outlined in **Fig. 1.49**. The microscopic appearance of chronic active gastritis is shown in **Fig. 1.50**.

A summary of the 'Sydney' classification of gastritis

Endoscopic appearances	Aetiology	Histological features	Topography
Erosive	*H. pylori*	Acute vs chronic	Prepyloric
Exudative	NSAID	Activity	Antral
Friability	Alcohol	Atrophic changes	Corpus
Erythema	Others	Intestinal metaplasia	Pangastritis
		Histological severity	
		Oedema	
		Presence of bacteria	
		Eosinophilia	
		Granulomata	
		Haemorrhage	

The gastritic process is described using combinations of terms from the four columns above; for example, a moderately active erosive chronic gastritis of the prepyloric region with HLOs (*Helicobacter*-like organisms) present. The term 'reactive' gastritis is sometimes used to denote drug-induced changes.

Fig. 1.49 *A summary of the 'Sydney' classification of gastritis.*

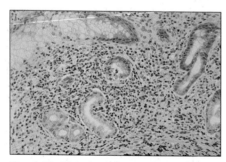

Fig. 1.50 *Chronic active gastritis. H&E-stained antral biopsy specimen showing the typical appearance of chronic active gastritis.*

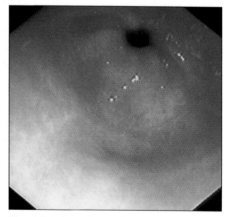

Fig. 1.51 *Antral gastritis. Erythematous gastric antrum in a patient with Helicobacter pylori infection.*

H. pylori infection is the main cause of chronic gastritis and antral erythema is a typical finding (**Fig. 1.51**). Diagnosis is confirmed on histological examination of biopsy material (see **Fig. 1.21**). NSAIDs cause an acute gastritis, while chronic gastritis may be granulomatous secondary to conditions such as Crohn's disease, tuberculosis (**Fig. 1.52**) or sarcoidosis. Causes of gastritis are:

Common
- *H. pylori*
- Drugs and other irritants – alcohol, NSAIDs, cytotoxics, corrosive agents
- Bile reflux

Less common
- Autoimmune disease
- Irradiation
- *Staphylococcus aureus* – food poisoning
- Opportunistic infections – cytomegalovirus, *Herpes simplex*, fungi, tuberculosis
- Crohn's disease
- Eosinophilic gastritis
- Lymphocytic gastritis
- Sarcoidosis
- Idiopathic

Chronic gastritis, particularly that associated with alcohol abuse, may lead to 'watermelon stomach' (**Fig. 1.53**). This form of gastric vascular ectasia can lead to chronic blood loss and anaemia.

Atrophic gastritis and pernicious anaemia

Autoimmune chronic gastritis is characterised by circulating autoantibodies to gastric parietal cells and to intrinsic factor. However, only a minority of those with gastric parietal antibodies actually develop any demonstrable disease in the form of atrophic gastritis of the body and fundus of the stomach (**Fig. 1.54**) or full-blown pernicious anaemia. There is an association with autoimmune thyroiditis and other autoimmune conditions including vitiligo.

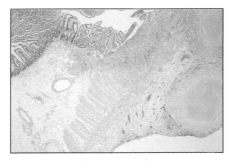

Fig. 1.52 *Gastric tuberculosis. Histological appearance of tuberculous gastritis showing granuloma.*

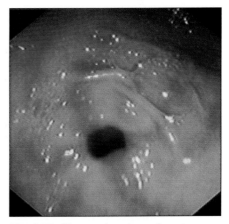

Fig. 1.53 *Watermelon stomach. Endoscopic view, showing streaks of gastric vascular ectasia radiating out from the pylorus.*

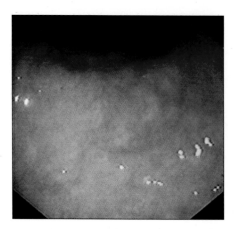

Fig. 1.54 *Atrophic gastritis. This view of the gastric body reveals that the normally thick, longitudinal folds (rugae) have been lost and replaced with a smooth, atrophic mucosa.*

These patients present with symptoms of anaemia and those more specific to vitamin B_{12} deficiency (owing to malabsorption secondary to binding or blocking intrinsic factor antibodies), such as a painful glossitis and paraesthesiae. Owing to the presence of hypochlorhydria or achlorhydria, colonisation of the stomach with *H. pylori* is very uncommon, presumably because these conditions are unfavourable for the organism.

The Schilling test is abnormal (in patients who have received presaturation of their vitamin B_{12} stores), with less than 10% of a dose of oral [58]Cobalt-labelled vitamin B_{12} being excreted in the urine. This corrects in the second part of the test when intrinsic factor is added, unlike causes of terminal ileal disease where there is no correction (see chapter 2). Following initial dosing of six injections on alternate days, regular 3-monthly intramuscular vitamin B_{12} injections should be given.

Ménétrier's disease

This is hyperplasia of the gastric mucosa, particularly in the fundus, and body of the stomach. Highly convoluted gastric rugal folds are seen. The cause is unknown, but men are more commonly affected. There is no clear relationship with *H. pylori* infection.

Patients usually complain of dyspepsia, but anorexia, nausea and bleeding may occur. Vomiting may sometimes occur, caused by obstruction from giant rugal folds.

There is a protein-losing enteropathy and patients may occasionally present with oedema and ascites as a result of hypoproteinaemia. Gastric acid secretion is decreased, owing to a reduction in parietal cell mass.

Treatment consists of high-protein meals or supplements to correct the hypoproteinaemia. Full acid suppression may sometimes be helpful if there is bleeding. Surgical resection is rarely necessary, except in cases of persistent symptomatic hypoproteinaemia.

Gastric ulcers

Benign peptic ulceration of the stomach cannot be distinguished from gastric malignancies or duodenal ulceration on purely clinical grounds. Patients usually complain of epigastric pain. If the lesion has been slowly oozing blood, iron deficiency anaemia and tiredness may be presenting features, rather than frank haematemesis or melaena.

H. pylori, NSAIDs, aspirin, corticosteroids and smoking are amongst the aetiological factors. Less commonly, gastric ulcers may result from Crohn's disease, tuberculosis or vasculitides.

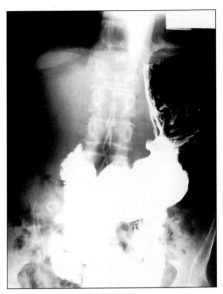

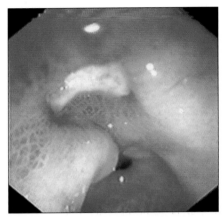

Fig. 1.56 *Gastric ulceration. The white, sloughy base of this large prepyloric gastric ulcer can be clearly seen. Gastric ulcers should be biopsied to exclude neoplasia and the endoscopy repeated after a course of antisecretory therapy to ensure healing has occurred. Incidentally, this patient also had alcoholic cirrhosis and the mucosa surrounding the ulcer has the characteristic 'snakeskin' appearance of portal hypertensive gastropathy.*

Fig. 1.55 *Gastric ulceration on barium meal. A large gastric ulcer on the lesser curve is visible as a protrusion of the barium with surrounding rolled edges.*

The characteristic appearances of ulceration may be seen on barium meal (**Fig. 1.55**) but endoscopy is more commonly performed (**Fig. 1.56**), where biopsy for histological analysis can be from the ulcer edge.

Management of gastric ulceration

- Exclude gastric cancer
- Acid suppression (H$_2$ antagonist proton pump inhibitor) for 4–6 weeks
- Eradicate *Helicobacter pylori* if present
- Stop smoking
- Stop or reduce non-steroidal anti-inflammatory drugs, if possible
- Check ulcer healing at repeat endoscopy and continue acid suppression until healed
- Consider surgery for resistant ulcers

It has become standard practice to repeat the endoscopy after 4–6 weeks of acid suppression, in order to check that the gastric ulcer has healed or is healing, because occasionally malignant lesions can be missed. With the advent of H$_2$ antagonists and PPIs, the need for surgery has considerably diminished, now being largely reserved for complications such as perforation or uncontrolled bleeding. The association of *H. pylori* with gastric ulceration is weaker than with duodenal ulceration, but appropriate eradication regimes may prevent recurrence.

The gastrointestinal effects of NSAIDs are discussed in detail in chapter 7.

Gastric cancer

Gastric adenocarcinoma is the commonest tumour of the stomach. Patients are often asymptomatic until the disease is relatively advanced.

Benign	Malignant
• Hyperplastic polyps	• Adenocarcinoma
• Adenomatous polyps	• Primary gastric lymphoma
• Leiomyoma	• Carcinoid
• Lipoma	• Leiomyosarcoma
• Neurofibroma	• Secondary lymphoma
• Glomus tumour	• Secondary carcinoma
	• Plasmacytoma
	• Choriocarcinoma
	• Leukaemic infiltration

Weight loss, early satiety, a more generalised anorexia or, if the lesion has ulcerated the mucosa, epigastric pain which may be indistinguishable from benign peptic ulceration are presenting features. If the tumour is in the prepyloric region, patients may present with vomiting from gastric outlet obstruction, although this can occur with benign ulceration. Atrophic gastritis predisposes to gastric cancer and dietary factors including nitrite and aflatoxin contamination have also been implicated, along with cigarette smoking.

The incidence of gastric adenocarcinoma has decreased in recent years, but it remains one of the leading causes of cancer deaths worldwide. The condition has a marked geographic variation (**Fig. 1.57**) and is particularly common in Japan, where there are mass population screening programmes to detect early disease. In most other countries, emphasis has been placed on the early investigation of symptomatic patients, such as those with dyspepsia, as gastric cancer is relatively less common.

This contrasting approach to diagnosing the condition may account, at least in part, for the international differences in prognosis. In Japan the 5-year survival rate for patients with early gastric cancer is more than 90%, whereas survival rates in the UK are currently 17% at 2 years and 12% at 5 years. This reflects the fact that such tumours have often metastasised to regional lymph nodes, if not the liver, before a diagnosis is made. Patients with early gastric cancer have a good prognosis provided the tumour is confined to the mucosa and submucosa.

Diagnostically, a barium meal may help delineate the anatomy, but endoscopy enables biopsies to be taken. At endoscopy, tumours may appear exophytic (**Fig. 1.58**) or ulcerated with a raised, rolled edge (**Fig. 1.59**). Occasionally, extensive submucosal infiltration leads to the development of *linitis plastica*, a diffuse narrowing of the gastric lumen.

Surgery provides the only chance of cure if there is no metastatic spread and can offer important palliation for complications such as gastric outlet obstruction.

Chemotherapy is frequently used as an adjunct to surgery, but results with single agents (most commonly 5-fluorouracil) or combinations of cytotoxic drugs have generally been disappointing. Controlled trials are continuing.

As a result, the emphasis remains on improving the early diagnosis and perhaps even the prevention of stomach cancer. The world has seen a steady fall in gastric cancer mortality rates since the 1950s. The precise reasons for this are unknown and the rate of decline has been similar in most countries, including Japan with its screening programmes. Increased early detection is therefore probably not the main factor in this phenomenon.

The most common form of stomach cancer, the 'intestinal type' distal adenocarcinoma, seems related to the development of atrophic gastritis with intestinal metaplasia and particularly to infection with 'cag positive' strains of *H. pylori*. In the future, primary

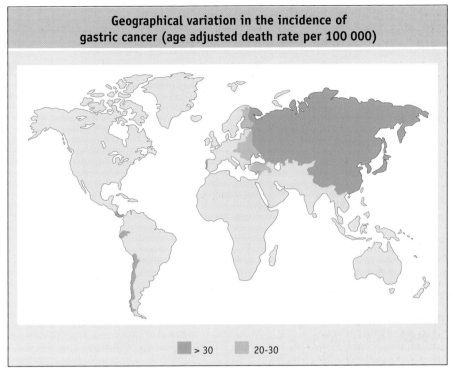

Geographical variation in the incidence of gastric cancer (age adjusted death rate per 100 000)

> 30   20-30

Fig. 1.57 *Geographical variation in the incidence of gastric cancer. Gastric adenocarcinoma is relatively uncommon in North America, Western Europe and Australasia. The areas with the highest incidence rates are Russia, Japan, China, South America and certain parts of Eastern Europe.*

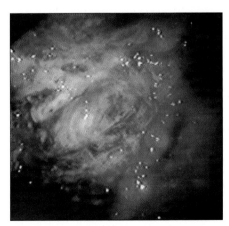

Fig. 1.58 *Exophytic gastric cancer. The fundus of this patient's stomach contained an extensive, bleeding, ulcerative area due to an adenocarcinoma.*

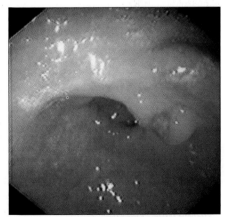

Fig. 1.59 *Gastric ulceration. This prepyloric ulcer has a heaped-up, rolled edge. Histological biopsy confirmed a gastric adenocarcinoma.*

41

prevention may be possible, perhaps by modification of dietary factors or possibly by eradication of *H. pylori*. Interestingly, although the incidence of the common distal gastric cancer has fallen dramatically, several western nations have recently reported a rise in the numbers of proximal (cardia) stomach cancers. The reason for this is unknown, but it presumably reflects an environmental influence.

The decreasing incidence of adenocarcinoma of the distal is one recent trend in foregut disorders in the developed nations. Others include:

Decreasing incidence
- New acquisition of *Helicobacter pylori*
- Duodenal ulceration
- Gastric ulceration

Increasing incidence
- Gastro-oesophageal reflux disease
- Barrett's oesophagus
- Adenocarcinoma of the distal oesophagus and gastric cardia

Gastric polyps

Benign gastric polyps are not uncommon endoscopic findings (**Fig. 1.60**). The commonest histological diagnosis is the hyperplastic or regenerative polyp seen in around 70% of cases (**Fig. 1.61**). It is important to know the histology, because although hyperplastic polyps have low malignant potential, benign adenomatous gastric polyps which arise from glandular tissue in the antrum are associated with a higher risk of gastric cancer. This varies in published series from 3% to 38%, with lesions > 2 cm providing a bigger risk. Further investigations should include barium follow-through and colonoscopy to delineate polyps at other sites in the gastrointestinal tract.

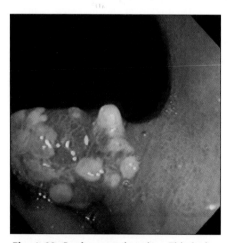

Fig. 1.60 *Benign gastric polyp. This lesion was present high on the lesser curve of the stomach, close to the oesophagogastric junction. Despite its macroscopic appearance, histology of the completely excised polyp revealed it to be benign in nature.*

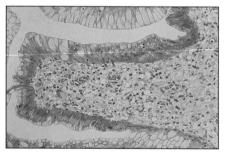

Fig. 1.61 *Histological appearance of gastric polyp. The polyp shown in Fig. 1.60 was excised using a diathermy snare. The lesion consisted of a hyperplastic glandular mucosa.*

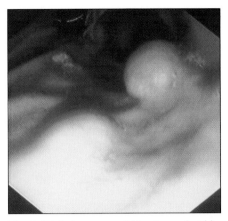

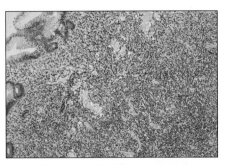

Fig. 1.63 *Gastric 'MALToma'. Histology of a gastric mucosa-associated lymphoma, with an obvious diffuse infiltration of lymphoid cells. This patient's tumour regressed when his* H. pylori *infection was eradicated.*

Fig. 1.62 *Leiomyoma of the stomach. This 'J' manoeuvre shows the endoscope looking back on itself towards the fundus. A gastric leiomyoma can be seen bulging beneath the mucosa.*

Other tumours of the stomach

Other tumours of the stomach consist of gastric carcinoid tumours, leiomyomas (**Fig. 1.62**), leiomyosarcomas and lymphomas, including lymphomas of mucosa-associated lymphoid tissue (MALT) – so-called 'MALTomas' (**Fig. 1.63**). Although the stomach does not normally contain significant quantities of lymphoid tissue, *H. pylori* infection stimulates its growth and may lead to the development of these low-grade B cell tumours. The eradication of an *H. pylori* infection can lead to MALToma regression or disappearance.

Leiomyomas, which are benign smooth muscle tumours, have a characteristic umbilicated appearance at endoscopy. This is caused by central ulceration which may give rise to bleeding. Biopsy of these lesions at endoscopy is usually unrewarding since they are submucosal. Endoscopic ultrasound may reveal the extent of each lesion, but surgery rather than endoscopic excision is required to remove them. Leiomyomas may also occur in the oesophagus and throughout the small intestine.

Developmental abnormalities such as heterotopic pancreatic rests in the stomach may have similar appearances to leiomyomas, being submucosal and appearing as a mound-like area in the prepyloric region.

Bezoars

These lesions in the stomach are either composed of vegetable fibre (phytobezoar) in those vegans or vegetarians with a high indigestible fibre content to their diet or else they are composed of ingested hair (trichobezoar), usually in long-haired individuals who absentmindedly chew their own hair. Treatment usually involves breaking up the bezoar at endoscopy in order to facilitate passage through the pylorus. Prokinetic agents should be administered to facilitate gastric emptying.

DISEASES OF THE DUODENUM

Duodenal ulcer disease

Epidemiology and aetiology. Peptic ulcer disease, affecting the stomach or duodenum, is an extremely common problem. Estimates suggest that some 4 million Americans have active peptic ulceration and about 10% of the adult population will develop an ulcer during their lifetime. In most countries, including the United States, United Kingdom and Australia, duodenal ulcers are about twice as common as gastric ulcers. However, in Japan, Turkey, Peru and Finland it is gastric ulceration which is most frequent.

Duodenal ulceration has been variously linked to low socio-economic status, cigarette smoking, NSAIDs, psychological stress and blood group O, but the most significant pathogenic risk factor is infection with the bacterium *H. pylori*. Chronic infection may lead to increased secretion of gastric acid, the duodenal mucosa itself being more vulnerable to acidic damage if there is concomitant infection of duodenal mucosal islands of gastric metaplasia.

H. pylori is responsible for a spectrum of disease from duodenitis to frank duodenal ulceration (see p. 36) and is present in 95–100% of duodenal ulcer patients. Individuals with *H. pylori* gastritis are 14 times more likely to develop an ulcer compared to controls. Host factors are also influential, however, an example being the wide disparity seen in Africa between almost universal carriage rates of *H. pylori* and a relatively low incidence of duodenal ulcer disease.

Clinical features and diagnosis. Patients with duodenal ulcers may complain of recurrent epigastric pain or can present with acute bleeding. There are characteristic appearances on barium meal (**Fig. 1.64**), but the presence of ulceration is confirmed at endoscopy (**Fig. 1.65**). *H. pylori* status may be determined by rapid urease testing or histological examination of gastric antral or corpus biopsies. Complications of duodenal ulcer disease include bleeding, perforation (**Fig. 1.66**) and scarring of the duodenal cap (**Fig. 1.67**), which may lead to pyloric stenosis and gastric outlet obstruction (**Fig. 1.68**).

Management. The advent of H_2 antagonists or proton pump inhibitors has meant that surgery for duodenal ulceration is rarely required. The various surgical options are shown in **Fig. 1.69** and their endoscopic appearances post-surgery in **Fig.1.70**.

Effective *H. pylori* eradication with a combination of acid suppression and antibiotics results in cure not only of any acute ulcers, but also of the recurrent symptoms. Guidelines

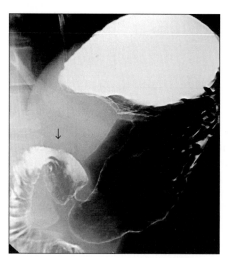

Fig. 1.64 *Duodenal ulceration. Barium meal showing an ulcer in the duodenum (arrowed).*

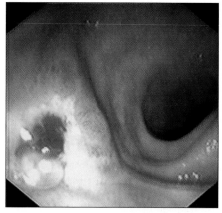

Fig. 1.65 *Duodenal ulceration. Large anterior ulcer in the first part of the duodenum, with evidence of recent haemorrhage.*

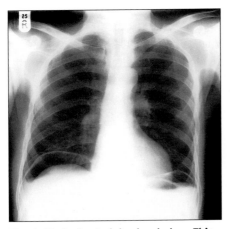

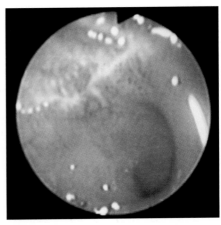

Fig. 1.66 *Perforated duodenal ulcer. This 36-year-old man presented with an acute abdomen. His chest X-ray clearly shows air under both sides of the diaphragm, the result of a perforated duodenal ulcer found at laparotomy.*

Fig. 1.67 *Duodenal scarring. Chronic ulceration has led to scarring and distortion of the duodenal cap in this elderly man. In some cases, gastric outlet obstruction may be the result.*

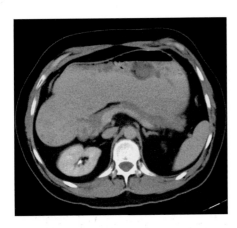

Fig. 1.68 *Pyloric stenosis. This patient had a long history of duodenal ulcer disease. His abdominal CT scan shows a grossly dilated stomach, the result of gastric outlet obstruction due to pyloric stenosis.*

for treating *H. pylori* are often confusing, since the merits of different combinations of drugs have been reported over the years. A typical regimen consists of concurrent treatment with omeprazole, amoxycillin and metronidazole for 1 week, although in inner city areas in the UK there is increased incidence of *H. pylori* metronidazole resistance. An alternative antibiotic such as clarithromycin should therefore be substituted in these circumstances. Two recommended regimens are shown here, both of 1 week's duration. Patients taking metronidazole must be warned to avoid alcohol, in view of its disulfiram-like reaction:

OAC 500 (LAC 500)
- Omeprazole 20 mg b.d. (or lansoprazole 30 mg b.d.)
- Amoxycillin 1 g b.d.
- Clarithromycin 500 mg b.d.

OMC 250 (LMC 250)
- Omeprazole 20 mg b.d. (or lansoprazole 30 mg b.d.)
- Metronidazole 400 mg b.d.
- Clarithromycin 250 mg b.d.

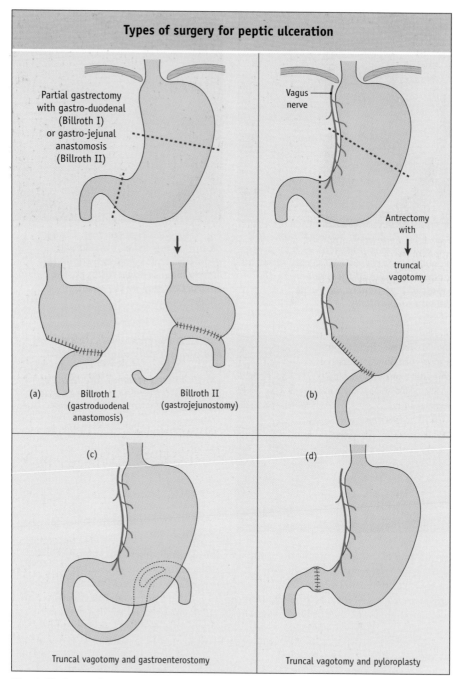

Fig. 1.69 *Types of surgery for peptic ulceration. (a) Partial gastrectomy with gastroduodenal or gastrojejunal anastomosis (Billroth I or II). (b) Truncal vagotomy and antrectomy with gastroduodenal anastomosis. (c) Truncal vagotomy and gastroenterostomy. (d) Truncal vagotomy and pyloroplasty.*

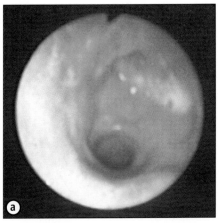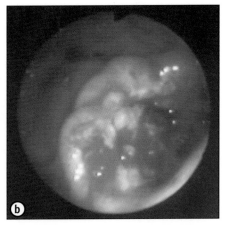

Fig. 1.70 *Endoscopic appearances after surgery for duodenal ulceration. (a) The normal appearance of a Polya-type gastrectomy, with the two gastric 'outlets' visible. (b) Post-gastrectomy malignancy. This 74-year-old man presented with weight loss and anaemia. Some 30 years previously he had had an antrectomy (Billroth I gastrectomy) for peptic ulceration. At endoscopy, a malignant tumour can be seen around his anastomotic site.*

Should one of these fail, it is worth trying a course of the alternative regimen in view of the possibility of infection with a drug-resistant strain. Occasionally, neither is effective and a more prolonged course of multidrug therapy is required. For example, a 1-week regimen consisting of omeprazole 20 mg b.d., tetracycline 500 mg q.d.s., bismuth subcitrate 120 mg q.d.s. and metronidazole 400 mg b.d. may be effective. However, it is always worth bearing in mind that inadequate compliance with therapy is the commonest cause of treatment failure.

Other causes of duodenal ulcer and duodenitis. H. pylori is not the only cause of duodenitis. Other causes of duodenal inflammation and ulceration include:

- Coeliac disease
- Non-steroidal anti-inflammatory drugs
- Tuberculosis
- Crohn's disease
- Giardiasis
- Ankylostomiasis
- Vasculitides
- Zollinger–Ellison syndrome
- Systemic mastocytosis
- Ischaemia
- *Herpes simplex*
- Cytomegalovirus
- Cryptosporidiosis
- Renal failure

Brunner's gland hyperplasia and benign nodular lymphoid hyperplasia

Brunner's gland hyperplasia may just be an incidental finding at endoscopy; it causes a nodular appearance in the duodenum which looks like duodenitis at endoscopy or on barium meal. Similar appearances may be seen with benign nodular lymphoid hyperplasia. Neither diagnosis is of any importance and the two can be differentiated on histological analysis of duodenal biopsy material.

Zollinger–Ellison syndrome

Multiple duodenal ulcers (**Fig. 1.71**) which appear to be resistant to standard treatment measures should raise the possibility of Zollinger–Ellison syndrome, where the presence of a pancreatic or duodenal gastrinoma leads to hypersecretion of gastrin which constantly stimulates the production of high basal gastric acid output from the gastric parietal cells.

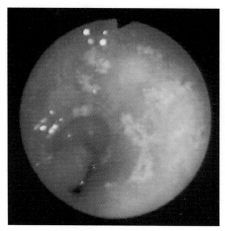 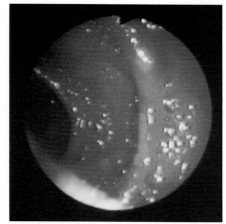

Fig. 1.71 Multiple duodenal ulcers. Numerous white ulcer bases can be seen in the first part of this patient's duodenum.

Fig. 1.72 Distal duodenal ulceration. As well as multiple ulcers in the duodenal bulb, this patient with a gastrinoma had ulceration extending down into the second and third parts of the duodenum.

Patients often complain of diarrhoea which may be the only presenting symptom. This is caused by acid deconjugation of bile salts and inactivation of lipases, causing fat malabsorption. Vitamin B_{12} deficiency may also be a feature. The syndrome is probably underdiagnosed, but these tumours are malignant in more than 60% of cases.

Features of the Zollinger–Ellison Syndrome may be summarised as follows:

* Multiple or unusually persistent ulcers.
* Diarrhoea
* Jejunal ulceration
* Elevated serum gastrin (in the absence of achlorhydria or hypercalcaemia)
* Basal acid output > 60% of peak stimulated output
* Rise in serum gastrin level of > 50% and rise of acid output of > 18 mmol/hour following intravenous secretin

At endoscopy, ulceration may be seen right along the duodenum (**Fig. 1.72**) and also in the stomach and oesophagus. Ulceration may even have spread into the jejunum. Hypertrophy of the gastric body mucosa is also a characteristic feature.

Fasting serum gastrin levels are high and radioisotope scans using the labelled somatostatin analogue octreotide may show hot spots of tumours expressing somatostatin receptors, but localisation of the gastrinoma is often difficult. Spiral CT scanning with contrast agents or MRI may be helpful, but the pickup is often disappointingly low since the tumours are usually very small. Selective angiography may be helpful, and selective venous sampling of gastrin levels at portography can be valuable in deciding if the tumour is pancreatic or duodenal.

Large doses of PPIs keep symptoms at bay, so that surgery is rarely required on a routine basis. Octreotide may damp down gastrin secretion. Partial pancreatectomy or duodenal resection should not be undertaken lightly and, furthermore, survival in malignant disease with hepatic metastases can be many years, since the tumours are slow-growing.

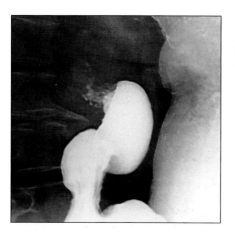

Fig. 1.73 *Duodenal carcinoma. Barium meal showing a post-bulbar stricture in a patient with duodenal adenocarcinoma.*

Carcinoma of the duodenum

Adenocarcinoma of the duodenum is extremely rare, but the second part of the duodenum is the commonest site for cancer anywhere in the small intestine (**Fig. 1.73**). Patients usually present with weight loss, anorexia and nausea or with epigastric pain if the lesion has ulcerated. Slow blood loss may result in anaemia, whereas frank bleeding is unusual. If periampullary, then jaundice may be a presenting feature, but it is not invariable.

Treatment usually involves a Whipple's procedure (partial pancreatoduodenectomy), but exophytic lesions can be excised at endoscopy, provided that the stalk does not show any evidence of invasion.

Duodenal diverticula

These are not an uncommon finding at endoscopy and are usually located in the second part of the duodenum, particularly around the ampulla of Vater, which may empty into a diverticulum in some individuals. Duodenal diverticulosis may be a focus for bacterial overgrowth and can be an endoscopic hazard, particularly at endoscopic retrograde cholangiopancreatography (ERCP), where a side-viewing endoscope is used.

FUNCTIONAL DISEASE: NON-ULCER DYSPEPSIA (NUD)

This term refers to chronic, recurrent, often meal-related discomfort in the epigastrium, which is initially thought to be caused by peptic ulceration, but at subsequent endoscopy no ulcer can be found. The condition is sometimes referred to as 'functional dyspepsia' and implies the persistence of a cluster of symptoms (**Fig. 1.74**) despite normal endoscopic findings.

It is difficult to give exact figures on the prevalence of NUD, but a number of population surveys undertaken in Europe and the USA suggest that it may affect up to 30% of the adult population.

Symptoms may vary. Some patients have classical ulcer-type dyspepsia with epigastric pain that can be pinpointed with great accuracy. The pain may be relieved by food or antacids and may be worse on lying flat in bed at night. Other patients may have predominantly reflux symptoms with heartburn, eructation (belching), retrosternal pain and acid reflux. Some may develop dysmotility symptoms such as early satiety after meals, intolerance of fatty foods, generalised anorexia and the sensation of abdominal bloating.

Symptom patterns in non-ulcer dyspepia	
Ulcer-type symptoms	Epigastric pain Relief with food or antacid medications Pain worse at night
Reflux symptoms	Acid regurgitation Heartburn Upper gastrointestinal flatulence Retrosternal pain
Dysmotility symptoms	Anorexia Early satiety Postprandial bloating Generalised upper abdominal discomfort Nausea and/or vomiting
Miscellaneous	Non-specific malaise Combinations of above symptoms

Fig. 1.74 *Symptom patterns in non-ulcer dyspepia.*

There is a relationship between NUD and the irritable bowel syndrome, particularly in the subgroup of patients with bloating. Both of these conditions are functional gastrointestinal disorders with no demonstrable structural disease and may reflect regional variations of the same pathophysiological mechanisms. Certainly there is often overlap between these two 'foregut' and 'hindgut' disorders, with population studies showing that around 30% of patients with NUD also have the irritable bowel syndrome.

The role of *H. pylori* in the genesis of NUD remains controversial. *H. pylori* infection and NUD are relatively common, but no direct causal link has been demonstrated. Some studies have suggested that infection rates are higher in NUD patients than the general population, but trials documenting the effect of eradication therapy have so far been conflicting. This may be due to the difficulties in documenting fluctuations in dyspeptic symptomatology in the absence of any demonstrable physical disease. Large-scale trials of eradication therapy for NUD are continuing.

The current treatment of patients with NUD is mostly empirical and depends to a large extent on the predominant symptoms. A suggested algorithm for treatment is shown in Fig. 1.75.

If reflux symptoms predominate then acid suppression with a PPI or H_2 antagonist may be appropriate. Prokinetic agents such as cisapride may also be effective, especially if bloating or other dysmotility symptoms are present. If these drugs fail to provide benefit, *H. pylori* eradication therapy may improve symptoms in patients with a positive test for the organism, although there is currently little hard evidence to support this practice (see above). Patients with severe, recurrent or resistant symptoms should be considered for further investigation with gastric emptying studies or oesophageal pH monitoring.

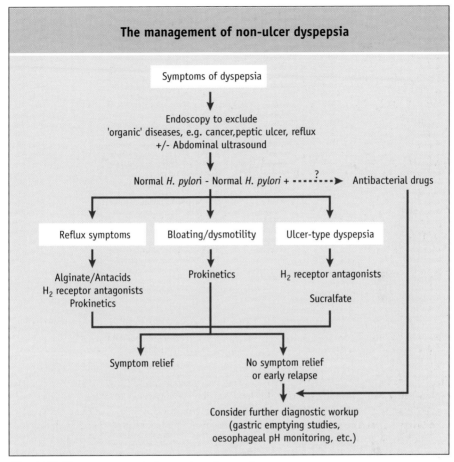

Fig. 1.75 *The management of non-ulcer dyspepsia.*

chapter 2

The Midgut

STRUCTURE AND FUNCTION

EMBRYOLOGY

The midgut extends from the distal half of the second part of the duodenum to the distal third of the transverse colon (see **Fig. 1.1**). *In utero*, from the 6th week onwards, the midgut develops to a large extent outside the abdominal cavity, owing to encroachment from rapidly enlarging organs such as the liver and kidneys which force the midgut through a widely patent umbilicus (**Fig. 2.1**). Blood supply to the midgut is from the superior mesenteric artery. The midgut rotates around 90° in an anticlockwise position along an axis formed by the vascular supply, before returning to the abdominal cavity by the third month *in utero*. In doing so, the gut rotates by a further 180°. The caecum and ascending colon lengthen to occupy their adult positions only once this anticlockwise rotation has taken place. Most of the duodenum is subsequently retroperitoneal – the duodenojejunal flexure is fixed to the posterior abdominal wall by the suspensory ligament of Treitz. Apart from the ascending colon which also becomes retroperitoneal, the rest of the midgut is attached to a relatively mobile mesentery which provides the blood supply.

Congenital abnormalities of the midgut include absence of rotation or malrotation of the midgut loop. This usually presents as bowel obstruction in the first few weeks of life, owing to band-like adhesions which may be fairly restrictive. Causes of neonatal intestinal obstruction may be summarised as follows:

- Intestinal atresia
- Intestinal duplication
- Malrotation with or without small bowel volvulus
- Meconium plug syndrome
- Meconium ileus
- Absent distal ileal musculature
- Hirchsprung's disease

Small bowel atresia and duplication of segments of the gut may present in a similar fashion, although the latter may not present until much later in life as a focus for intussusception or volvulus. Congenital abnormalities associated with intestinal atresia include:

- Malrotation
- Ectopic anus
- Annular pancreas
- Omphalocoele
- Gastroschisis
- Congenital heart disease
- Down's syndrome
- Cri-du-chat syndrome

Surgical correction is required for all these congenital abnormalities and may also be necessary for associated malformations elsewhere.

ANATOMY

Although embryologically part of the midgut, the ascending and proximal two-thirds of the transverse colon will be considered with the hindgut (see chapter 3). The small intestine from the latter part of the duodenum to the ileocaecal valve is dealt with here.

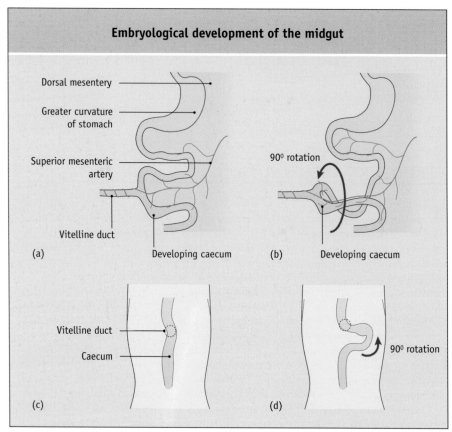

Embryological development of the midgut

Dorsal mesentery

Greater curvature
of stomach

Superior mesenteric
artery

90° rotation

Vitelline duct

(a)   Developing caecum   (b)   Developing caecum

Vitelline duct

Caecum

90° rotation

(c)   (d)

Fig. 2.1 *Embryological development of the midgut. The developing midgut undergoes an anticlockwise rotation of 90° while growing in the extra-embryonic coelom of the umbilical cord. (a) and (b) Left-side views. (c) and (d) Front views.*

The approximate length of the small intestine is about 6 m when measured post-mortem but the multiple loops of jejunum and ileum are usually a lot shorter in reality, owing to muscular tone and peristaltic waves which are continually changing the conformation in which the bowel is held. Following on from the duodenum, the next two-fifths of the small intestine is jejunum, with ileum composing the remainder. There is no definite transition from jejunum to ileum, but the transverse folds in the jejunum tend to be more pronounced and the ileum is somewhat thinner than the jejunum.

The bowel wall consists of a longitudinal and circular muscle layer, surrounded by serosa and lined by a mucous membrane containing both circular folds and villi to increase the surface area for nutrient absorption. There are also lymphoid aggregates throughout the small intestine which are best developed in the ileum (Peyer's patches).

The villi are lined on their luminal surface by enterocytes which compose a columnar epithelium and contain lymphatic and vascular supplies within the lamina propria (**Fig. 2.2**).

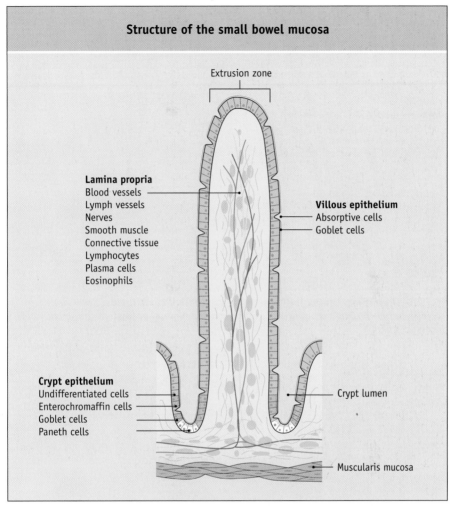

Structure of the small bowel mucosa

Extrusion zone

Lamina propria
Blood vessels
Lymph vessels
Nerves
Smooth muscle
Connective tissue
Lymphocytes
Plasma cells
Eosinophils

Villous epithelium
Absorptive cells
Goblet cells

Crypt epithelium
Undifferentiated cells
Enterochromaffin cells
Goblet cells
Paneth cells

Crypt lumen

Muscularis mucosa

Fig. 2.2 *Structure of the small bowel mucosa: the small intestinal villi and crypts. There is a rapid turnover of cells, with crypt enterocytes frequently showing active mitoses. Apoptotic cells are eventually shed from the apices of the villi. The absorptive functions of each villus are complemented by a rich supply of blood vessels and lymphatics.*

PHYSIOLOGY

The main function of the small intestine is to absorb nutrients and its mucosal surface area is adapted maximally for this purpose with folds and villi which increase the interface for absorption more than 20-fold. The particular sites of absorption of dietary constituents are shown in **Fig. 2.3**; most occur in the proximal small bowel. Specific enterocyte membrane transport proteins exist for many dietary constituents. As electrolytes and glucose are absorbed (**Fig. 2.4**), luminal water is drawn passively across the epithelium. This cotransport of glucose and sodium is particularly relevant to rehydration therapy, where the most efficient correction of fluid depletion is achieved by giving rehydration solutions based on salt, sugar and water.

Sites of maximal absorption for various dietary constituents

Substance	Proximal	Small intestine Mid	Distal	Colon
Sugars (glucose, galactose, etc)	++	+++	++	0
Amino acids	++	+++	++	0
Water-soluble and fat-soluble vitamins except vitamin B_{12}	+++	++	0	0
Antibodies in neonates	+	++	+++	?
Long-chain fatty acids absorption and conversion to triglyceride)	+++	++	+	0
Bile salts	+	+	+++	
Vitamin B_{12}	0	+	+++	0
Ca^{2+}	+++	++	+	?
Cl^-	+++	++	+	+
Fe^{2+}	+++	++	+	?
K^+	+	+	+	Sec
Na^+	+++	++	+++	+++
SO_4^{2-}	++	+	0	?

Fig. 2.3 *Sites of maximal absorption for various dietary constituents. Sec = net secretion of potassium occurs in the colon when the luminal potassium concentration is below 25 mmol/l.*

Protein digestion

Protein digestion begins in the acidic environment of the stomach, where pepsin begins the hydrolysis of proteins into smaller peptide units. Luminal digestion continues in the proximal small bowel, chiefly mediated by pancreatic peptidase enzymes (**Fig. 2.5**). These proteases are secreted as inactive precursors or proenzymes. After release from the pancreas, they are converted to their active forms in the duodenal lumen by enterokinase (also known as enteropeptidase), the secretion of which is controlled by cholecystokinin (**Fig. 2.6**). The small intestine is able to absorb the products of protein digestion either as amino acids or as oligopeptides, which may be further hydrolysed by brush-border enzymes immediately prior to entering the cell. Once inside the enterocyte, the amino acids can be utilised by the cells themselves or, for the vast majority, transported across the basolateral membrane and into the bloodstream.

Carbohydrate digestion

Dietary polysaccharides (starches, glycogen and glucose polymers) are broken down by the action of salivary and pancreatic amylases to α-limit dextrans and disaccharides. Specific brush-border disaccharidases further digest these into absorbable monosaccharides (**Fig. 2.7**). Glucose and galactose are absorbed by the secondary active transport mechanism shown in **Fig. 2.4**, while fructose enters the epithelial cell by facilitated diffusion.

The overall process is not completely efficient, however. Up to 20% of the potentially digestible carbohydrate in the diet may reach the colon, where it is metabolised by colonic bacteria. The main products generated are fatty acids that are easily absorbed, but large amounts of methane and hydrogen gases may be produced and passed as flatus (see over). The commonest cause of carbohydrate malabsorption is lactase deficiency (see pp 71, 75).

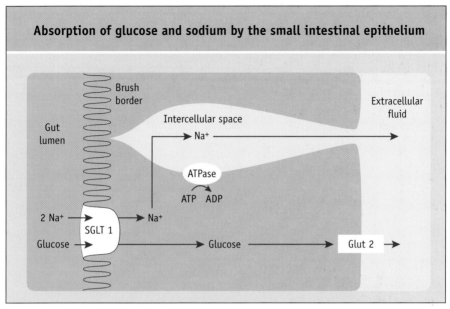

Fig. 2.4 *Absorption of glucose and sodium by the small intestinal epithelium. Both glucose and sodium are carried across the luminal membrane by the SGLT-1 sodium-dependent glucose transporter, with two Na+ ions absorbed for every glucose molecule. At the basolateral surface, sodium is extruded by adenosine triphosphate (ATP)-sensitive active transport, which maintains the low intracellular sodium concentration and hence the downward gradient for SGLT-1 to be effective (ADP = adenosine diphosphate). Meanwhile, glucose enters the interstitial space by facilitated diffusion using the GLUT-2 transport protein. Therefore, the absorption of glucose occurs by secondary active transport, the energy being used indirectly in the maintenance of the sodium gradient.*

Fat digestion

Fats are emulsified by the combined detergent action of bile salts, lecithin and monoglycerides in the small intestine. Pancreatic lipase hydrolyses fat to free fatty acids and 2-monoglycerides which are absorbed passively. Cholesterol esters are hydrolysed by pancreatic esterase. Around 95% of dietary fat is absorbed under normal circumstances. Medium chain fatty acids (C8–12) are absorbed directly into the portal vein, but other fatty acids are resynthesised into triglycerides in the enterocytes and carried by lipoproteins (chiefly chylomicrons) into the lymphatic circulation.

The digestion and absorption of fats is summarised in **Fig. 2.8,** together with some of the defects that may lead to malabsorption.

Absorption in the terminal ileum

The terminal ileum is specialised for the absorption of bile salts (see chapter 4) and also of vitamin B_{12}, a complex undertaking also involving the 60 000 molecular weight glycoprotein, intrinsic factor, which is secreted by gastric parietal cells. Intrinsic factor probably stimulates endocytosis of vitamin B_{12} by the terminal ileal enterocytes.

The successful absorption of B_{12} also requires a normally functioning pancreas. Human saliva contains a specific B_{12}-binding protein, known as R protein, that has a greater affinity for the vitamin than intrinsic factor. The R protein remains bound to the vitamin

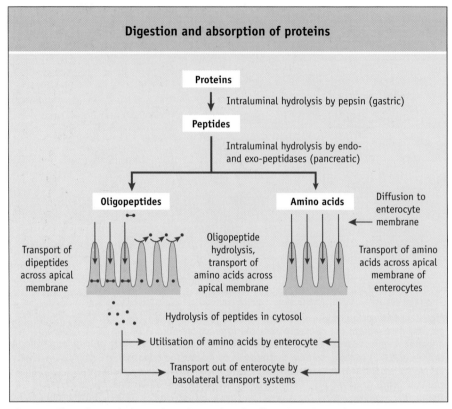

Fig. 2.5 *Digestion and absorption of protein. The digestion of proteins and oligopeptides is achieved by a combination of gastric pepsin, pancreatic peptidases and brush-border enzymes.*

until it reaches the duodenum, where it is hydrolysed by pancreatic enzymes, allowing intrinsic factor to bind to B_{12} so that the complex may be absorbed. Hence, patients with exocrine pancreatic deficiency may develop vitamin B_{12} deficiency.

Gut hormones

The integration of digestive processes such as motility, secretion and absorption is closely regulated by the autonomic nervous system and the effects of enteric hormones. The small bowel itself contains many endocrine and neuroendocrine cells, whose secretions may exert localised paracrine or distant hormonal effects. In addition to the control of digestion, these same mechanisms regulate epithelial growth and development, appetite and inflammatory responses. The actions of the principal gut hormones are summarised in Fig. 2.9.

Small bowel immunology

Mucosa-associated lymphoid tissue (MALT) contributes around 80% of the body's immunocytes. These lymphoid areas are to be found in the respiratory system, urogenital tract and conjunctiva, but principally in the digestive system and the small bowel. This should not be surprising, given that the small intestine is frequently exposed to a wide

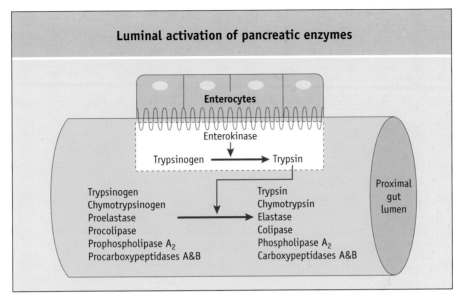

Fig. 2.6 *Luminal activation of pancreatic enzymes. The exocrine pancreas secretes digestive enzymes as inactive precursors. They are converted to their active forms in the intestinal lumen by the enzyme enterokinase, which is produced by the small bowel mucosa.*

Fig. 2.7 *Carbohydrate digestion by brush-border enzymes.*

Carbohydrate digestion by brush-border enzymes

Enzyme	Substrate	Products
Sucrase	Sucrose	Glucose Fructose
Lactase	Lactose	Glucose Galactose
Maltase	α_1-linked oligosaccharides (< 10 residues in size)	Glucose
Isomaltase	α-limit dextrans	Glucose
Trehalase	Trehalose (disaccharide)	Glucose

range of potential antigens from sources as diverse as normal dietary constituents, commensal bacteria and potentially harmful pathogens.

Peyer's patches, aggregates of MALT, can be found throughout the small bowel and, at lower frequencies, elsewhere in the gastrointestinal tract. The patches themselves have two main, lymphoid constituents – B cell follicles and parafollicular T cell areas. The mucosal 'dome' of Peyer's patches (**Fig. 2.10**) also contain specialised 'M' cells of epithelial origin that have phagocytic and antigen-presenting functions.

It is now becoming apparent, however, that Peyer's patches are not the sole site of immune regulation in the intestine. The normal surface enterocytes themselves can have vital roles in influencing the balance between immunity and tolerance, not least by their

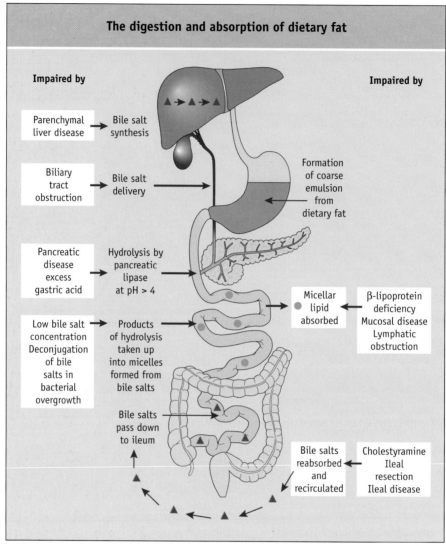

The digestion and absorption of dietary fat

Impaired by

Parenchymal liver disease → Bile salt synthesis

Biliary tract obstruction → Bile salt delivery

Pancreatic disease excess gastric acid → Hydrolysis by pancreatic lipase at pH > 4

Low bile salt concentration Deconjugation of bile salts in bacterial overgrowth → Products of hydrolysis taken up into micelles formed from bile salts

Bile salts pass down to ileum

Impaired by

Formation of coarse emulsion from dietary fat

Micellar lipid absorbed

β-lipoprotein deficiency Mucosal disease Lymphatic obstruction

Bile salts reabsorbed and recirculated ← Cholestyramine Ileal resection Ileal disease

Fig. 2.8 *The digestion and absorption of dietary fat. The priority in fat digestion is to try to convert insoluble lipids into water-soluble forms that can be absorbed and transported around the body. Hence, emulsified fats are mixed with detergent-like bile salts and pH-sensitive pancreatic lipases in the alkaline environment of the upper small bowel. Impairment of the digestive processes shown here may lead to fat malabsorption and steatorrhoea.*

own expression of cytokines and costimulatory molecules. It seems that cross-talk between M cells, enterocytes and antigen-presenting cells (such as dendritic cells) is a vital part of the immune response. This aspect of small bowel physiology continues to be intensively studied, with relevance to fields as diverse as vaccine development, food allergy, tumour immunology and infectious diseases.

The major gastrointestinal hormones

Hormone	Main site of distribution	Major physiological roles
Gastrin	Gastric antrum – G cells	Stimulates gastric acid secretion ? Trophic to gastric mucosa
Cholecystokinin	Upper small intestinal mucosa – I cells	Stimulates pancreatic secretion Stimulates gall-bladder contraction
Secretin	Upper small intestinal mucosa – S cells	Stimulates pancreatic secretion
Motilin	Duodenal mucosa and more distally – M cells	Regulates interdigestive complex of intestinal motility
GIP (gastric inhibitory polypeptide or glucose-dependent insulinotropic peptide)	Upper small intestinal mucosa – K cells	Stimulates insulin secretion Inhibits acid secretion
VIP (vasoactive intestinal peptide)	Nerve fibres of gastrointestinal tract	Regulator of blood flow and secretion
Neurotensin	Distal small intestinal and colonic mucosa – N cells	? 'Ileal brake'
Somatostatin	Mucosal D cells and nerves throughout gastrointestinal tract	Inhibits secretion and motility widely in gastrointestinal tract
Peptide YY	Distal small intestinal and colonic mucosa – L cells	'Ileal brake'. Inhibition of gastric emptying, pancreatic secretion and intestinal transit
Pancreatic polypeptide	Pancreas	? Feedback inhibition of pancreatic and biliary secretion
Enteroglucagon	Distal small intestinal colonic mucosa – L cells	? Trophic to intestine

Fig. 2.9 *The major gastrointestinal hormones.*

The functions of mucosa-associated lymphoid tissue may be summarised as follows:
- Protection against invasion by pathogenic organisms
- Prevention of the uptake of undigested potential antigens, including proteins from food and commensal bacteria
- Avoidance of the development of potentially harmful immune responses to 'non-threatening' substances.

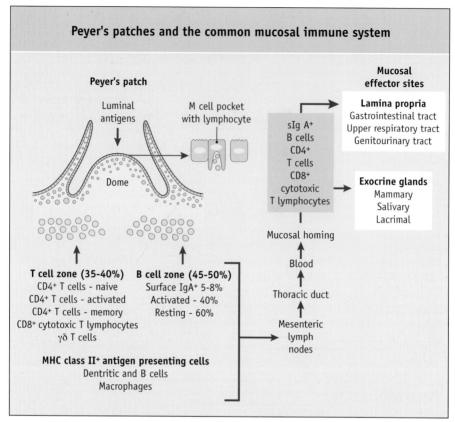

Fig. 2.10 *Peyer's patches and the common mucosal immune system. Peyer's patches are enteric collections of lymphoid tissue. Their epithelial 'dome' contains specialised M cells, whose basal surface is invaginated to allow close contact with lymphocytes, so that antigens may be easily presented. Microorganisms such as Salmonellae may gain access to the host by this route, but can also directly invade enterocytes. The gut mucosa also contains many dendritic cells, efficient at processing and presenting antigens to lymphocytes, as well as B cells that are the source of secretory immunoglobulin A (sIgA).*

SYMPTOMS AND SIGNS

SYMPTOMS OF SMALL BOWEL DISEASE

Diarrhoea

It is important to establish what the patient means by diarrhoea and what the previous pattern of normality was. Some patients may be used to having their bowels opened every other day, while others find movements three times daily normal. Affected individuals may therefore be passing normal stool volumes, but have an increase in stool frequency. It is important to establish whether bowel movement is watery or fatty. If patients are unsure, direct questioning as to how easily stool is flushed away is helpful. Those with steatorrhoea usually have floating stools which may be so oily that a thin, immiscible film is formed on the surface of the water in the toilet pan. The passage of red blood or mucus points to a colonic aetiology rather than small bowel pathology. The causes of diarrhoea are as follows:

Increased fluid secretion
- Bacterial toxins
- Hormones
- Prostaglandins
- Neurotransmitters
- Bile acid and fatty acid malabsorption
- Viral enteritis
- Coeliac disease
- Intestinal obstruction
- Immunosensitisation
- Laxatives

Exudative diarrhoea
- Colitis
- Rectal carcinoma
- Villous adenoma

Reduced fluid absorption
- Motility effects
  Irritable bowel syndrome
  Vagotomy and gastrectomy
  Autonomic neuropathy
  Drugs and hormones
- Osmotic effects
  Laxative ingestion
  Monosaccharide or disaccharide
  intolerance
  Congenital chloridorrhoea
- Mucosal defects
  Intestinal resections and bypass
  Intestinal mucosal diseases
  Enteropathogenic microorganisms

A diagnostic approach to diarrhoea involves:

Initial steps
- Confirm loose stools
- Exclude infection
- Assess whether watery, bloody or fatty

If watery:
- Check drugs
- Check diet (e.g. excessive sorbitol)
- Sigmoidoscopy
- Assess whether functional or organic
- Exclude colonic disease (colonoscopy or barium enema)
- Exclude hypolactasia (breath test)
- Exclude secretory diarrhoea (large volume persisting despite fasting and intravenous fluids)
- Exclude endocrine causes

If bloody:
- Sigmoidoscopy
- Exclude colonic disease (colonoscopy or barium enema)

If fatty:
- Exclude coeliac disease (endoscopic-duodenal biopsy)
- Exclude other small bowel disease (small bowel barium meal)
- Exclude bacterial overgrowth (lactulose or ^{14}C-glycocholate breath test or trial of tetracycline)
- Exclude pancreatic disease (pancreatic ultrasound)

Questioning about alcohol intake, drug ingestion (including over-the-counter remedies such as laxatives) or other precipitating factors such as sorbitol-containing mints and chewing gums is important.

The irritable bowel syndrome (see chapter 3) is a functional rather than an organic cause of diarrhoea. Pointers in the history include intermittent nature, often alternating with constipation. The patients are physically healthy with no weight loss and are usually under the age of 40 years at first presentation. They often complain of abdominal bloating which can be the salient feature. Careful questioning regarding stressful lifestyle and any known precipitating factors is required.

Abdominal pain

Colicky abdominal pain accompanied by distension and/or vomiting is suggestive of intestinal obstruction which may occur in stricturing processes in the small intestine, such as Crohn's disease. Similar symptomatology may be part of the irritable bowel syndrome, but in the latter condition patients are systemically well. Pain, typically 15–30 minutes after meals, may indicate mesenteric angina, particularly if investigation of the foregut, biliary tree and pancreas is unrevealing.

Weight loss

Causes of weight loss are as follows:

- Malignant disease
- Hyperthyroidism
- Adrenal insufficiency
- Diabetes
- Hyperparathyroidism
- Hypercalcaemia
- Crohn's disease
- Coeliac disease
- Intracranial lesions, particularly hypothalamic
- Anorexia nervosa
- Intestinal parasitosis

Direct questioning should explore whether there is a family history of malabsorptive complaints such as Crohn's or coeliac disease. A careful dietary history must be obtained; where there is doubt about nutritional intake, an assessment should be made by a trained dietician, since eating disorders such as anorexia nervosa and bulimia may present with weight loss.

A suitable approach to investigating the 'organic' causes of weight loss includes a meticulous history and physical examination, full blood count, serum biochemistry (including calcium), thyroid function tests and erythrocyte sedimentation rate (ESR). Assessment should also include testing for faecal occult blood, a chest X-ray and an abdominal ultrasound; consideration should be given to upper and lower gastrointestinal endoscopy with histological biopsy of the small bowel.

Wind

Various studies have shown that it is normal to pass up to 2 litres of flatus per day with a widely variable anal emission rate. Excessive wind may be a presenting syndrome of malabsorptive conditions such as hypolactasia or may result from a high dietary intake of poorly absorbed fibre such as leguminous vegetables (peas, beans and pulses). The odiferous component of flatus is related to the levels of sulphur-containing substances such as methanethiol and hydrogen sulphide. The troublesome sensation of abdominal bloating, particularly in young, otherwise fit people is often a good indication of irritable bowel syndrome.

The sources of gases present in flatus are:

- Swallowed air → nitrogen, oxygen
- Neutralisation of gastric acid by small intestinal bicarbonate → carbon dioxide
- Colonic bacterial metabolism → methane, hydrogen sulphide, carbon dioxide

Bleeding

Bleeding from the small intestine may be acute or chronic and present as frank melaena or as an iron deficiency anaemia. Altered blood from the small intestine may have the appearance of dark blackcurrant jelly, but if bleeding is very brisk, fresh blood may be passed, particularly if the pathology is in the terminal ileum.

PHYSICAL SIGNS OF SMALL BOWEL DISEASE

Careful physical examination may point to anaemia (mucosal pallor), hypoalbuminaemia (leuconychia, peripheral oedema), vitamin B_{12} deficiency (glossitis, angulostomatitis) or iron deficiency (koilonychia, glossitis). Digital clubbing can be a feature of malabsorptive states such as Crohn's disease. Patients with malabsorption may also have skin pigmentation. Specific gastrointestinal diseases have manifestations beyond the gut (see chapter 6) which may be found on examination (for example, perioral freckling is a feature of the Peutz–Jeghers syndrome), while known systemic diseases can present with small intestinal pathology (for example, polyarteritis nodosa or Behçet's disease can cause small intestinal ulceration, while the itchy skin rash, dermatitis herpetiformis, is associated with gluten sensitivity). These systemic manifestations are documented in chapter 7.

INVESTIGATIONS

An algorithm for the investigation of diarrhoea and suspected malabsorption is shown on page 63.

DIAGNOSTIC RADIOLOGY

Plain radiography

The plain abdominal X-ray is invaluable in investigating the acute abdomen, potentially revealing small bowel obstruction or extra-intestinal gas due to perforation. It is less useful in the assessment of chronic disorders such as malabsorption.

Barium studies

A radiological assessment of the small bowel may be performed with a small bowel follow-through (Fig. 2.11). Barium is swallowed rapidly and images are taken every 10–30 minutes until barium has reached the caecum. The technique is useful for showing areas of

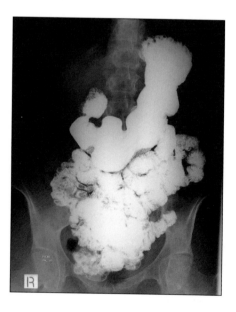

Fig. 2.11 *Barium meal and follow-through. Normal stomach and small bowel.*

ulceration, stricturing and dilatation (in Crohn's disease, for example), and other structural abnormalities such as fistulae or diverticula. An assessment can be made of bowel wall thickness, which may be increased as a result of a lymphoma or radiation damage.

A small bowel enema allows better views of the terminal ileum (**Fig. 2.12**). Barium is injected rapidly via a nasogastric tube into the small intestine. This procedure is called enteroclysis and distends the bowel with barium more readily than the standard barium follow-through. Although superior images are obtained, the need for intubation means this is not a very pleasant investigation for the patient.

Nuclear medicine studies

Radiolabelled white cell scintigraphy with ^{99m}Tc can delineate areas of inflammation such as the terminal ileum in Crohn's disease (**Fig. 2.13**), while ^{99m}Tc-labelled pertechnetate can highlight ectopic gastric mucosa in the small intestine – in a Meckel's diverticulum (**Fig. 2.14**). However, a negative scan does not exclude this diagnosis.

Radiolabelled red cell scintigraphy may be of use in localising bleeding points in the small intestine, but there usually has to be fairly brisk bleeding before a positive result is obtained.

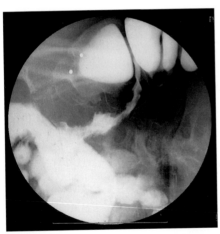

Fig. 2.12 *Small bowel enema. This patient with Crohn's disease has terminal ileitis, as demonstrated by the thin ileal segment showing classic 'rose-thorn' ulceration. The caecum (left) is normal.*

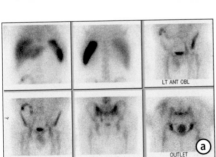

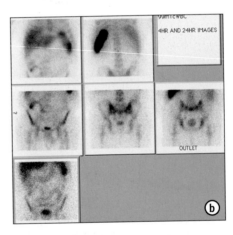

Fig. 2.13 *White cell scanning using ^{99m}Tc scintigraphy in a patient with Crohn's disease. (a) On the scans taken 1 hour after intravenous injection of the labelled white blood cells, there is a visible loop of bowel on the right side of the abdomen. (b) The images acquired at 4 and 24 hours post-injection further define this area as the terminal ileum and adjacent caecum.*

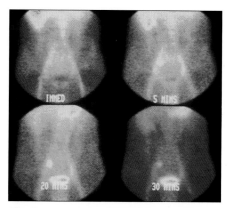

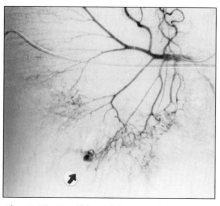

Fig. 2.14 *Meckel's diverticulum. These scintigraphic images, using intravenous ^{99m}Tc pertechnetate to visualise acid-secreting mucosa, were obtained from a patient with occult gastrointestinal bleeding. As well as the expected delineation of the stomach and bladder, there is an obvious 'hot spot' in the right iliac fossa.*

Fig. 2.15 *Small bowel haemorrhage. Super-selective angiography of the small intestine, with an area of active bleeding (arrowed).*

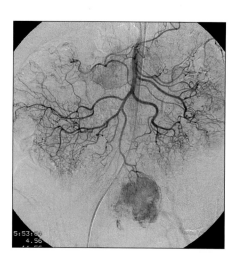

Fig. 2.16 *Small intestinal tumour blush. An abnormal area of circulation, known as a 'tumour blush', is clearly visible in the lower part of this small bowel angiogram. The tumour was excised at laparotomy and found to be of neuroendocrine origin.*

Visceral angiography

This technique is useful in localising bleeding sources which have eluded endoscopic diagnosis (**Fig. 2.15**). Abnormal vasculature can be seen, although an experienced radiologist is needed. Other pathology may be seen including tumour blushes (**Fig. 2.16**) and even areas of intussusception (**Fig. 2.17**).

Computed tomography (CT) and magnetic resonance imaging (MRI)

Both these techniques can reveal small intestinal pathology, but the advent of three-dimensional reconstructions of helical CT and MRI allows a virtual enteroscopy in a

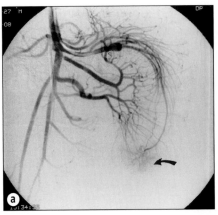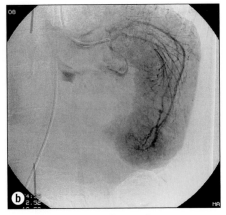

Fig. 2.17 *Small bowel intussusception. Selective superior mesenteric arteriograms, demonstrating jejuno-jejunal intussusception due to a hamartomatous polyp. (a) The arterial phase shows the typical crowding of the blood vessels caused by the intussusception (top). Additionally, there is a particularly prominent arterial branch that is supplying a 3 cm mass (the hamartoma itself, arrowed). (b) In the venous phase two prominent early-filling veins can be seen draining the hypervascular mass.*

totally non-invasive fashion. MR angiography is useful for looking at the major blood vessels, but at present resolution is not good enough to demonstrate small vessel abnormalities in the gut. Standard visceral angiography therefore remains the mainstay of investigation of small intestinal bleeding points.

ENDOSCOPY

The majority of the small intestine cannot be reached using a standard endoscope, although most of the duodenum can be routinely inspected (**Fig. 2.18**). However, longer specialised *enteroscopes* have been developed in order to visualise the jejunum and ileum.

The Sonde-type enteroscope is long and thin, and may be passed deep into the small bowel, being aided in its progression by peristalsis. The bowel wall is usually inspected on withdrawal of the instrument, although this can give rise to difficulties in determining whether or not any bleeding point is actually due to trauma from the intubation.

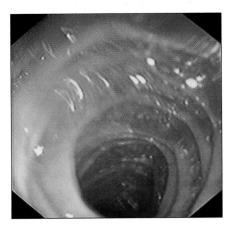

Fig. 2.18 *Normal appearance of the small intestine. Endoscopic view of the distal duodenum, showing the typical array of transverse mucosal folds.*

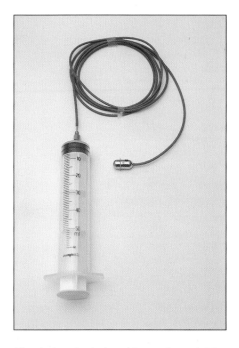

Fig. 2.19 *Crosby–Kugler biopsy capsule. A suction-guillotine mechanism is used to obtain small intestinal biopsies. The patient, having fasted overnight, swallows the capsule. Movement into the small bowel can be facilitated by lying patients on their right side and by administering an intravenous promotility drug such as metoclopramide. Radiographic screening ensures the capsule is in the jejunum. The biopsy specimen is obtained by rapidly sucking a piece of mucosa into the guillotine using the 20 ml syringe attached to the connecting tube.*

The device also lacks a biopsy channel. More recently, 'push enteroscopy' has been developed, using an instrument that has both a biopsy channel and some of the handling characteristics of a normal endoscope, allowing a more detailed inspection of the jejunum and proximal ileum. The role of enteroscopy remains relatively limited.

Crosby–Kugler biopsy capsules

Small intestinal biopsies can be obtained using these metal capsules (**Fig. 2.19**).
A combination of peristalsis and feeding of the capsule down into the intestine ensures that it arrives in the correct position. With the advent of endoscopy, the procedure can be foreshortened by passing the capsule down the small intestine under direct vision. The capsule is threaded up the endoscope's biopsy channel in a retrograde fashion prior to intubation of the patient. Nevertheless, if adequate biopsies have been taken from the second part of the duodenum with a standard endoscope and biopsy forceps, then the need for the time-consuming Crosby capsule is largely obviated.

TESTS FOR BACTERIAL OVERGROWTH

Jejunal aspiration

Only relatively scant numbers of bacteria are present in the upper jejunum under normal circumstances. Assessments of bacterial overgrowth can be made by microbiological examination of jejunal aspirates, collected through the biopsy channel at upper gastrointestinal endoscopy. Bacterial numbers in excess of 10^6 per ml are abnormal. This technique can also be used to culture specific pathogens such as *Giardia* and *Strongyloides* spp.

Breath tests

These non-invasive methods of assessing bacterial overgrowth in the small intestine (**Fig. 2.20**) are based on the excess numbers of bacteria producing gases that are absorbed

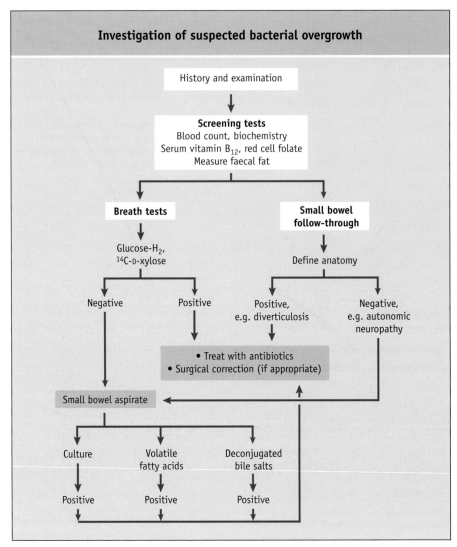

Fig. 2.20 *Investigation of suspected bacterial overgrowth.*

into the bloodstream and then exhaled. Several different tests are available. Radiolabelled ^{14}C tests rely on the measurement of $^{14}CO_2$ in the breath following oral administration of either ^{14}C-xylose or ^{14}C-glycocholate. Both these agents will be metabolised by gut bacteria if present in the jejunum, but remain unaltered in the normal subject.

A glucose-hydrogen breath test involves detecting a rise in hydrogen exhaled in the breath after an oral glucose load, but there is a significant false positive rate. Patients should have good oral hygiene and avoid eating peas, beans and pulses for 48 hours before the test in order to ensure a low basal hydrogen measurement. Smoking during the test gives an artificially elevated hydrogen level, while antibiotics up to 3 weeks beforehand can give a false negative result.

TESTS OF ABSORPTION

Assessment of carbohydrate malabsorption

Lactose tolerance test and lactose-hydrogen breath test. Deficiency of the mucosal disaccharidase, lactase, leads to colicky abdominal pain, flatulence and diarrhoea after eating dairy products. This is not uncommon in Chinese and South Asian adults on a western European diet (there is a prevalence of 90–100% and 60–90% respectively, compared to 15–30% for Europeans).

In the lactose intolerance test a rise in blood glucose of less than 1.1 mmol/l, with serial blood estimations made every 30 minutes for 2 hours following the oral administration of lactose, suggests hypolactasia. The lactose-hydrogen breath test is similar to the glucose-hydrogen breath test (for bacterial overgrowth) and is subject to the same strict conditions for interpretation. Lactase-deficient individuals fail to digest the disaccharide and so it remains available for luminal metabolism by hydrogen-producing bacteria.

Similar tests can be performed to investigate sucrose malabsorption. These may also be a sensitive method of assessing gut permeability in coeliac disease, where mucosal damage and consequent loss of the brush-border disaccharidases can lead to absorption of unaltered sucrose, which can then be measured in the urine.

Assessment of fat malabsorption

Up to 95% of dietary fat is absorbed in healthy people and the average normal stool fat content is less than 7 g in 24 hours. Patients with coeliac disease, tropical sprue and other small intestinal conditions may have some degree of steatorrhoea of between 10 and 20 g in 24 hours, but those with pancreatic insufficiency can have frank steatorrhoea of the order of 30–50 g or more in 24 hours.

Three-day faecal fat tests. This is still the gold standard for the measurement of fat malabsorption. Patients should eat at least 100 g of fat per day for the week leading up to and including the 3 test days. The main inaccuracy is incomplete stool collection, usually because of patient non-compliance. Other tests include direct stool microscopy to look for fat droplets, while the addition of Sudan III dye makes this more apparent by staining fat an orange colour.

Radiolabelled ^{14}C fat breath tests. The measurement of $^{14}CO_2$ in the breath, following ingestion of labelled fats such as ^{14}C-triolein, may be more acceptable to the patient than a 3-day faecal fat collection. Patients with malabsorption have delayed $^{14}CO_2$ excretion, while pancreatic insufficiency may be demonstrated in those patients with low breath $^{14}CO_2$, who correct to normal levels after oral pancreatic enzyme supplementation.

Assessment of vitamin B$_{12}$ malabsorption

This can be assessed using the Schilling test. First, the patient's bodily stores of vitamin B$_{12}$ are saturated by parenteral injection of the vitamin. An oral dose of ^{58}Co-labelled vitamin B$_{12}$ is then given. If less than 10% of the administered dose is excreted in a 24-hour urine collection, this indicates deficient absorption and the test should be repeated with supplementation of intrinsic factor.

Individuals with terminal ileal disease will not increase their urinary excretion of the labelled B$_{12}$ when intrinsic factor is added, unlike those with pernicious anaemia. A variation of the test involves giving ^{57}Co-labelled B$_{12}$ attached to intrinsic factor and ^{58}Co-labelled vitamin B$_{12}$ at the same time. This method enables both parts of the test to be performed at once.

Assessment of bile acid malabsorption

Bile salts are normally absorbed in the terminal ileum. Malabsorption results in diarrhoea. If this is suspected, then a therapeutic trial should be carried out using cholestyramine, which binds bile salts. The specific SeHCAT (selenium homocholic acid taurine) test, which relies on ^{75}Se-labelled bile salt, is expensive and rarely indicated. Normal subjects retain up to 90% of the γ-emitting bile salt used in the latter test in the body after a week, because of an efficient enterohepatic circulation. With terminal ileal disease, however, less than 2% remains.

STUDIES OF SMALL BOWEL MOTILITY

Motility can be assessed by ingesting radio-opaque beads and taking serial plain abdominal radiographs. Alternatively, radiolabelled meals can be given in the nuclear medicine department and the rate of progress through the bowel monitored with scintigraphy (see **Fig. 7.7**).

DIFFERENTIAL DIAGNOSIS

COELIAC DISEASE

This is the commonest cause of malabsorption in people of northwest European, especially Celtic, ancestry. There is a genetic predisposition, the strongest human leucocyte antigen (HLA) associations being HLA B8 DQW2. The condition is also called gluten-induced enteropathy, non-tropical sprue or coeliac sprue.

Affected individuals develop an immunological response to the four water-insoluble β, γ, φ and particularly α-gliadin fractions of gluten protein found in wheat, rye and barley. Rice and maize do not contain toxic gluten proteins, but oats may possibly have an adverse effect in a minority of patients. Recent research has identified a single transglutaminase-modified peptide as the dominant T-lymphocyte epitope that is derived from α-gliadin.

Gluten sensitivity leads to a lymphocytic enteritis and villous atrophy when gluten is present in the diet. The classical consequence of this is malabsorption of the dietary constituents that are absorbed in the proximal small bowel (see **Fig. 2.3**), particularly iron, folate, calcium, fats and amino acids. There may also be extrusion of protein and calcium from the affected mucosal surface.

The histological hallmark of the condition is partial or subtotal villous atrophy, most evident in the upper small intestine (**Fig. 2.21**). Jejunal biopsy with a Crosby–Kugler capsule (see **Fig. 2.19**) before and after a gluten-free diet has been the traditional method of diagnosis, but good-quality specimens may be obtained from the second part of the duodenum at endoscopy.

The key points to remember for coeliac disease are:
- Affects around 1 in 200 of the general population
- Concept of coeliac 'iceberg': only a small proportion of those with gluten sensitivity have clinically overt disease
- Most cases are diagnosed in adulthood – peak incidence is in the fifth decade
- Should be part of the differential diagnosis in a wide range of clinical situations, such as anaemia, osteoporosis or with associated diseases (see below)
- Serological diagnosis is improved by availability of anti-endomysial antibody tests
- Treatment requires completely gluten-free diet

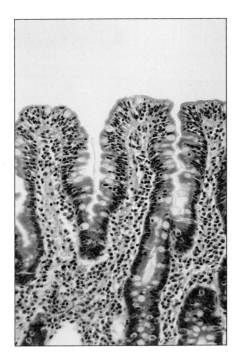

Fig. 2.21 *Villous atrophy in coeliac disease. Distal duodenal biopsy showing severe villous atrophy with intraepithelial lymphocytosis and crypt hyperplasia.*

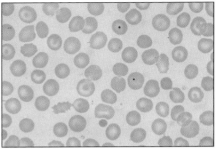

Fig. 2.22 *Hyposplenism in coeliac disease. Blood film from a patient with gluten-sensitive enteropathy, demonstrating Howell–Jolly bodies (the small nuclear remnants visible in some erythrocytes), poikilocytosis and target cells.*

Clinical features and diagnosis

The clinical features of coeliac disease are as follows:

Common	Uncommon
• Weight loss	• Digital clubbing
• Pallor	• Bruising
• Oedema	• Ascites
• Angular stomatitis	• Peripheral neuropathy
• Glossitis	• Tetany
• Aphthous ulceration	
• Abdominal distension	
• Skin pigmentation	
• Muscle wasting	

Physical examination, however, is frequently normal. Patients may present with tiredness, weight loss and anaemia due to iron and/or folate deficiencies, but vitamin B_{12} deficiency is relatively uncommon. Hypoproteinaemia causes peripheral oedema but rarely ascites. Steatorrhoea is not uncommon, but bruising or overt bleeding, because of accompanying malabsorption of the fat-soluble vitamin K, is fairly rare. Osteomalacia secondary to vitamin D and calcium malabsorption is a particular risk in the elderly.

Investigations may reveal a microcytic, macrocytic or normocytic anaemia depending on the underlying iron and folate deficiencies. Splenic atrophy, occurring in up to 30%, may result in thrombocytosis and the appearance of Howell–Jolly bodies and abnormally shaped erythrocytes on blood film examination (**Fig. 2.22**). If there is a vitamin B_{12} deficiency, it is worth performing a Schilling test. Hypoproteinaemia, hypocalcaemia and hypomagnesaemia are often present and the alkaline phosphatase may be elevated if there is osteomalacia. Occasionally there may be an IgA deficiency on serum protein electrophoresis, but usually the IgA is increased with a decreased IgM. The prothrombin time may be prolonged if there is a vitamin K deficiency. Small bowel barium follow-through examinations may show coarsening of the normal feathery appearance of the small intestinal mucosa with a featureless appearance in severe cases.

Diagnosis rests on demonstrating the typical histological features on small bowel biopsy, ideally supported by a favourable response to gluten restriction and relapse on subsequent gluten challenge. Many gastroenterologists consider this latter challenge unnecessary for most patients.

In recent years, serological tests for the diagnosis of coeliac disease have become more widely available. Both anti-gliadin and anti-endomysial antibody tests are available, the latter having the highest sensitivity and specificity. Indeed, anti-endomysial antibodies parallel uncontrolled gluten sensitivity so closely that a positive result is almost 100%-specific. However, the test is based on the detection of immunoglobulin A (IgA) and so sensitivity is lower, at around 80–6%. Indeed, anti-endomysial antibodies may be absent altogether in cases of IgA deficiency. The additional use of anti-gliadin antibodies may be helpful in this situation and the serial estimation of antibody titres can be used as a method of monitoring response to gluten-free diets.

Management
Initial management consists of:
- Full explanation of the condition, its significance and the importance of adhering to the dietary restrictions
- Consider liaison with patient support group (e.g. Coeliac Society in the UK)
- Maintain strict gluten-free diet
- Monitor progress regularly, ideally in a specialised coeliac disease clinic
- Ensure regular consultation with a dietician
- Consider nutritional supplements – iron, folic acid, calcium as appropriate
- Monitor dietary compliance by serial estimation of anti-endomysial and anti-gliadin antibodies
- If clinical response suboptimal, consider repeat small bowel biopsy or imaging to exclude neoplasia, particularly in older patients.

Another important aspect of management is to search for disease associations and complications. Associated conditions include dermatitis herpetiformis, an itchy bullous eruption occurring on extensor surfaces and other pressure areas (see chapter 7). There is also an increased incidence of small intestinal lymphoma or carcinoma, usually in those individuals who have not kept to a gluten-free diet or who have presented late in life. The small bowel neoplasm may be readily apparent on barium studies or CT scanning (Fig. 2.23), but can be very difficult to diagnose, particularly in the early stages. Other adult diseases associated with coeliac disease include:
- Type I diabetes mellitus
- Thyrotoxicosis
- Immunoglobulin A deficiency
- Primary biliary cirrhosis
- Diuresis
- Sjögren's syndrome
- Epilepsy
- Osteoporosis

TROPICAL SPRUE
Patients with a history of travel, particularly to southeast Asia and the Caribbean littoral of Central and South America, can present with this post-infective malabsorption

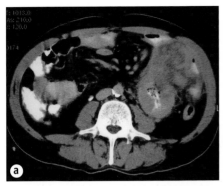 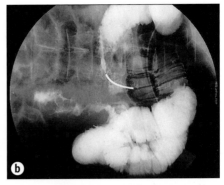

Fig. 2.23 *Small intestinal lymphoma in coeliac disease. This patient with gluten-sensitive enteropathy developed severe weight loss and anaemia. A large lymphoma can be seen arising from the small intestine. (a) Abdominal CT scan. (b) Small bowel enema.*

syndrome. Clinical features are similar to coeliac disease with anaemia, glossitis, folic acid deficiency and steatorrhoea. There has usually been an episode of travellers' diarrhoea. Persisting bacterial overgrowth with organisms such as *Escherichia coli* and *Klebsiella* spp. is not uncommon. Therefore, jejunal aspiration is a useful diagnostic test and also rules out infection with other organisms such as *Giardia* or *Strongyloides* spp. Partial or even subtotal villous atrophy is seen on histological examination of biopsies from the second part of the duodenum provided at endoscopy.

Treatment involves tetracycline for up to a month and folic acid supplementation. Response is generally swift, but avoidance of dairy products is also important because there is an associated lactose intolerance which can persist until there has been complete regeneration of the small intestinal mucosa. If untreated, the condition may persist for months or even years.

POST-INFECTIVE MALABSORPTION

There may be persistent hypolactasia following recovery from any infectious cause of diarrhoea, because of inflammation or destruction of the small intestinal enterocyte brush-border and consequent loss of the brush-border disaccharidases. Unless dairy products are avoided, abdominal bloating, flatulence and diarrhoea may be persisting symptoms for up to a month after the initial infection.

INFECTIOUS DIARRHOEA

Most infectious agents do not neatly confine themselves to the small intestine or colon and any level of the gut may be affected. Common causes of infectious diarrhoea which affect the small intestine are summarised in **Fig. 2.24**. Infective colitis is discussed in chapter 3.

Cholera

Vibrio cholerae is a Gram-negative, enterotoxin-producing, flagellated, comma-shaped bacillus which is the cause of a severe small intestinal secretory diarrhoea. It causes waterborne disease and is endemic in South Asia, particularly the Ganges flood plain. However, since the 1960s a pandemic has occurred involving Africa, the countries of the Mediterranean littoral and, most recently, South and Central America, where it has spread rapidly in countries such as Peru and Bolivia.

Common worldwide causes of infectious diarrhoea with small intestinal involvement	
Viral	Rotavirus Norwalk agent Adenovirus
Bacterial toxin	Enterotoxigenic *E. coli* *Vibrio cholerae* *Vibrio parahaemolyticus* *Clostridium* spp. *Bacillus cereus*
Bacterial invasion	Entero-invasive *E. coli* *Campylobacter jejuni* *Shigella* spp. *Salmonella* spp. including typhoid *Yersinia enterocolitica*
Parasitic	*Giardia lamblia* *Cryptosporidium* spp. *Strongyloides stercoralis* *Capillaria philippensis*

Fig. 2.24 *Common worldwide causes of infectious diarrhoea with small intestinal involvement.*

The incubation period is usually 24–72 hours, before the abrupt onset of painless, watery diarrhoea. It is usually contracted through drinking water or eating poorly prepared foods which have been washed in or contain infected water. Shellfish are also a notable reservoir of *Vibrio* spp., including the related but less severe *V. parahaemolyticus*. The organisms are susceptible to gastric acid which presents some line of defence in healthy people, but in those individuals with any cause of hypochlorhydria or achlorhydria, infection takes hold much more easily.

Once the organisms have colonised the small bowel, an enterotoxin is produced with five B (binding) subunits which attach irreversibly to the GM-1 monosialoganglioside molecule in the enterocyte cell wall, and two A (activating) subunits which migrate into the enterocyte to activate adenylate cyclase and switch on cyclic adenosine 3′, 5′-monophosphate (cAMP) production (**Fig. 2.25**). This leads to rapid secretion of electrolytes into the small bowel and the production of the characteristic diarrhoea, which has been termed 'rice-water stool'. The organisms are obvious on stool microscopy, but in the differential diagnosis it should be remembered that *Plasmodium falciparum* malaria can occasionally present with watery diarrhoea.

Treatment is supportive, with oral rehydration using sugar/salt solutions. A convenient recipe consists of 40 g of sucrose or 20 g of glucose and 3.5 g of salt per litre of clean drinking water. If disease is severe, intravenous rehydration is required. Tetracycline may reduce the organism load in the small intestine and shorten the duration of diarrhoea, but the focus should be on primary prevention. Vaccination provides limited protection, but basic public health measures and avoidance of suspect foodstuffs, including ice in drinks, are most important.

Typhoid

Typhoid or enteric fever is caused by the Gram-negative, entero-invasive *Salmonella typhi*. A severe systemic illness results from ingestion of contaminated food, including shellfish

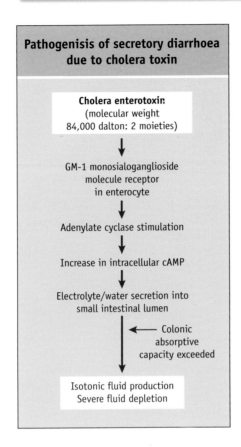

Fig. 2.25 *Pathogenesis of secretory diarrhoea due to cholera toxin.*

Pathogenisis of secretory diarrhoea due to cholera toxin

Cholera enterotoxin
(molecular weight
84,000 dalton: 2 moieties)

↓

GM-1 monosialoganglioside
molecule receptor
in enterocyte

↓

Adenylate cyclase stimulation

↓

Increase in intracellular cAMP

↓

Electrolyte/water secretion into
small intestinal lumen

← Colonic
absorptive
capacity exceeded

↓

Isotonic fluid production
Severe fluid depletion

and poultry, and also drinking water. The systemic manifestations are detailed in chapter 6. The main site of gut involvement is the ileum, particularly the Peyer's patches. Deep ovoid ileal ulcers develop during the course of the illness. Constipation is an early symptom, but watery diarrhoea supervenes as small bowel involvement becomes more pronounced.

Diagnosis is obtained from blood, bone marrow or stool culture, depending on the stage of the disease. Chloramphenicol, cotrimoxazole, amoxycillin or ciprofloxacin are amongst the effective antibiotic treatments. However, prevention should be stressed; prophylactic vaccination confers partial immunity, but sensible precautions such as not drinking water or eating salads, unpeeled fruit, ice-cream and raw shellfish in endemic areas should be paramount.

Infection with *S. paratyphi* and other *Salmonella* spp. is less severe, but is none the less an important cause of travellers' diarrhoea.

Travellers' diarrhoea

Travellers' diarrhoea is very common, affecting 30–50% of visitors from developed to developing countries. In most cases it results from bacterial pathogens, the most frequent being colonisation with enterotoxigenic *E. coli* (ETEC):

- Enterotoxigenic *E. coli* (ETEC) (frequency 40%)
- *Shigella* spp. and/or enterohaemorrhagic *E. coli* (EHEC) (10%)
- *Salmonella* spp. (10%)
- Viruses (5%)

- *Aeromonas/Plesiomonas* spp. (5%)
- Protozoa (5%)
- *Campylobacter jejuni* (3%)
- No pathogen isolated (22%)

Dysentery (i.e. bloody stool) occurs in less than 10% of cases and the disorder is self-limiting (lasting a median of 2 days) in most patients. Prolonged diarrhoea is rare, occurring in less than 1% of cases, and is usually due to non-bacterial causes such as *Giardia*, other protozoa or occasionally helminths.

Viruses account for less than 10% of cases.

Routine laboratory investigation is not required in most patients, but if the illness is prolonged or there is dysentery, stools should be sent for microscopy and culture along with histological analysis of a rectal biopsy.

Serology in acute dysentery is not usually helpful, with the exception of amoebic colitis, in which 75% of patients express specific IgG antibodies against *Entamoeba histolytica*.

Risk factors for developing travellers' diarrhoea include:
- Travel originating from highly industrialised region
- No travel to tropical area in previous 6 months
- Failure to avoid contaminated food or water
- Age < 5 years
- Immunodeficiency
- Achlorhydria
- Standard of drinking water supply, sewage disposal and food preparation in host country
- Local prevalence of microbial pathogens

The mainstay of treatment is ensuring appropriate hydration and electrolyte balance during the illness. A 3–5-day course of an antibiotic (e.g. doxycycline, trimethoprim, cotrimoxazole or a quinolone) has been shown to shorten the duration of illness. A single dose of ciprofloxacin 500 mg has recently been shown to be effective. However, treatment of a predominantly self-limiting condition with antibiotics poses a real risk of encouraging resistant organisms, particularly in the developing world, and should be reserved for immunocompromised patients or for those with severe disease (more than six stools per day, or the presence of dysentery).

Other causes of bacterial food poisoning

The various strains of *E. coli* (enterotoxigenic, entero-invasive, enteropathogenic, enterohaemorrhagic) are responsible for sporadic outbreaks of food poisoning. There are two *E. coli* enterotoxins, heat-labile and heat-stable, the former produces a secretory diarrhoea in a similar way to *V. cholerae*.

Other *Vibrio* species such as *V. parahaemolyticus* can be contracted from eating foods such as shellfish and cause a watery diarrhoea similar to cholera but much less severe. *Campylobacter jejuni* and *Salmonella* spp. have reservoirs of infection in poultry and other animals. Drinking water may become contaminated too. The incubation period can be up to 10 days in both *C. jejuni* and *Salmonella* infections with ensuing diarrhoea, vomiting, fever and colicky abdominal pain. Colonic involvement may also occur, causing bloody diarrhoea which may mimic or exacerbate ulcerative colitis (see chapter 3).

Staphylococcus aureus causes precipitate vomiting rather than diarrhoea, only hours after ingestion of contaminated foods such as meat and dairy products, whereas *Clostridium perfringens* is classically contracted from rewarmed foods. Again, there is a very short incubation period, but diarrhoea is the most important symptom. Botulism is a much more serious condition, caused by a neurotoxin produced by *C. botulinum*.

The systemic manifestations of this rare condition, which is typically contracted from poorly canned or vacuum-packed foods, are discussed in chapter 6.

Bacillus cereus is a Gram-positive, aerobic, spore-forming, enterotoxigenic organism which causes two syndromes, one similar to clostridial diarrhoea and the other similar to staphylococcal vomiting. The latter was first recognised in the UK in rewarmed rice from take-away food outlets.

These infections are self-limiting and therefore only supportive measures are required, but in severe *C. jejuni* infection treatment with erythromycin may be effective.

Giardiasis

The flagellated protozoan, *Giardia lamblia*, causes acute diarrhoea and flatulence. However, there may be a spectrum of symptoms ranging from asymptomatic chronic infection to marked malabsorption, similar to tropical sprue, with weight loss, steatorrhoea and foul-smelling flatus. Giardiasis is usually contracted from infected drinking water; it is a disease not only of tropical countries, but can also be caught in temperate zones including the UK and notably the area around St Petersburg in Russia. Infection may complicate the course of disease in individuals infected with human immunodeficiency virus (HIV).

The giardial trophozoites can be seen on microscopy of jejunal aspirates or biopsies (Fig. 2.26). Other diagnostic tests include the string test, where a gelatin capsule attached to a nylon line is swallowed and retrieved 4 hours later. If parasites are present, they can be observed at microscopy, adherent to the string. A short course of treatment with metronidazole or tinidazole is usually effective.

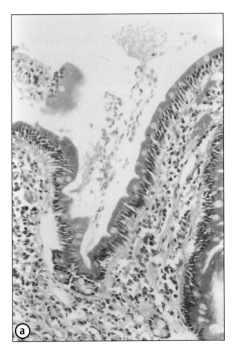 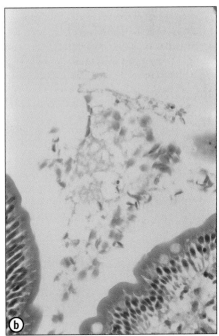

Fig. 2.26 *Giardiasis. Haematoxylin and eosin (H & E) stained duodenal biopsies, demonstrating multiple Giardia organisms in the intestinal lumen. (a) Lower power view. (b) High-power view.*

Strongyloides

A spectrum ranging from chronic infection through to overt malabsorption can be caused by the nematode, *Strongyloides stercoralis*. It is a common infection in tropical countries, mainly southeast Asia and the Caribbean. It is a cause of iron deficiency anaemia, in common with all other hookworms, which are contracted by larval penetration of the skin, usually the feet. Diagnosis is obtained on microscopic examination of small bowel aspirate or biopsy, although a reasonably sensitive serological test based on enzyme-linked immunosorbent assay (ELISA) is also available. As with giardiasis, the string test is useful. Treatment with thiabendazole for 3 days is usually effective.

WHIPPLE'S DISEASE

This rare condition most frequently affects middle-aged men. It is characterised by partial villous atrophy seen on histological analysis of biopsies at endoscopy from the second part of the duodenum (**Fig. 2.27**). However, the hallmark is the presence of macrophages which stain magenta with periodic acid-Schiff. This is due to the presence of Gram-positive bacilli, which have only recently been cultured for the first time. The organism was previously identified by polymerase chain reaction (PCR) analysis and was given the name *Tropheryma whippelii*.

Patients typically have diarrhoea and may also have a wide range of clinical features such as lymphadenopathy, fever, a flitting arthritis which affects both large and small joints, and also skin pigmentation. The organism may be a cause of endocarditis and valvular thickening can occur. Rarely, there may be involvement of the central nervous system (CNS), with cranial nerve lesions and an encephalopathy which includes behavioural disturbances and memory loss. The organism may be seen in the cerebrospinal fluid on lumbar puncture (see chapter 6).

Various antibiotic regimes have been recommended, but most include cotrimoxazole for up to 1 year in addition to initial treatment with penicillin, streptomycin or tetracycline for the first 2 weeks or so. There is usually a good response to treatment, except if there is CNS involvement because any neurological damage is usually irreversible.

IMMUNODEFICIENCY SYNDROMES

Any person with an impaired immune system is susceptible to opportunistic infections. The majority of patients with HIV have diarrhoea complicating the course of their disease at some stage. The causal pathogens are protean; some of the most common are listed in

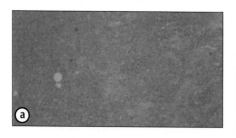
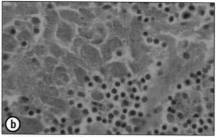

Fig. 2.27 *Histology of Whipple's disease. A mesenteric lymph node from a patient with Whipple's disease. The specimens have been stained with PAS, demonstrating abundant magenta-coloured macrophages. (a) Low-power view. (b) High-power view.*

Infective agents in HIV-positive patients with diarrhoea	
Protozoal	*Cryptosporidium*
	Microsporidium
	Isospora belli
	Giardia lamblia
	Entamoeba histolytica
Viral	Human immunodeficiency virus
	Cytomegalovirus
	Herpes simplex
Bacterial	*Salmonella* spp.
	Campylobacter jejuni
	Shigella spp.
	Atypical mycobacterial spp. including *M. avium intercellulare*

Fig. 2.28 *Infective agents in HIV-positive patients with diarrhoea.*

Fig. 2.28. Despite repeated stool cultures, duodenal aspirates or duodenal (and rectal) biopsies for culture and histological examination, often no causal organism is isolated in these diarrhoeal episodes. However, it should be remembered that HIV itself can activate vasoactive intestinal polypeptide (VIP) receptors in the gut and cause an intrinsic watery diarrhoea.

Chapter 7 contains details of further gastrointestinal manifestations of acquired immunodeficiency syndrome (AIDS).

Protozoal infections

Coccidian protozoa include *Cryptosporidium*, *Microsporidium* and *Isospora* spp. They can all cause malabsorption in immunosuppressed patients.

Cryptosporidium This coccidian protozoan causes a severe, watery, cholera-like diarrhoea. Colicky abdominal pain, nausea and vomiting may be features. *Cryptosporidium* is a common animal pathogen and causes a self-limiting illness, including travellers' diarrhoea, in the normal human host, but a much more severe and prolonged illness in patients with AIDS or in other immunosuppressed states. It may be a cause of AIDS-related sclerosing cholangitis. The organism can be seen on stool microscopy or small bowel biopsy (**Fig. 2.29**). Symptomatic treatment including rehydration and antidiarrhoeal agents is the mainstay because the organism is otherwise difficult to treat. However, spiramycin may be effective.

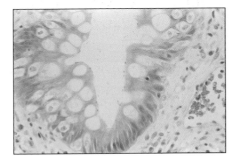

Fig. 2.29 *Intestinal cryptosporidiosis. Jejunal biopsy (longitudinal view) of the small intestinal crypts. The* **Cryptosporidia** *can be seen as the tiny red-stained spherical organisms adherent to the luminal surface of the epithelial cells.*

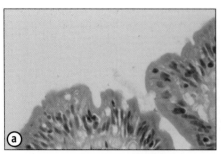

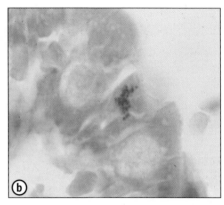

Fig. 2.30 *Intestinal microsporidiosis. Duodenal biopsies from a patient with AIDS and microsporidiosis. (a) H & E stain. (b) Giemsa stain. The spores are revealed as small, dark-blue oval shapes within the enterocyte.*

Microsporidia There are numerous species of this spore-forming protozoan, which causes similar symptoms to cryptosporidiosis in HIV-positive and other immunosuppressed patients. It has been reported to cause a spectrum of other conditions including conjunctivitis, hepatitis and sclerosing cholangitis. Diagnosis can be difficult, as there are no specific lesions to be found at endoscopy. Light microscopy of biopsy specimens may also be unrevealing, although certain stains such as PAS or Giemsa may visualise the organisms better (**Fig. 2.30**). Electron microscopy is the most specific method of detecting the spores in intestinal biopsies. As with cryptosporidiosis, the treatment is difficult, but agents such as albendazole may be effective.

Isospora This parasite is similar in its presentation to cryptosporidial infections, but the *Isospora* oocysts are much larger and are easily seen on stool microscopy. Cotrimoxazole may be effective in treatment.

Viral infections

Cytomegalovirus (CMV) and *Herpes simplex* virus (HSV) can cause ulceration of any part of the gastrointestinal tract. If the small intestine is affected, diarrhoea and malabsorptive symptoms predominate, whereas pain is the predominant symptom in the oesophagus or the rectum (see chapters 1 and 7). Treatment is usually with ganciclovir for CMV and aciclovir for HSV, but for those patients with AIDS who are on combination treatment with reverse transcription inhibitors such as zidovudine, foscarnet is a useful alternative for both because it does not exacerbate neutropenia.

Atypical mycobacteria

These opportunistic pathogens, such as *Mycobacterium avium intercellulare*, can be widely disseminated in patients with AIDS (**Fig. 2.31**), but when they affect the small intestine the predominant symptoms are diarrhoea, weight loss, fevers and malabsorption. It should be noted that the histological appearances of the small intestine on PAS staining may mimic Whipple's disease with an abundance of magenta-staining PAS-positive macrophages. However, diagnosis is made on Ziehl–Neelsen staining of biopsy material or stool samples. Combination treatment usually includes agents such as clofazimine and azithromycin.

OTHER SMALL INTESTINAL PARASITIC INFECTIONS

Common parasitic infestations which do not cause diarrhoea are outlined below.

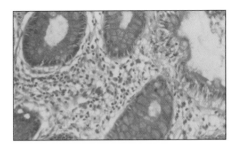

Fig. 2.31 *Atypical mycobacteria visible on rectal biopsy from a patient with AIDS.*

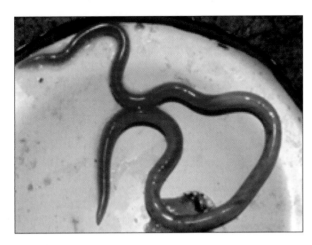

Fig. 2.32 *Large adult roundworm (Ascaris lumbricoides) passed per rectum.*

Hookworms

Infestation with *Ankylostoma duodenale* or *Necator americanus* is an important cause of iron deficiency anaemia worldwide. As with *Strongyloides*, infection is through the skin, particularly via bare feet. All these worms have complex life cycles, with a migratory phase from the gut via the bloodstream to the lungs and thence back to the small intestine where the adults then live. They can be seen on microscopy of jejunal aspirates obtained at endoscopy, and the eggs can be seen on microscopy of fresh stool samples. Correction of iron deficiency and treatment with either mebendazole or albendazole is appropriate.

Roundworms

Ascaris lumbricoides is a large roundworm (**Fig. 2.32**), often more than 20 cm long, with a worldwide distribution; the highest incidence is in the tropics. After the host has ingested ova in contaminated food or water, larvae emerge in the duodenum and migrate into the bloodstream before maturing in the lung. There is often an accompanying pneumonitis and larvae are coughed up into the pharynx and swallowed. Mature male and female roundworms then become established in the intestine. As well as hypersensitivity reactions, the worms may cause physical complications such as obstruction or perforation and may migrate into the ampulla of Vater, causing jaundice or pancreatitis. Large numbers of worms may lead to malnutrition simply by competing with the host for ingested food. Diagnosis requires demonstrating the eggs in stool samples, or passing the worms themselves, and barium imaging may reveal nests of worms in the small or large bowel. Treatment is usually with pyrantel pamoate, albendazole or mebendazole.

Tapeworms

Infestation with the segmented cestodes *Taenia solium* (pork tapeworm), *T. saginata* (beef tapeworm) and *Diphyllobothrium latum* (fish tapeworm) is usually asymptomatic, but with a high worm load there may be small intestinal obstruction. Eggs or segments of the adult may be seen on stool microscopy. Treatment with the antihelminthic, praziquantel, is effective.

Anisakiasis

Anisakis spp. are common fish parasites and are often found in fish-eating whales and dolphins. These roundworms are becoming more common in the western world with the increased popularity of Japanese-style sushi bars where raw fish is eaten. Nausea, vomiting and epigastric pain are presenting symptoms, but the worm also causes enteric ulceration, with the ileocaecal area most frequently involved. This may mimic appendicitis. Drug treatment of this parasite is difficult.

CROHN'S DISEASE

Crohn's disease is a chronic inflammatory condition that can affect any part of the gastrointestinal tract from mouth to anus (see chapter 3), but in the small intestine the terminal ileum is most commonly involved. Inflammation affects the whole of the bowel wall and the characteristic histological finding is non-caseating granuloma formation (**Fig. 2.33**). Initial mucosal ulceration may lead to fibrosis, stricturing and fistula formation.

Presenting symptoms depend on the extent of the disease and its complications, but include diarrhoea, colicky abdominal pain due to partial obstruction, anorexia, weight loss and pyrexias. The causes of diarrhoea in small intestinal Crohn's disease are as follows:

- Extensive mucosal involvement causing generalised malabsorption
- Bacterial overgrowth
- Bile acid malabsorption from terminal ileal involvement or excision
- Entero-enteric fistulae
- Short bowel syndrome following multiple excisions
- Secondary intestinal infections
- Amyloidosis

On investigation, patients are often anaemic (iron and less often folate deficiencies) with a high ESR and C-reactive protein. Significant terminal ileal disease may be reflected in vitamin B_{12} deficiency which does not correct when intrinsic factor is given in the second part of the Schilling test. The diagnostic test of choice is the small bowel enema which highlights terminal ileal involvement (**Fig. 2.34**).

Maintenance treatment with 5-aminosalicylic acid derivatives such as mesalazine and management of acute exacerbations with steroids and steroid-sparing agents still do not

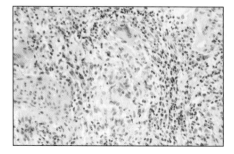

Fig. 2.33 *Small intestinal granuloma in Crohn's disease.*

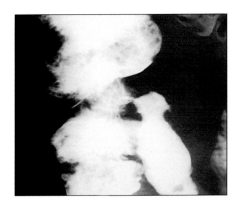

Fig. 2.34 *Terminal ileitis in Crohn's disease. Right iliac fossa view of a small bowel enema in a patient with ileocaecal Crohn's disease, demonstrating a narrowed terminal ileum with typical 'rose-thorn' ulceration. Another example is shown in Fig. 2.13.*

obviate the need for surgery in some, particularly for stricturoplasty or resection and treatment of fistulae. Elemental diets may be as effective as steroids in calming down an exacerbation of small intestinal Crohn's disease.

Differential diagnosis

Ileocaecal tuberculosis. Tuberculosis can affect any part of the gut, but the terminal ileum is the most commonly affected part. The condition usually presents like Crohn's disease and it has similar radiological appearances. The usual agent is M. *tuberculosis*, which may have spread from the lungs in swallowed sputum, although ingestion of unpasteurised milk may lead to infection with M. *bovis*. The condition is commoner in South Asian populations. Treatment should involve standard triple antituberculous therapy for 18 months.

Yersinial infections. *Yersinia enterocolitica* is a Gram-positive organism which causes ulceration in the small intestine, but it primarily affects the terminal ileum and colon. Yersinial infections can present acutely with watery diarrhoea and abdominal pain, or with an enteric fever syndrome similar to typhoid. Chronic infection can mimic Crohn's disease with similar appearances on small bowel enema. Stool or blood cultures may be positive. The organism is sensitive to a wide range of antibiotics including tetracycline, cotrimoxazole and chloramphenicol.

Other causes of ulcerative jejunoileitis. Ulceration in the small intestine may be caused by a wide variety of conditions, some of which are listed below:

- Crohn's disease
- Coeliac disease*
- Chronic infections
  Ileocaecal tuberculosis
  Yersinia enterocolitica
- Intestinal ischaemia
- Vasculitic conditions
  Polyarteritis nodosa
  Wegener's granulomatosis
  Behçet's disease

- Drugs
  Non-steroidal anti-inflammatory agents
  Enteric-coated potassium preparations
- Neoplasia
  Lymphoma*
  Leiomyoma
- Excessive gastric or ectopic acid production
  Zollinger–Ellison syndrome
  Meckel's diverticulum

* Most important

Patients may present with abdominal pain and malabsorptive symptoms. As in Crohn's disease, complications may occur such as bleeding, stricture or fistula formation or perforation. Barium studies show similar appearances. Endoscopic biopsy is important and direct visualisation with enteroscopy may occasionally have a role.

NECROTISING ENTERITIS

This small intestinal infection, also known as pigbel, is caused by *Clostridium perfringens* in malnourished populations, particularly in the Papua New Guinea Highlands, where it is associated with ingestion of poorly prepared pork. A spectrum from acute diarrhoea to extensive small intestinal necrosis with vomiting, abdominal distension and systemic collapse is usual. Treatment is supportive with rehydration. There is a high mortality, but tetracycline or chloramphenicol may be effective. A similar condition may be caused by *Bacillus anthracis* (anthrax), but this is extremely rare.

PROTEIN-LOSING ENTEROPATHY

This is not a single disease, since any number of conditions which cause small intestinal inflammation may cause an exudative protein loss:

- Crohn's disease
- Ileocaecal tuberculosis
- Yersinial enterocolitis
- Coeliac disease
- Tropical sprue
- Whipple's disease
- Giardiasis
- Ménétrier's disease
- Giant gastric ulcers
- Intestinal lymphoma
- Lymphatic obstruction
- Intestinal lymphangiectasia
- Congestive cardiac failure

In some patients the cause may be obvious, e.g. Crohn's disease, but in other individuals there may be an isolated hypoproteinaemia. Other potential sources of protein loss should be investigated (such as the urinary tract in nephrotic syndrome).

The condition may be diagnosed by measuring faecal clearance of α_1-antitrypsin or with nuclear medicine studies where faecal loss of $^{51}CrCl_3$, which binds to plasma albumin, can be measured. The source of gastrointestinal protein loss may be localised by scintigraphy, using radiolabelled transferrin.

MECKEL'S DIVERTICULUM

This is the most common congenital malformation of the gastrointestinal tract and results from incomplete closure of the embryonic vitelline duct. It is present in about 2% of the population, located about 60–100 cm proximal to the ileocaecal valve. Ectopic gastric mucosa may line the Meckel's diverticulum if it does not contain normal ileal epithelium. Most diverticula are completely asymptomatic. However, ulceration may occur in the diverticulum itself or in adjacent mucosa if there is significant acid production.

Patients can present with abdominal pain which mimics appendicitis, and overt or chronic gastrointestinal bleeding. The diverticulum can be difficult to spot on barium studies, but may be picked up on angiography (**Fig. 2.35**) which is performed if there has been bleeding. ^{99m}Tc-labelled pertechnetate scintigraphy can highlight ectopic acid-secreting mucosa (see **Fig. 2.14**). Treatment involves excision of the diverticulum at laparotomy.

TUMOURS OF THE SMALL INTESTINE

Although the mucosal surface area of the small intestine makes up over 80% of the total luminal surface from mouth to anus, small bowel tumours are rare, accounting for around 1% of gastrointestinal malignancies. These tumours often present late and their rarity often leads to a delay in diagnosis, since the small bowel can be relatively difficult to investigate. In **Fig. 2.36**, the different types of tumour are listed.

Gastrinomas are discussed in chapter 1 and the carcinoid syndrome in chapter 6. The Peutz–Jeghers syndrome is described, along with other familial polyposis syndrome, in chapter 3.

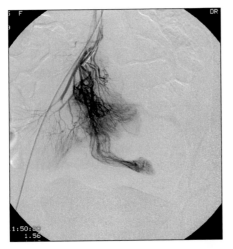

Fig. 2.35 *Meckel's diverticulum on arteriography. Selective, superior mesenteric arteriogram from a patient being investigated for occult gastrointestinal bleeding. The Meckel's diverticulum can be clearly seen as a pouch-like projection directed downwards, away from the main arterial branches.*

Fig. 2.36 *Small intestinal tumours.*

Small intestinal tumours	
Benign tumours	Lipoma Adenoma Leiomyoma Fibroma Neurofibroma
Hamartomas	Peutz–Jeghers polyp Angioma
APUDomas (APUD = amine precursor uptake and decarboxylation)	Gastrinoma Carcinoid tumour
Primary malignant tumours	Adenocarcinoma Lymphoma Leiomyosarcoma Sarcoma Kaposi's sarcoma
Secondary malignant tumours	Carcinoma Melanoma Lymphoma

Adenomas

These are commonest in the proximal part of the duodenum and the villous type has the greatest potential for malignant change. They may occur sporadically or as part of familial adenomatous polyposis (see chapter 3) and may be a source of iron deficiency, but more often than not these tumours are incidental findings at endoscopy. They must be removed in a similar fashion to colonic polyps (see chapter 3) and patients should undergo a similar surveillance programme. A follow-up endoscopy every 3 years is generally recommended. Screening colonoscopy is also appropriate, as is the investigation of near blood relatives.

Adenocarcinomas

Carcinomas may be associated with malignant change in isolated or multiple adenomatous polyps or with specific syndromes such as Gardner's syndrome (see chapter 3). Patients with poorly controlled or untreated coeliac disease have an increased risk, but more so with the development of lymphomas. Peutz–Jeghers syndrome (hamartomatous polyps) has rarely been associated with duodenal carcinoma, while jejunal and ileal carcinomas have been linked to the chronic inflammation of coeliac disease and Crohn's disease.

Presenting symptoms depend on the site of the lesion, but weight loss and obstructive symptoms such as colicky abdominal pain and vomiting are not uncommon. Iron deficiency anaemia is more common than frank haemorrhage. Lesions may be seen on small bowel enema or on CT or MRI of the abdomen. Actively bleeding lesions can be delineated at visceral angiography, but laparotomy with or without 'on-table' enteroscopy is required for definitive diagnosis and resection provides the only chance of 'cure'.

Lymphomas

These present in a similar fashion to adenocarcinomas and should always be considered in patients with coeliac disease who develop abdominal pain or weight loss (see **Fig. 2.23**). Investigation is the same as for adenocarcinomas. Primary gut lymphomas should be resected and various chemotherapy or combined chemotherapy and radiotherapy regimens exist, but 5-year survival is poor.

α-chain disease and Mediterranean lymphomas

Diffuse plasma cell infiltration of the small intestine is associated with repeated enteric bacterial or helminthic infections and is characterised by circulating α heavy chains. This has been termed immunoproliferative small intestinal disease (IPSID). The 'benign' form of the condition is called α-chain disease and the more aggressive variety is termed Mediterranean lymphoma, because the highest incidence is in countries of the Mediterranean littoral. Patients are usually young men and they present with symptoms of malabsorption, weight loss, fever, chronic diarrhoea and abdominal pain. Digital clubbing may be present. Treatment is with tetracycline, metronidazole, cytotoxic agents and sometimes radiotherapy, but prognosis for the aggressive forms is poor. If there is an intercurrent worm infestation, the addition of antihelminthics to the regimen may help.

Leiomyomas and leiomyosarcomas

These can be difficult to distinguish histologically. Patients usually present with bleeding or obstructive symptoms (**Fig. 2.37**). Smooth muscle tumours, like other mass lesions, may be a focus for intussusception (see **Fig. 2.17**). Resection offers the best chance of cure in the malignant forms.

SURGICAL CAUSES OF MALABSORPTION

Iatrogenic causes of malabsorption should not be forgotten. Jejuno-ileal bypass used to be a popular treatment for morbid obesity, but bacterial overgrowth can occur in the blind loop and specific deficiencies such as vitamin B_{12} occur unless the appropriate replacement is given. Other areas of fluid stasis – as in jejunal diverticulosis (**Fig. 2.38**), for example – can prove suitable sites for bacterial overgrowth.

Short gut syndrome may occur after significant intestinal resection – for example, after radiation enteritis or Crohn's disease. Octreotide may be helpful in stemming the high-output diarrhoea.

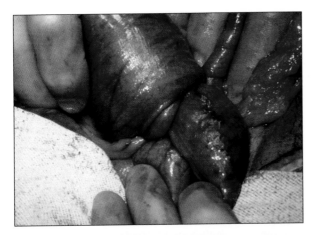

Fig. 2.37 *Small intestinal leiomyoma. Identification of a small bowel leiomyoma at laparotomy in a patient with recurrent intestinal obstruction.*

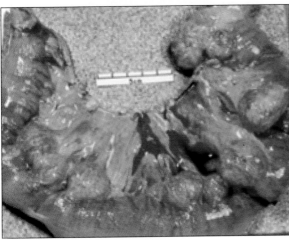

Fig. 2.38 *Jejunal diverticulosis. Resection specimen showing multiple rounded diverticulae extruding from the jejunal mucosa. This patient had developed chronic malabsorption due to persistent bacterial overgrowth.*

RADIATION ENTEROPATHY

Radiation-induced bowel damage is a complication of radiotherapy for pelvic and abdominal malignancies. The terminal ileum and the rectum have been commonly affected by irradiation of gynaecological tumours due to their anatomical position. The condition is now less common because of tailoring of radiotherapy regimes, including dose fractionation.

Acute irradiation enteritis occurs at the time of the radiotherapy and resolves on completion of the regime. All rapidly dividing cells are susceptible and in the small intestine this leads to enterocyte damage, manifesting as mucosal ulceration with resultant diarrhoea and malabsorptive symptoms. However, this is usually overshadowed by the bloody diarrhoea of radiation proctitis, if present.

Chronic irradiation enteritis occurs 5–6 years after radiotherapy and patients may not connect their symptoms to their previous history. The pathological hallmarks (**Fig. 2.39**) are the development of marked fibrosis with the presence of abnormal, large collagen-containing 'radiation fibroblasts' and also an obliterative endarteritis. This may lead to ulceration of the mucosa, bleeding, stricturing and fistula formation, or occasionally

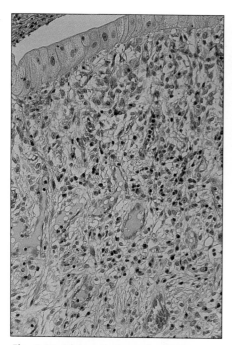

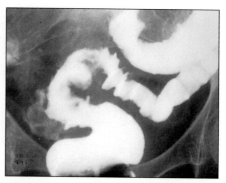

Fig. 2.40 *Radiation colitis. Irradiation may cause similar damage to the colon as well as small bowel involvement. This barium enema demonstrates severe colonic ulceration with some stricturing in an elderly female previously treated with pelvic radiotherapy.*

Fig. 2.39 *Histopathology of radiation enteritis. This high-power view shows the presence of radiation-induced granulation tissue in the lamina propria with an excess of fibroblasts.*

infarction or perforation of the small intestine due to ischaemia. An increased incidence of malignancy in radiation-induced bowel is also reported.

Functional changes include bowel obstruction or pseudo-obstruction and varying degrees of malabsorption with diarrhoea which may involve frank steatorrhoea. Since the terminal ileum is often worst affected, vitamin B_{12} and bile acid malabsorption is a common feature. Bacterial overgrowth is also not uncommon. There are often characteristic features on small bowel radiology (**Fig. 2.40**).

Treatment should be supportive. Lactose-free and low-residue diets are important, while cholestyramine may be helpful to reduce bile salt-induced diarrhoea. Occasionally, intractable high-output diarrhoea may need to be treated with octreotide if all other measures fail. Surgery should be avoided unless absolutely necessary, since anastomoses in radiation-damaged bowel can fall apart due to poor wound healing.

MESENTERIC ISCHAEMIA

Atherosclerosis of the visceral arteries is not an uncommon post-mortem finding, but critical stenosis causing mesenteric angina is comparatively rare. Classically, there is central abdominal pain 15–30 minutes after meals. Affected individuals may be afraid to eat and weight loss and malabsorption can be part of the presenting picture. Stenoses in the coeliac axis or the superior mesenteric artery can be demonstrated on angiography. Vascular reconstruction or angioplasty is required before total occlusion supervenes with potentially devastating consequences.

NUTRITION AND MALNUTRITION

The systemic manifestations of malnutrition are discussed in chapter 6, together with the specific eating disorders, anorexia nervosa and bulimia nervosa. Food allergies and food intolerance are discussed in chapter 7.

IRRITABLE BOWEL SYNDROME

This is an extremely common functional disorder of the bowel which affects at least 50% of patients attending gastroenterology clinics. A significant percentage of people in the general population of western countries have symptoms consistent with the irritable bowel syndrome at some stage in their lives. Colicky abdominal pain, abdominal distension and watery diarrhoea alternating with constipation are typical symptoms. The condition is frequently exacerbated by stress or anxiety. Its diagnosis and management are considered in more detail in chapter 3.

The Hindgut

Disorders of the colon, rectum and anus are extremely common clinical problems. Each year, Americans spend an estimated $800 million on over-the-counter laxatives in an effort to treat the most frequent gastroenterological symptom of all – constipation.

The symptoms of the irritable bowel syndrome (IBS) have a prevalence of about 20% in the 'normal' populations of Europe and North America. IBS is said to account for over 3.5 million doctor–patient consultations each year in the USA and represents about a quarter of the workload of gastroenterologists in the western world.

Adenomatous colonic polyps can be found in about half of the population over the age of 60 years, while colorectal malignancy is second only to bronchial carcinoma as a cause of cancer death in the USA and Europe.

Furthermore, many large bowel disorders may be considered to be of relatively low pathological significance, but nonetheless account for a great deal of discomfort and embarrassment.

STRUCTURE AND FUNCTION

EMBRYOLOGY

Strictly speaking, the embryological hindgut extends from the distal third of the transverse colon to the anus. However, in functional and pathological terms, we should consider the large bowel as a whole, beginning at the ileocaecal valve (**Fig. 3.1**).

ANATOMY AND PHYSIOLOGY

The colon has two layers of smooth muscle, an inner matrix of circular fibres and an outer layer of longitudinal fibres that are concentrated into three streaks, known as the *taeniae coli*.

Colonic motility is still poorly understood. Unlike the stomach and small bowel, the colon does not have a single migratory motor complex (MMC) that travels its length. Instead there seem to be multiple contractile patterns, which are often poorly coordinated in the interdigestive period.

The colonic response to eating seems to be largely neurally mediated, albeit with a lesser hormonal component. Distension of the stomach with food leads to an immediate increase in colonic contractions, a phenomenon known as the 'gastrocolic reflex', which can be diminished by muscarinic antagonists. It is impaired in patients with autonomic neuropathy.

The arterial supply to the midgut is from the superior mesenteric artery (SMA), while that of the hindgut is from the inferior mesenteric artery (IMA). Consequently, the colon receives blood from both systems, the SMA supplying the ascending and transverse colon,

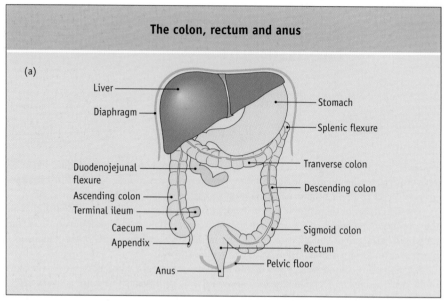

The colon, rectum and anus

(a)

Liver

Diaphragm

Stomach

Splenic flexure

Duodenojejunal flexure

Tranverse colon

Descending colon

Ascending colon

Terminal ileum

Caecum

Appendix

Sigmoid colon

Rectum

Pelvic floor

Anus

Fig. 3.1 *The colon, rectum and anus. (a) The anatomy of the large bowel. The transverse colon and sigmoid colon are always attached to a mesentery. However, the ascending colon is mesenteric in only 10% of individuals and the descending colon in 20%. (b) Arterial blood supply and lymphatic drainage. (c) Venous drainage of the large bowel.*

and the IMA nourishing the bowel distal to the splenic flexure. The SMA is effectively an end-artery, with inadequate collateral supply in the event of an acute occlusion. The colon is therefore vulnerable to ischaemia, particularly around the splenic flexure, where the two blood supplies meet.

The rectum receives blood from the IMA as well as from an anastomosis with branches of the internal iliac arteries.

The colon and electrolyte balance

The colon has a key role in maintaining adequate fluid and electrolyte balance. The liquid small-bowel contents are converted into solid, formed bowel motions by its ability to reabsorb water and electrolytes. Patients in whom this mechanism is defective (for example, after total colectomy with ileostomy) can become fluid-depleted very easily, although the kidney and small bowel adapt accordingly to its loss.

Under normal conditions, the colon reabsorbs 95% of the sodium and water presented to it (**Fig. 3.2**). Experimental perfusion studies have shown that the colon is capable of absorbing up to 6 litres of water and 800 mmol of sodium a day, which makes for a useful reserve in case of impaired absorption by the small intestine.

The anus and rectum: sphincter mechanisms and continence

A normally functioning hindgut is essential for maintaining faecal continence. The rectum effectively acts as a reservoir, storing faeces until defaecation is appropriate. The arrival of faeces in the rectum triggers an 'accommodation' response, relaxing its musculature to accommodate the bowel motion.

The colon, rectum and anus

(b)

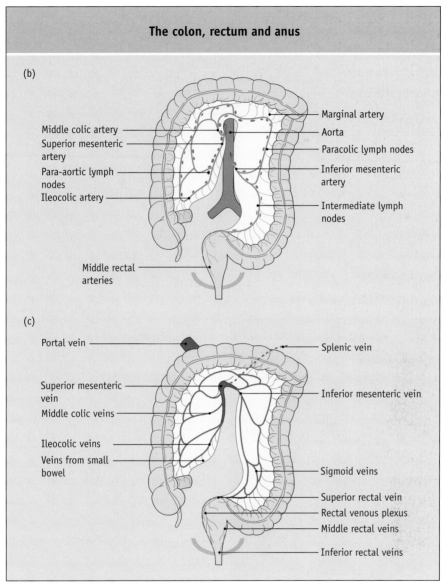

Middle colic artery

Superior mesenteric artery

Para-aortic lymph nodes

Ileocolic artery

Middle rectal arteries

Marginal artery

Aorta

Paracolic lymph nodes

Inferior mesenteric artery

Intermediate lymph nodes

(c)

Portal vein

Superior mesenteric vein

Middle colic veins

Ileocolic veins

Veins from small bowel

Splenic vein

Inferior mesenteric vein

Sigmoid veins

Superior rectal vein

Rectal venous plexus

Middle rectal veins

Inferior rectal veins

Fig. 3.1 (cont) *The colon, rectum and anus. (b) Arterial blood supply and lymphatic drainage. (c) Venous drainage of the large bowel.*

The rectum is richly innervated with nerves sensitive to stretching and distension, but is relatively anaesthetic for pain due to heat or sharp objects (a feature which allows colonoscopic biopsies and diathermy-polypectomy to be well tolerated). Progressive distension of the rectum results in the urge to defaecate and, eventually, pain.

The anal canal, however, is much more sensitive to light touch, pain and temperature. Its innervation is adept at distinguishing between solid, liquid and gaseous bowel contents.

Fluid balance and the gut

Volume of fluid entering GI tract (MI)		Sodium content (mmol)
Diet	2000	150
Saliva	1000	50
Gastric juice	2000	100
Bile	1000	200
Pancreatic juice	2000	150
Enteric secretion	1000	150
Total	9000	800
Volume of fluid leaving region (ml)		**Amount of sodium leaving region (mmol)**
Duodenum	9000	800
Jejunum	5000	700
Ileum	1500	200
Colon	100	3
Whole gut	100	3

All the figures given in these tables refer to a 24-hour period.

Fig. 3.2 *Fluid balance and the gut.*

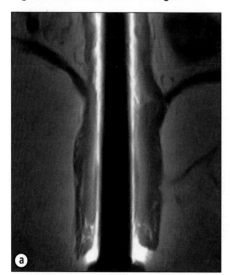

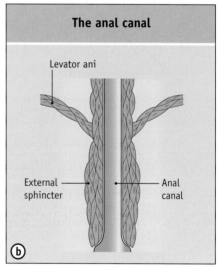

The anal canal

Levator ani

External sphincter

Anal canal

Fig. 3.3 *The anal canal. (a) Endoanal magnetic resonance image of the sphincter muscles. High-definition images can be obtained by using an endoanal MRI coil. (b) Explanatory diagram (coronal view in a normal patient).*

The anal canal is approximately 4 cm long and is surrounded by the anal sphincter mechanism (**Fig. 3.3**). Histologically, the upper half of the canal is lined by a rectal-type columnar mucosa that is abruptly replaced by squamous epithelial cells from the dentate line downwards. The upper half of the anal mucosa is folded longitudinally into the 'columns of Morgagni', which contain prominent venous plexi. Like the lower end of the oesophagus, this is one of the sites where the portal venous system can communicate with the systemic circulation if there is portal hypertension (hence the presence of anorectal varices in some patients with cirrhosis of the liver). As well as the vascular supply, the dentate line also separates lymphatic drainage; the upper half of the anal canal drains to the pelvic and abdominal lymph nodes, whilst the lower half drains externally to the inguinal nodes.

The sphincter mechanism consists of internal and external sphincter muscles, augmented by the anal cushions. The internal sphincter is tonically active at rest, keeping the anus and perianal skin dry, under the control of intramural enteric nerves and some intrinsic myogenic activity. It accounts for the majority of resting anal tone. Distension of the rectum with faeces triggers a brief relaxation of the internal sphincter (via the myenteric nerves) which is rapidly followed by restoration of the normal tone. This reflex continues with progressive rectal distension, but eventually the relaxation phase increases, so that faeces progress into the anal canal and continence is maintained by the external sphincter.

The external sphincter muscle differs in that it consists largely of type I skeletal muscle fibres. These have a higher content of oxidative enzymes than most skeletal muscles, which allows the sustained contraction necessary to maintain faecal continence. This is supported by the puborectalis muscle (part of levator ani) which forms a sling derived from the pelvic floor. The 'anorectal angle' caused by the puborectalis muscle seems to aid continence although its relative importance is debated.

Experimental studies of the wall tension produced by the sphincter muscles suggests that they alone would not be sufficient to close the anal canal completely. This deficit in sphincter function appears to be corrected by the anal cushions, submucosal pads of vascular tissue that surround the anus and seem to provide an overlapping sealing mechanism. Evidence supporting this role comes from the incidence of faecal soiling in patients who have had radical haemorrhoidectomy operations, where the cushions are removed.

SYMPTOMS AND SIGNS

Most symptoms of large bowel disease relate to alterations in bowel habit. But what is a *normal* bowel habit? To some extent the definition depends on geography and dietary intake (stool weight and volume varying in different parts of the world). In Europe and North America, only 1% of the population opens their bowels less often than three times a week or more often than three times a day, and deviations from this are taken to be abnormal. As well as its amount, alterations in the consistency of stool are important.

Constipation

The use of the term 'constipation' by patients is very subjective, but in general patients consider themselves constipated if not opening their bowels on most days. There are many related symptoms, including the passage of small, hard stools (regardless of frequency), feelings of incomplete evacuation, difficulty in initiating a bowel movement, straining at stool and feelings of abdominal 'bloating'.

Causes of constipation are legion (**Fig. 3.4**). Most commonly, it will be a result of diet, lifestyle and motility changes (such as the irritable bowel syndrome). However, a change in bowel habit may be the first sign of colorectal malignancy or, less commonly, another serious medical condition. Consequently, a detailed history and full examination, including rectal, are mandatory procedures. Specific enquiry should be made for 'worrying symptoms' such as weight loss, rectal bleeding, tenesmus and pain. A suggested diagnostic work-up is shown in **Fig. 3.5**.

Causes of constipation	
Dietary	Low consumption of fibre Poor fluid intake
Lifestyle	Lack of exercise Sedentary occupation Long-distance travel Pregnancy Ageing

Structural	Strictures – carcinomatous
	    diverticular inflammatory
	Rectocoele
	Prolapse
	Anal fissure
	Post-hysterectomy
	    (or other pelvic surgery)
	Hirchsprung's disease

Metabolic	Diabetes mellitus Hypokalaemia Hypothyroidism Hypercalaemia Porphyria
Drug-induced	Chronic laxative abuse Opiates Aluminium compounds Anticholinergics Iron supplements Antidepressants Calcium channel antagonists Bismuth chelate
Neurological	Cerebral palsy Stroke Multiple sclerosis Parkinson's disease Spinal cord injury
Others	Irritable bowel syndrome Depression Pseudo-obstruction syndromes Endometriosis Systemic sclerosis Inflammatory proctitis

Fig. 3.4 *Causes of constipation.*

Most patients with 'simple' constipation will improve with lifestyle modification – a higher intake of fluids and dietary fibre or regular exercise. Dietary fibre:

- Consists of plant cell-wall polysaccharides, e.g. cellulose, pectin
- Is easily obtained in wholemeal bread, wholegrain cereals, unpeeled fruit and vegetables, pulses, brown rice and sweetcorn
- May be partly fermented by colonic bacteria, producing short-chain fatty acids, methane, carbon dioxide and hydrogen

Diagnostic work-up for the constipated patient	

1. Exclude or identify systemic illness	Take a history
	Full physical examination
	Blood tests as indicated
	    (e.g. thyroid function, urea and
	    electrolytes, calcium, full blood
	    count, glucose)

2. Perform digital rectal examination	Inspection – fissures, prolapse Check perianal sensation Assess sphincter tone Feel for anorectal masses
3. Further investigations as appropriate	Sigmoidoscopy Double-contrast barium enema Colonoscopy (if history of rectal bleeding or if anaemic) Anorectal manometry

Fig. 3.5 *Diagnostic work-up for the constipated patient.*

- Increases stool mass
- Speeds up intestinal transit time
- Acts as a faecal softener (less time for water reabsorption)
- Increases the amount of colonic bacteria
- Reduces the incidence of diverticular disease and colorectal cancer

Compliance can be aided by patient education about the mechanisms involved, as well as discouraging unnecessary laxative abuse.

For the remainder, treatment should be of the underlying cause, where appropriate. In the absence of a specific cause, after the investigations in **Fig. 3.5**, or failure to respond to lifestyle modification, a trial of laxative therapy may be necessary. However, laxative treatment should be kept as brief as possible as long-term use can lead to hypokalaemia and an atonic, non-functioning colon. A classification of laxatives is included in **Fig. 3.6**, although this disguises the fact that some have a complex action. All have their drawbacks. Bulking agents require a high fluid intake to avoid obstruction. Non-absorbable sugars (such as lactulose) can cause troublesome flatulence and bloating. Stimulant laxatives may cause abdominal cramp and can eventually lead to an atonic bowel. Finally, danthron preparations are recommended only for the terminally ill or those with opiate-induced constipation because of fears of carcinogenicity with long-term use. Bowel preparation for colonoscopy or barium enema examinations may involve cathartic solutions of polyethylene glycol. These are *not* suitable as first-line treatments for constipation.

Diarrhoea

Diarrhoeal illnesses are a significant health problem worldwide, accounting for the deaths of some 5–8 million infants and small children each year in many developing nations. Diarrhoea is one of the most common symptoms in gastroenterology and every physician needs to have an understanding of its pathophysiology and management.

Like constipation, the definition of diarrhoea is influenced by cultural factors regarding appropriate stool output. For instance, the average normal daily stool output is about 500 g in rural Uganda, versus just 100–200 g per day in Europe and North America.

Treatment of constipation	
1. Non-pharmacological	Patient education Improve intake of dietary fibre Increase fluid intake Bowel retraining (e.g. not avoiding urge to defaecate)

2. Laxative therapy	Bulking agents: methylcellulose, ispaghula husk, bran
	Osmotic laxatives: lactulose, lactitol, sorbitol,
	    magnesium sulphate, magnesium citrate,
	    magnesium hydroxide
	Stimulant laxatives: senna, bisacodyl, docusate
	    sodium, danthron, sodium picosulphate
	Faecal softeners: docusate sodium, paraffin

3. Enemas and suppositories	Sodium acid phosphate Arachis oil Sodium citrate Glycerol
4. Surgical approaches	For anorectal fissure: anal stretch, sphincterotomy For rectal prolapse: rectal fixation, rectopexy For pelvic floor descent: pelvic floor support

Fig. 3.6 *Treatment of constipation.*

Consequently, most gastroenterologists in the western world would define diarrhoea as a stool output of more than 200 g per day. From the patient's perspective, however, a useful definition is that diarrhoea is 'the too rapid evacuation of too fluid stools'.

In many patients, taking a full history will allow discrimination between diarrhoea due to disease affecting the small or large intestine. Small bowel diarrhoea is often associated with a central abdominal ache that is unrelated to defaecation; colonic diarrhoea, however, may be accompanied by pain in the left iliac fossa, which is often relieved by passing a bowel motion. A pale, fatty, offensive stool that may be difficult to flush away suggests malabsorptive small bowel diarrhoea. Colonic diarrhoea is more likely to occur with blood and mucus per rectum, or may be very watery in nature. In some patients, the distinction is blurred, often because the underlying pathology affects both small and large bowel. In the case of bile salt malabsorption, for example, due to defective reabsorption in the terminal ileum, bile salts pass into the colon causing a secretory (choleretic diarrhoea).

As a basic minimum, patients with suspected colonic diarrhoea should have a sigmoidoscopy with rectal biopsy and stools should be sent for microscopy and culture. Even if the mucosa is macroscopically normal, histological examination can reveal evidence of inflammatory bowel disease, melanosis coli (suggestive of laxative abuse, see **Fig. 3.60**), collagenous colitis or infectious pathogens such as amoebae in tropical travellers. The investigation and management of diarrhoea are dealt with in more detail in chapter 2.

Rectal bleeding

Patients who present with rectal bleeding require careful assessment. Often the cause is a haemorrhoid or small anal fissure, but the doctor should not attribute bleeding to local causes without considering the possibility of more proximal bowel disease. Particularly if there are associated symptoms such as tenesmus, alteration in bowel habit, abdominal pain or weight loss, consideration must be given to the possibility of colorectal malignancy. The causes of rectal bleeding are:

- Bleeding from the foregut
  - Peptic ulcer disease
  - Severe haemobilia
- Diverticular disease
- Colorectal neoplasia
  - Adenocarcinoma
  - Colonic polyps
- Inflammatory bowel disease
  - Ulcerative colitis
  - Crohn's disease
- Anorectal conditions
  - Anal fissure
  - Haemorrhoids
  - Solitary rectal ulcer
- Ischaemic colitis
- Vascular abnormalities
  - Anorectal varices
  - Telangiectasia (e.g. Osler–Weber–Rendu)
  - Amyloidosis
- Infective colitis
  - Shigellosis
  - Campylobacteriosis
  - Amoebiasis
- Radiation enteritis
- Intussusception
- Meckel's diverticulum

Enquiry should be made about the appearance of the blood. If it is bright red and fresh (haematochezia), this usually suggests an anorectal cause, whereas darker, altered blood may be of more proximal origin. Likewise, blood that is mixed in with the stool may point to a colonic source, while haemorrhoids may give rise to blood that is passed after a normal bowel motion.

Digital rectal examination should be performed in all patients and a proctoscopy carried out to look for haemorrhoids or a fissure. In those patients in whom malignancy is suspected (the middle-aged or elderly, or those with the associated symptoms listed above) a colonoscopy is necessary.

Massive, acute rectal bleeding is fortunately uncommon. However, bleeding into the gastrointestinal tract at any level may result in blood per rectum, particularly where bleeding is brisk. Usually, rectal bleeding implies a lesion distal to the ligament of Treitz, but foregut lesions may bleed too rapidly for the blood to be 'altered' before reaching the anus. Consequently, patients must be asked about upper gastrointestinal symptoms and most gastroenterologists would recommend a gastroscopy to exclude foregut bleeding where haematochezia is severe.

There are relatively few prospective, randomised studies to support either colonoscopy or angiography in acute, haemodynamically significant rectal bleeding. The investigation of choice will largely depend on local facilities and expertise. Colonoscopy can be technically difficult to perform where bleeding is copious, but some authorities have used nasogastric-colonic lavage to cleanse the bowel rapidly before the procedure. Without bowel preparation, colonoscopy is rarely helpful.

Arteriography may show extravasation of contrast medium into the bowel lumen, but this only occurs in 60–70% of patients as bleeding is often intermittent. Associated vascular abnormalities, however, such as angiodysplasia or early venous return from arteriovenous communications, may be detected. Coil embolisation of bleeding lesions may be offered, although care must be taken to ensure that an adequate collateral circulation maintains the integrity of the gut wall.

Lower abdominal pain

As with pain elsewhere in the abdomen, the history is all-important, including the site, severity, character, duration, periodicity, associated symptoms and exacerbating or relieving factors.

It is possible, to some degree, to localise pain to particular viscera, although the non-specific nature of innervation and the frequency of referred pain may make this difficult. In general, pain in the right iliac fossa suggests pathology arising from the caecum and appendix (the latter when the parietal peritoneum is involved), ovary, mesenteric adenitis or the right pelviureteric urinary tract.

Suprapubic discomfort is often a feature of cystitis or pain arising from the uterus and adnexae, although colonic pain may also manifest itself here as well as in the central abdominal area.

Pain from the left kidney and ureter, as well as being felt in the loin area, may radiate into the left iliac fossa, a site where pain (particularly related to defaecation) is commonly felt from diseases of the sigmoid colon. The irritable bowel syndrome, constipation and diverticulosis are also frequently associated with left iliac fossa pain, as are lower bowel strictures due to neoplasia or inflammatory bowel disease.

Anal pain

The two most frequent causes of a painful anus are haemorrhoids (or 'piles') and anal fissures.

Haemorrhoids. Haemorrhoids occur when the anal vascular cushions protrude and become congested because of pressure exerted by the anal sphincter. They often cause perianal discomfort, but may become acutely painful if thrombosed or strangulated. Affected patients are usually constipated and the passage of hard stools, associated with straining, exacerbates the problem. Bleeding may result, especially post-defaecation.

If haemorrhoidal thrombosis occurs, it may give rise to an acutely painful swelling that protrudes from the anal canal, known as a 'thrombosed external pile'. This usually resolves spontaneously over 1 or 2 weeks.

Haemorrhoids can be treated by minimising straining at stool, using the dietary and lifestyle treatments mentioned in **Fig. 3.6.** Definitive treatment of the piles themselves involves the injection of sclerosants or the use of band ligation, either of which can easily be performed in the proctologist's outpatient clinic. Radical surgical treatment (haemorrhoidectomy) may be necessary in severe cases.

Anal fissures. The development of an anal fissure is also associated with constipation. This lesion is essentially a split in the skin of the anus, usually orientated in the midline, extending outwards from the dentate line. The lesion can be exquisitely painful, so much so that a rectal examination may be impossible. Secondary spasm of the anal sphincter exacerbates the problem further. There may be an associated oedematous skin tag, known as a 'sentinel pile'.

Many acute anal fissures will heal with conservative management, faecal softening and pain relief. Topical treatment with glyceryl trinitrate 0.2% ointment (twice daily for 6–8 weeks) has shown some success in lowering anal canal pressures and allowing healing to occur in around 50% of patients. However, chronic fissures are unlikely to heal spontaneously and surgical intervention is usually required. Operative techniques include anal stretch procedures or lateral internal sphincterotomy. Both procedures carry a small risk of inducing incontinence.

Proctalgia fugax. Acute anorectal pain may also result from the syndrome of proctalgia fugax. This tends to cause a sudden, sharp, fleeting rectal pain that may last for a few minutes or a few hours. Its cause is unknown, although it may be associated with psychological stress or functional gastrointestinal disorders. The pain can be very severe. Care should be taken to exclude other causes of pain in the region, such as anal fissures, thrombosed piles, coccydynia or colorectal strictures. The precise origin of the pain is unknown, although some authors have suggested a spasm of the pubococcygeus muscle in the pelvic floor. Treatment relies on excluding the 'organic' conditions above, reassuring the patient that attacks become less frequent with age and by the use of hot baths or, occasionally, muscle relaxant drugs.

Pruritus ani

The unpleasant sensation of perianal itching and irritation may be the result of the same dermatological and medical disorders that cause itching elsewhere in the body. However, more commonly, the cause of isolated pruritus ani is difficult to determine, not least because patients may have entered a cycle of itch-scratch-itch long after the initial trigger has disappeared.

Local causes include discharging sinuses or fistulae, prolapsing haemorrhoids, skin tags, fissures, warts, poor hygiene (or, conversely, over-zealous hygiene with excessive application of soaps), dermatophytosis, candidiasis, lice, worm infestations (particularly threadworms in children) and contact dermatitis due to medicinal creams and ointments. No cause is found in about 50% of patients.

Tenesmus

The sensation of incomplete anorectal evacuation is known as tenesmus. It is an important symptom, as it can be the result of a mass in the anus, rectum or distal colon. Proctitis may also cause the same feeling, especially where there is faecal urgency. In some patients, the feeling of incomplete evacuation can be a manifestation of the irritable bowel syndrome, but tenesmus should always prompt a search for an underlying colorectal lesion.

INVESTIGATIONS

DIAGNOSTIC RADIOLOGY

Plain radiography

A plain film of the abdomen is often useful in large bowel disorders. It may reveal colonic distension, as seen in toxic megacolon (see 'Acute colitis' below), or obstruction due to a stricture or, tumour. Patients with sigmoid volvulus may have spectacular dilatation of the large bowel on plain radiography (Fig. 3.7). Similarly, a faecally loaded colon can be demonstrated in the constipated patient. An abdominal X-ray also gives useful information about the bowel wall, which may be congested and oedematous in inflammatory colitis or intestinal ischaemia. Finally, the presence of intracolonic foreign bodies may be revealed.

Barium enema

Despite the widespread availability of colonoscopy, the double-contrast barium enema remains useful. The two investigations are often complementary, depending on the diagnostic information required (Fig. 3.8). Both require bowel preparation with strong laxatives and cause a certain amount of patient discomfort during the procedure.

Wherever possible, the double-contrast barium enema should be performed rather than single-contrast, as the former is much more sensitive in detecting mucosal lesions (Fig. 3.9).

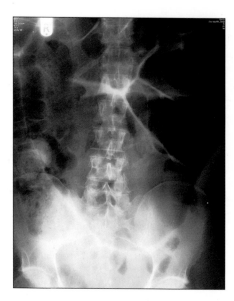

Fig. 3.7 *Sigmoid volvulus. In this condition, a loop of sigmoid colon becomes twisted around its mesentery to form a closed-loop obstruction. It often occurs in elderly patients with long, redundant sigmoid loops and a history of chronic constipation. Occasionally, the mass of a sigmoid carcinoma may destabilise a loop of bowel so that it wraps around itself. This figure shows a grossly dilated segment of colon arising from the pelvis in an inverted 'U' shape. If left untreated, the volvulus can develop venous infarction, followed by perforation and life-threatening faecal peritonitis. Treatment involves relieving the obstruction by inserting a rigid sigmoidoscope. A flatus tube is then carefully manipulated into the twisted loop and the bowel contents are allowed to rush out. If this procedure is unsuccessful (and even if successful, the volvulus may recur), then surgery is usually required.*

The double-contrast method involves rapidly infusing the contrast medium into the rectum, allowing it to reach the splenic flexure. 'Spot' images of the rectosigmoid area are taken and the barium is allowed to drain out, before volumes of air or carbon dioxide are insufflated and used to propel the remaining barium around the colon, leaving a thin coating of barium in the gas-filled bowel. The patient's posture is changed several times to allow a number of different radiological views to be taken. As a rule, all the mucosal surfaces of the colon should be demonstrated before the examination can be said to be complete.

Comparative studies with colonoscopy have shown that a double-contrast barium enema is able to detect 98% of neoplastic lesions greater than 1 cm in diameter and about 70% of those less than 1 cm. Unfortunately, radiological artefacts (**Fig. 3.10**) may be generated by overlapping loops of colon, faecal residue and diffuse mucosal abnormalities such as diverticular disease. In these circumstances, a colonoscopy is usually necessary.

Defaecating proctogram

In patients who have disorders of the anal sphincter or pelvic floor, it is possible to image the defaecating process by introducing a barium paste plug into the rectum and taking radiological pictures as the plug is voided into a specially adapted commode. An alternative approach is the use of dynamic magnetic resonance imaging (MRI) techniques, which can give even more detailed views (**Fig. 3.11**).

Computerised tomography (CT)

The CT scanner remains very valuable for delineating abdominal masses (see **Fig. 1.8**). In colorectal malignancy, it can be very useful in detecting not only hepatic metastases, but also enlarged local lymph nodes and extramural infiltration of adjacent tissues. Unfortunately, 'conventional' CT can be quite limited in detecting subtle invasion of the bowel wall and the presence of tumour in normally sized lymph nodes. Other areas where

Barium enema versus colonoscopy

	Advantages	Disadvantages
Barium enema	Does not require sedation Better at demonstrating fistulae Demonstrates motility Demonstrates subtle strictures Cheaper than colonoscopy	Bowel preparation still necessary Faecal residue may cause artefacts Mucosal vascular lesions less visible Overlapping loops may obscure views Biopsy not possible

Most useful indications: Abdominal pain, altered bowel habit, suspected fistulae

	Advantages	Disadvantages
Colonoscopy	Therapeutic potential (e.g. polypectomy) Allows tissue biopsies to be taken Angiodysplasia may be seen Terminal ileum may be intubated Usually needed if barium enema abnormal	Sedation; bowel preparation Small (but significant) perforation risk Small fistulae often missed Difficult to see behind mucosal folds More expensive to perform

Most useful indications: Rectal bleeding, anaemia, biopsy or therapeutic procedure, surveillance

Fig. 3.8 *Barium enema versus colonoscopy.*

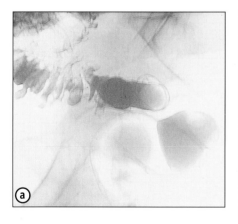 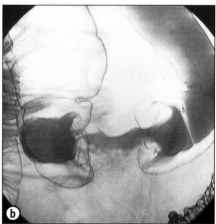

Fig. 3.9 *Double-contrast barium enema. (a) Multiple colonic diverticula. (b) An 'apple-core' stricture due to colonic adenocarcinoma.*

abdominal CT is useful include the detection of abscesses, particularly those associated with colonic Crohn's disease, diverticulosis or psoas abscess formation.

The development of higher-resolution spiral CT scanning techniques has greatly increased the ability to detect mucosal pathology. With bowel preparation and intravenous contrast, the images obtained have been described as 'virtual colonoscopy' (**Fig. 3.12**) and can be particularly useful in the staging of tumours (**Fig. 3.13**). It is now possible to blend these images into three-dimensional luminal views similar to those obtained colonoscopically.

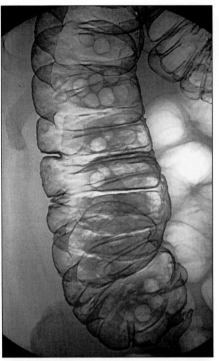

Fig. 3.10 *Barium enema – a polyposis syndrome? This double-contrast barium enema was performed on a young man with chronic abdominal pain. Multiple colonic filling defects are shown and were reported as suggesting a polyposis syndrome. A colonoscopic examination 1 week later found that they had all vanished – and the patient freely admitted to a diet rich in garden peas and sweetcorn!*

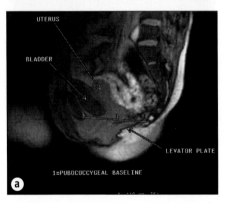
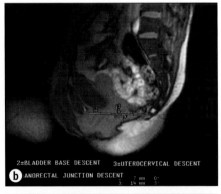

Fig. 3.11 *Dynamic pelvic floor imaging using MRI. MR sequences can now be acquired every half-second or so and this rapidity allows functional studies of the gastrointestinal tract to be undertaken. (a and b) These sagittal views can be used to measure pelvic floor descent as well as giving valuable information on the local anatomy. (c) Diagrammatic baseline sagittal view. (1 = pubococcygeal baseline; 2 = bladder base descert; 3 = uterocarvical descent; 4 = anorectal junction descent)*

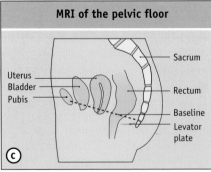

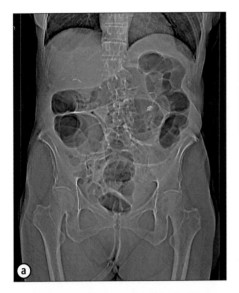

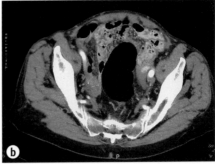

Fig. 3.12 'Virtual colonoscopy' demonstrating a sigmoid polyp. (a) After oral bowel preparation, a rectal tube is inserted and air insufflated. (b) An intravenous contrast agent is then given and the high-resolution spiral CT image demonstrates a large polyp in the sigmoid colon (marked with a white diagonal line).

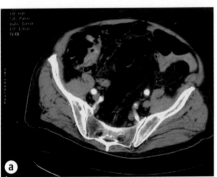 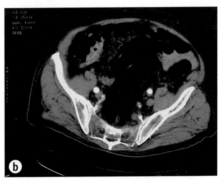

Fig. 3.13 'Virtual colonoscopy' detection of a caecal tumour. (a) A large irregular tumour in the caecum had been missed on an earlier, incomplete colonoscopy. (b) The tumour is marked with an 'X'.

Ultrasound

Ultrasound scanning is generally much better at imaging solid organs or fluid collections rather than gas-filled bowel. However, it can be of appreciable value in intestinal obstruction, where fluid-filled loops of intestine are visualised and real-time imaging allows the radiologist to distinguish a paralytic ileus from mechanical obstruction.

Abdominal masses are also amenable to visualisation, particularly in the iliac fossae, where there are wide differential diagnoses. An ultrasound can usually reveal whether a swelling is of gastrointestinal or gynaecological origin and one study has reported a 97% accuracy in determining the cause of a right iliac fossa mass.

Endoscopic ultrasound and MRI

By attaching ultrasonic probes to a colonoscope, it is possible to use endoscopic ultrasound to visualise the colon, rectum and anus. This technique can be useful in staging colorectal tumours, but has probably been most widely used to image the anal canal, sphincter mechanism and pararectal spaces.

107

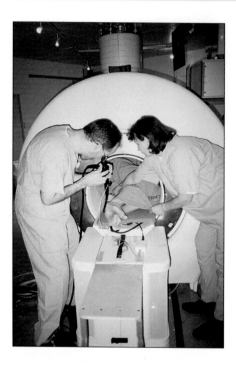

Fig. 3.14 *MRI colonoscopy.*

A more recent development has been the use of endoanal MRI to obtain high-quality images by inserting an MRI coil directly into the anus. Although still largely experimental, this technique does provide detailed views of anal and perianal structures (see **Fig. 3.3a**). MR-compatible colonoscopes have also been developed with radiofrequency coils incorporated into the tip of the instrument for high-resolution imaging of mucosal lesions (**Fig. 3.14**). Currently this imaging modality is a research tool, but the finely detailed views of mucosal and submucosal abnormalities that are obtained may make it useful in the surveillance of dysplastic changes, for example.

Nuclear medicine

Nuclear medicine techniques are often used to image the hindgut. White cell scans (scintigraphy), using [111]indium or [99]technetium, are very effective at identifying sites of inflammation. After reinfusing the labelled leucocytes, gamma camera images are recorded at set intervals (usually 1 and 4 hours later).

White cell scans are particularly useful in the diagnosis and monitoring of inflammatory bowel disease (**Fig. 3.15**) during acute exacerbations, when both barium studies and colonoscopy can be dangerous. By determining the site of inflammation, white cell scanning may distinguish Crohn's colitis from ulcerative colitis, demonstrating small bowel involvement or definite 'skip lesions'. It should be noted, however, that uptake of white cells does not only occur in inflammatory bowel disease and 'positive' scans may also be found with vasculitides, enteric infections and radiation enteritis.

Angiography

Contrast angiography to demonstrate blood vessels can be a valuable investigation. In the lower gastrointestinal tract, angiography may demonstrate numerous pathologies when a

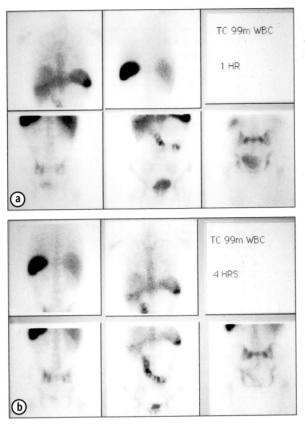

TC 99m WBC

1 HR

TC 99m WBC

4 HRS

(a)

(b)

Fig. 3.15 *White cell scintigraphy in inflammatory bowel disease. These images were recorded from a patient with inflammatory bowel disease after an infusion of ^{99}Tc-labelled white blood cells. (a) 1 hour afterwards. (b) 4 hours afterwards. There are separate areas of abnormally high leucocyte uptake in the transverse colon ('skip lesions'), a finding strongly suggestive of Crohn's disease rather than ulcerative colitis. The remaining colon and the small intestine are normal.*

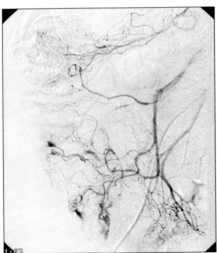

Fig. 3.16 *Large bowel angiodysplasia. Superior mesenteric angiography in an elderly woman with chronic iron deficiency anaemia. There are florid angiodysplastic areas in the caecum and ascending colon.*

skilled radiologist has cannulated the superior mesenteric and inferior mesenteric vessels. For instance, the abnormal circulation seen in areas of angiodysplasia (**Fig. 3.16**) may be

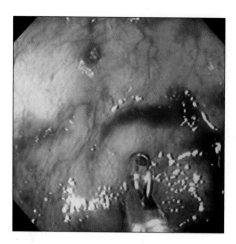

Fig. 3.17 *Flexible sigmoidoscopy. Normal sigmoid colonic mucosa with some adherent faeces. Biopsy forceps, as seen in the lower part of the picture, can be passed through the scope and used to obtain tissue for histology.*

evident, tumour circulation may be shown or the venous phase images may show abnormalities such as varices. Inflammatory bowel disease can give rise to subtle circulatory disturbances which can be recognised by the experienced observer.

PROCTOSCOPY AND SIGMOIDOSCOPY

Proctoscopy and rigid sigmoidoscopy are relatively simple procedures that can easily be carried out by the general physician. Bowel preparation is not required, although an enema may be useful if there is impacted stool. Proctoscopy allows inspection of the rectal mucosa, and therapeutic manoeuvres can be performed, including banding or injection of haemorrhoids. Rigid sigmoidoscopy is useful for assessing rectal and distal colonic mucosa and can easily be performed in the outpatient clinic. Up to 20 cm of mucosa may be seen. It is perhaps most useful in the investigation of diarrhoea, where a rectal biopsy is required. The presence of significant amounts of loose stool makes the examination difficult and mucosal views may be incomplete.

Flexible sigmoidoscopy provides much better imaging, without many of the 'blind spots' that may occur with the rigid instrument. Biopsies can easily be taken under direct vision (**Fig. 3.17**). Views can be obtained of about three times the penetration of a rigid sigmoidoscope. In many patients the instrument may be passed as far as the splenic flexure, although the lack of bowel preparation often prevents such advanced progress. As three-quarters of all colonic adenomas arise within 60 cm of the anus (the length of a fibreoptic sigmoidoscope), the examination has been proposed as a method of screening the population for colonic cancer. Several large-scale trials are currently under way, and initial reports suggest that even a single sigmoidoscopy to look for polyps, at the age of 50 years, may significantly reduce subsequent cancer risk.

COLONOSCOPY

In many respects, colonoscopy is the 'gold standard' investigation of the hindgut, offering an accurate macroscopic view of the whole colon and the distal terminal ileum. Furthermore, tissue biopsies may be taken and therapeutic procedures performed, including snare polypectomy (**Fig. 3.18**), balloon dilatation of strictures and haemostasis of bleeding lesions with laser or electrocoagulation.

The relative benefits of colonoscopy and double-contrast barium enema are shown in **Fig. 3.8**. It is worth bearing in mind that colonoscopy is potentially more hazardous than barium studies, with perforation rates of approximately 1 in 1700 and 1 in 25 000 procedures respectively. The combination of vagal stimulation and sedative drugs can lead

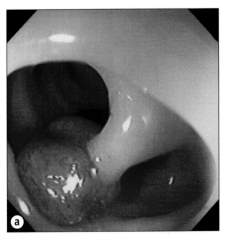 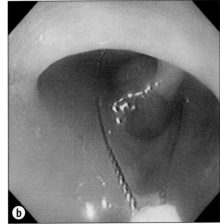

Fig. 3.18 *Colonoscopic polypectomy. (a) A pedunculated colonic polyp can be seen extending into the lumen. (b) A diathermy snare is passed down through the endoscope and the loop is encircled around the stalk of the polyp. The loop is tightened around the base of the stalk and an electrical current applied, coagulating the polyp's blood vessels and allowing its removal with little or no blood loss. With larger polyps, or those with very wide or long stalks, the risk of bleeding can be further reduced by prior injection of the stalk with adrenaline or sclerosant solutions.*

to hypotension, cardiac arrhythmia or respiratory depression. Bacteraemia is a common occurrence and prophylactic antibiotics should be used in those patients with prosthetic heart valves, previous endocarditis, immunosuppression or immunodeficiency. Where there is severe colonic inflammation (Crohn's disease, ulcerative colitis, bacterial colitis) and abdominal tenderness, there is a high risk of colonic perforation and the procedure should only be undertaken with extreme caution. The finding of severe ulceration in these circumstances should prompt curtailment of the examination for fear of perforating the weakened bowel wall.

In order to visualise the bowel lumen, the colon must be empty. Patients are usually prepared for the examination by taking a low-residue diet (or ideally only clear fluids) for the prior 24 hours. Iron preparations and constipating drugs should be stopped a week earlier. Laxative regimes vary but the two most widely used utilise either lavage with a polyethylene glycol balanced elecrolyte solution (on the day before the procedure) or a combination of sodium picosulphate and magnesium citrate. Bowel preparation regimes are unpopular with patients and poor compliance often leads to inadequate views being obtained at colonoscopy.

In trained hands, 'full' colonoscopy (i.e. at least to the caecum) is the norm in at least 90% of patients. The endoscopist can confirm that caecum has been reached by visualising the appendiceal orifice or caecal triradial fold, transilluminating the abdominal wall from within the bowel or by biopsying the terminal ileum (**Fig. 3.19**).

In some individuals, colonoscopy may be incomplete because of excessive looping and tortuosity of the bowel. These loops, principally in the sigmoid colon, may be difficult to dispel, leading to a painful and prolonged examination. Recent developments have led to the use of 'magnetic imaging' devices that give position-sensing information from special coils inserted into the colonoscope. Looping may also be reduced by the development of colonoscopes which allow the endoscopist to adjust the rigidity of the instrument. These innovations continue to be evaluated.

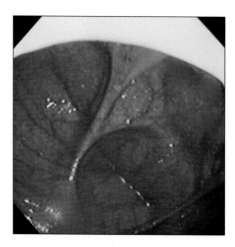

Fig. 3.19 *Normal caecum at colonoscopy. The triradial fold is clearly visible.*

It should be stressed that a normal colonoscopy does not fully exclude small focal lesions. Colonic polyps or vascular malformations may lie behind mucosal folds or be located at 'blind spots' on bends in the colon, particularly the splenic flexure. The colonoscopist needs to be vigilant both during the introduction of the colonoscope and its withdrawal. One recent study of consecutive 'back-to-back' colonoscopies by different operators suggested that up to 25% of small polyps may be missed.

Complications of colonoscopy are uncommon but well recognised. They include perforation of the colon, cardiac arrhythmias and splenic trauma.

MOTILITY STUDIES

Some patients with chronic idiopathic constipation may have an abnormally slow colonic transit time. It is possible to quantify this using scintigraphic techniques or radio-opaque markers.

Radioactive indium-labelling can be applied to polystyrene pellets and covered with a coating designed to release the pellets at the pH found in the terminal ileum. Gamma camera recordings are made of the pellets' progress through the colon.

Opaque markers can also be taken orally and their location assessed with fast-film (low radiation) plain radiography 4 days later. Transit times are compared with the mean values for the local population.

ANORECTAL MANOMETRY

Assessing the anorectal sphincter mechanism by manometry is often useful in patients with chronic constipation or faecal incontinence or soiling. The most common technique is the water-perfused catheter apparatus, whereby anorectal pressures are transmitted via a pneumohydraulic mechanism to an external pressure transducer. Sensors along the length of the catheter give a reading of the sequential pressure profile along the rectum and anus. Specific measurement can be made of the patient's sphincter 'squeeze pressure' during voluntary contraction, and the reflex responses to balloon distension of the rectum can be monitored.

Bowel preparation is usually unnecessary, although constipated patients may require an enema. The recordings may be obtained with the patient static; alternatively, an ambulatory apparatus is available for monitoring pressures during the patient's everyday activities. Readings give valuable information about rectal sensation, spinal reflexes and the integrity of the internal and external sphincters.

DIFFERENTIAL DIAGNOSIS

ACUTE COLITIS

Acute severe colitis is a medical (and potentially surgical) emergency. Patients presenting for the first time with severe inflammatory bowel disease and those with an infective colitis are often clinically indistinguishable.

Symptomatically, patients will usually have bloody diarrhoea, fever and abdominal discomfort. An accurate history, careful physical examination and a few simple investigations should clinch the underlying diagnosis in the majority of patients. In others, this may not be possible, not least because infectious and inflammatory colitis may coexist or because bacterial infections can precipitate acute presentations of ulcerative colitis (UC). Furthermore, patients with severe UC are often bacteraemic as a result of damage to colonic mucosa.

Although the two most common causes of acute colitis in developed nations are UC and bacterial infections, the differential diagnosis is wide and includes viral, amoebic and ischaemic colitis, along with Crohn's disease and rarer conditions such as irradiation colitis, Behçet's syndrome and the vasculitides.

Patients are usually very ill, often life-threateningly so. The key aspects to managing this disorder are performing an accurate (though rapid) initial assessment of the patient, prompt resuscitation and specific treatment of the underlying cause.

A few basic investigations are required. These should include sigmoidoscopy with rectal biopsy, stool microscopy and culture, a plain abdominal radiograph and taking blood for bacterial cultures, full blood count, biochemistry, albumin and inflammatory markers such as erythrocyte sedimentation rate (ESR) and C-reactive protein (CRP), if available. Barium enemas or colonoscopy carry appreciable risks in patients with acute colitis and should be deferred until the disease process is more quiescent.

Inspection of the rectal mucosa at sigmoidoscopy allows some grading of disease severity and may hint at the underlying cause (**Fig. 3.20**). Deep aphthous ulcers, relative rectal sparing or perianal disease may suggest Crohn's disease rather than UC; the distinction is largely academic, however, as the management of acute colitis is initially similar for both conditions.

Note should be made of any faeces, blood or mucus seen and the rigid sigmoidoscope can be utilised to obtain faecal specimens for analysis. A rectal biopsy should always be performed and sent for both histopathology and bacterial culture (the latter may yield a pathogen not detected on routine culture of faeces). Ischaemic colitis tends not to cause significant rectal involvement owing to the extensive collateral blood supply in this area.

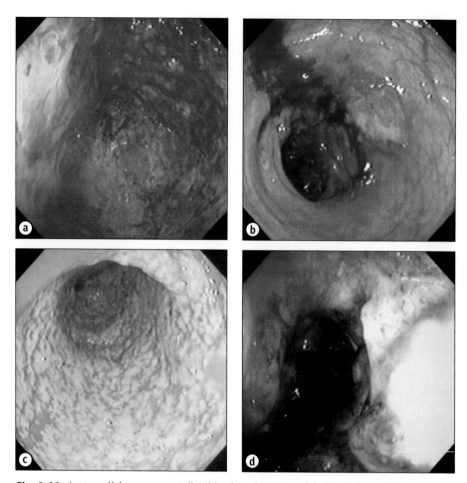

Fig. 3.20 *Acute colitis, as seen at flexible sigmoidoscopy. (a) Ulcerative colitis. Rectal view showing severe proctitis with hyperaemia, contact bleeding and ulceration. (b) Crohn's colitis often results in 'rectal sparing'. In the foreground, the rectal mucosa looks normal, but a distant area of sigmoid colon can be seen to be severely inflamed and bleeding. (c) Pseudomembranous colitis. This patient developed bloody diarrhoea after a course of broad-spectrum antibiotics. His stool cultures became positive for Clostridium difficile and this colonoscopic view demonstrates colitis with the typical pseudomembrane formation. (d) The rectum is usually also spared in ischaemic colitis, owing to its ample collateral blood supply. This view of the descending colon, however, shows severe inflammation, blue-purple discolouration and mucosal sloughing in a patient with significant mesenteric atheromatous disease.*

The causes of infective colitis are:

Bacterial
- *Campylobacter jejuni**
- *Salmonella**
- *Shigella**
- *Clostridium difficile**
- Enterohaemorrhagic *Escherichia coli*
- Entero-invasive *E. coli*
- Entero-aggregative *E. coli*
- *Aeromonas*
- *Staphylococcus aureus*
- *Yersinia*
- *Mycobacterium avium* complex
- *Neisseria gonorrhoea*
- *Treponema pallidum*
- *Chlamydia*

Protozoal
- *Entamoeba histolytica*
- *Balantidium coli*

Helminthic
- *Trichuris trichiura*
- *Strongyloides stercoralis*

Viral
- *Cytomegalovirus*
- *Adenovirus*
- *Herpes simplex*
- *Papillomavirus*

*Most common causes in immunocompetent individuals in temperate countries.

Patients with immunodeficiency states have a wider differential diagnosis, including some unusual protozoal and viral agents.

Fulminant colitis used to carry a mortality of 30–40% before the introduction of corticosteroid therapy in the 1950s. Progression to toxic dilatation, colonic dilatation and faecal perforation may occur whatever the aetiology.

Specific management aspects of the different types of acute colitis are detailed below.

ACUTE INFLAMMATORY BOWEL DISEASE

The important aspects of chronic ulcerative colitis and Crohn's disease, and their respective differences, are discussed elsewhere in this chapter. When severe colitis occurs as a result of either of these conditions, initial management is very similar.

Initial management and supportive treatment

In order to guide the treatment of this potentially life-threatening condition, various activity assessment indices have been developed, usually involving a combination of clinical and laboratory features. Perhaps the best known is the Truelove–Witts score.

All patients with severe disease should be admitted to hospital. Many gastroenterologists agree that it is safest to admit patients having their first acute presentation of UC, even if they do not meet the Truelove–Witts criteria of severe disease (more than six loose stools per day, macroscopic blood in stool, temperature over 37.5°C, tachycardia of more than 90 beats per minute, anaemia with a haemoglobin level below 9 g/dl, and an ESR above 30 mm/hour). This should at least allow monitoring of stool frequency and stabilisation of symptoms.

Patients require close monitoring, with regular assessment of temperature, pulse, blood pressure, stool output and meticulous attention to fluid balance. Daily plain abdominal X-rays should be performed during a severe attack to identify toxic dilatation of the colon. Phlebotomy with measurement of the full blood count, inflammatory markers (ESR, CRP), urea and electrolytes is essential, usually at daily intervals. Stool and blood specimens should be sent for culture.

Intravenous fluid resuscitation is usually necessary with crystalloids (supplemented with potassium to correct hypokalaemia), blood transfusion for anaemia and albumin infusion to correct hypoalbuminaemia.

Colitic patients are best managed as part of a multidisciplinary colitis team. Surgeons should be aware of the progress of patients who may be heading for colectomy and able to see the natural history of those who get better with medical treatment.

Some authorities have suggested a role for fasting to allow 'bowel rest' and feeding with parenteral nutrition. Recent trials appear to show this is unnecessary and patients who are capable of eating should be allowed to do so. Approximately 20% of individuals with severe colitis, however, will benefit from the withdrawal of dairy products as a result of the hypolactasia that may occur.

Severe inflammatory bowel disease is a prothrombotic state and most patients are potentially at risk from venous thromboembolic disease. Although the link is unproven, it is the authors' practice to give hospitalised colitic patients a regular prophylactic dosage of subcutaneous heparin.

Specific therapies

Many patients with acute colitis will receive antibiotic treatment. In the initial presentation of a febrile colitic illness, the differential diagnosis includes bacterial infection and so it is commonplace to give antibiotics along with steroids until the histological and bacteriological data are available to make a firm diagnosis. Ciprofloxacin and/or metronidazole are the usual blind treatments. The role of specific antibiotic treatment in UC is disputed, although it should be given to those who are bacteraemic. Controlled trials, however, have demonstrated a proven benefit for giving metronidazole in cases of Crohn's colitis.

Steroids are essential for the effective treatment of acute colitis. There is still some debate about the best route of administration, but evidence suggests that oral prednisolone's bioavailability is unpredictable in acute severe disease and so intravenous hydrocortisone is usually given (100 mg four times a day). If there is an adequate clinical response to this dose (as occurs in about 75% of cases), then after 7–10 days the patient can be weaned on to oral prednisolone at a dose of 40–60 mg a day, before starting a gradual reduction in dosage over subsequent weeks.

The 5-aminosalicylate (5-ASA) preparations are of more use in maintaining remission in chronic disease (see below) than in treating severe colitis, particularly when patients are already receiving an adequate dosage of corticosteroid. In those presenting for the first time, it is the authors' practice not to start a 5-ASA during an acute attack as some patients are hypersensitive to it and the resulting diarrhoea may cause diagnostic confusion. Once the acute episode is resolving, patients should be given a 5-ASA as maintenance treatment. There is no place for routine systemic corticosteroids in keeping patients in remission.

Importantly, patients should also avoid anti-diarrhoeal drugs during an acute attack, including anticholinergics and opioids. These drugs will slow colonic transit time leading to proximal constipation, may possibly increase the risk of toxic dilatation and, in any case, do not relieve the severe tenesmus that leads to stool frequency in patients with proctitis.

Failure to respond to intravenous hydrocortisone and/or the development of toxic dilatation of the colon are indications for more intensive immunosuppression or prompt surgical intervention.

A number of trials have now supported the use of intravenous cyclosporin in patients who have not responded to 7 days of steroid treatment. Although the majority (approximately 70%) of such patients did improve, there have been problems with relapse of colitis on cyclosporin withdrawal and the development of opportunistic infections or neurotoxicity. Those who fail to respond to a further 5–7 days of combined immunosuppression should be referred for surgery, although it is vital that potentially life-saving surgical intervention is not delayed to give failing medical treatment 'one more chance'.

The development of toxic dilatation of the colon (**Fig. 3.21(a)**), at any stage, used to be considered an absolute indication for surgery. Most gastroenterologists would advocate treatment with fluid resuscitation, antibiotics and continued steroids for a further 24 hours before surgical intervention, but this is obviously a hazardous process. Even with laparotomy, the mortality rate from a toxic colonic perforation can be as high as 40–50%. The physician should always be alert to the possibility, however, that perforation may occur without the development of a megacolon and any symptoms or signs of peritonism should be actively sought in all patients. The use of high-dose steroids may mask some of these findings and so regular abdominal films should be closely inspected.

Severe rectal haemorrhage may occur in acute colitis (**Fig. 3.21(b)**) but is relatively uncommon.

Some key differences between acute colonic Crohn's disease and UC are:
- Approximately 20–30% of patients presenting with acute severe colitis will eventually be diagnosed as having Crohn's rather than UC.
- Around 40–50% of those presenting with acute Crohn's will have some evidence of perianal disease.

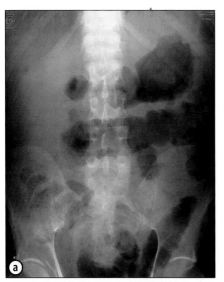 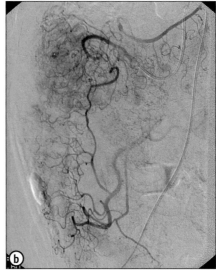

Fig. 3.21 *Complications of acute severe ulcerative colitis. (a) Toxic dilatation. Plain abdominal film of a patient with a pancolitis due to UC. There is dilatation of both the rectosigmoid and transverse colon, the diameter of the latter being just over 5.5 cm. The patient was febrile and tachycardic, features in keeping with the diagnosis of toxic megacolon, but improved over the subsequent 24 hours with steroid treatment and avoided a colectomy. Toxic dilatation is believed to be due to a combination of colonic bacterial fermentation and a degree of mucosal ischaemia, and may be further exacerbated by hypokalaemia, antidiarrhoeal drugs, barium enema or colonoscopy. (b) Severe colonic haemorrhage. Selective superior mesenteric arteriogram of a patient who had a severe right-sided colitis. There are widespread inflammatory changes, together with extravasation of contrast around the hepatic flexure, indicative of active bleeding into the colon. The patient required a colectomy in order to stop the bleeding.*

117

- Metronidazole is an effective adjunct to steroids for the treatment of colonic Crohn's disease.
- Toxic dilatation is more likely to occur in UC (10%) than in Crohn's colitis (2%)
- Colectomy is a 'curative' procedure for UC but not for Crohn's disease

Outcome of acute colitis

We have already stated that supportive treatment and steroid therapy are successful in about 75% of cases. Adding cyclosporin may help control resistant disease while a

Common causes of bacterial colitis			
	Source	**Natural history**	**Antibiotics**
Campylobacter jejuni	Poultry	Usually self-limiting Recovery in 7–10 days	Only if severe Ciprofloxacin
Shigella (spp).	Humans only Faeco-oral spread	Invasive and toxic Broad spectrum of severity May cause severe colitis, megacolon, perforation, haemolytic-uraemic syndrome	If systemic symptoms (or any *S. dysenteriae*) Ciprofloxacin Nalidixic acid
Salmonella spp.	Fresh and sea water Poultry, eggs Many animals	Variable (depending on type) May disseminate to blood, joints, heart, bones	Always treat if patient immunocompromised or there is chronic haemolysis Ciprofloxacin Cotrimoxazole Chloramphenicol All may prolong carrier state (1%)
Clostridium difficile	3% carriage rate rises to 20% after antibiotic course Widely distributed in hospitals	May occur after any antibiotic Pseudomembranous colitis If severe, toxic dilatation	Withdraw precipitant Supportive treatment Metronidazole Vancomycin Brewer's yeast Relapse common
Enterohaemorrhagic *E. coli* (EHEC)	Cattle gastrointestinal tract Beef, pork, lamb, poultry	Bloody diarrhoea in 30–95% Toxins damage endothelium 2–7% develop haemolytic-uraemic syndrome May be fatal, especially in children and the elderly	Supportive treatment Antibiotic therapy controversial

Fig. 3.22 *Common causes of bacterial colitis.*

patient's nutrition and fitness for surgery are optimised, or may enable the patient to avoid surgery altogether. However, those patients who have improved on medical treatment remain at risk of relapse and subsequent requirement for colonic resection – up to 47% in one follow-up study.

Surgery for inflammatory bowel disease is dealt with in more detail on page 128, but complicated reconstructive work is generally avoided in acute severe colitis. This is largely due to the risks of infection, comorbidity and the effects of imunosuppression on anastomoses and wound healing.

Most commonly, patients with fulminant colitis requiring surgery would have a colectomy performed, with formation of a Brooke ileostomy. The intention would be to perform an ileal pouch-anal anastomosis at a later stage once Crohn's disease has been excluded and the patient is in a healthier condition.

INFECTIVE (BACTERIAL) COLITIS

As detailed above, the mainstay of treatment of colitis of any aetiology is to resuscitate the patient adequately and restore salt and water homeostasis. Bloody diarrhoea may be sufficiently severe to require transfusion and correction of hypovolaemia.

Important aspects of the most common pathogens causing bacterial colitis are summarised in **Fig. 3.22**.

Pseudomembranous colitis due to *Clostridium difficile* is a not uncommon complication of antibiotic treatment, particularly amongst hospital inpatients, with significant morbidity and mortality in the elderly. Most patients will respond to a course of oral metronidazole or vancomycin, although relapse is common (about 20% of cases). Recent reports have described successful treatment with brewer's yeast, the active ingredient of which is *Saccharomyces cerevisiae*. The yeast is thought to act by altering the bowel flora, binding *C. difficile* toxin and increasing mucosal IgA production.

Chronic inflammatory changes in the colon may also occasionally be a feature of abdominal tuberculosis (**Fig. 3.23**).

ISCHAEMIC COLITIS

Pathogenesis

Some areas of the gut (such as the duodenum or the rectum) receive a rich blood supply from more than one source, whereas others (such as the distal small bowel and proximal colon) depend on the integrity of a single vessel, the superior mesenteric artery (SMA).

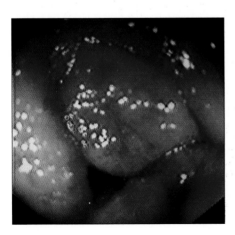

Fig. 3.23 *Chronic colitis due to Mycobacterium tuberculosis. Colonoscopic photograph of the ascending colon in a patient with abdominal tuberculosis. The mucosa appears inflamed, scarred and hypertrophic. The differential diagnosis of this focal appearance includes Crohn's disease and carcinoma.*

Hence, while occlusive disease of the SMA may lead to infarction of the ascending and transverse colon, the distal bowel, supplied by the inferior mesenteric artery (IMA), is better protected from infarction by its collateral supplies from the SMA and the haemorrhoidal arteries. The different patterns of colonic ischaemia are summarised in Fig. 3.24.

Colonic ischaemia		
	Aetiology	Natural history
Superior mesenteric artery Occlusive	1. Embolism – cardiac, aortic, mycotic sources	Overall 30–50% of mesenteric infarcts Severe abdominal pain Ischaemia followed by infarction
	2. Thrombosis of SMA	Potentially life-threatening
	3. Aortic dissection	
Non-occlusive	Diminished cardiac output Hypovolaemia Septic shock Stenotic atheromatous plaques Splanchnic arterial spasm	Causes up to half of all bowel infarcts Other viscera also ischaemic May be missed in acutely ill patient High mortality
Inferior mesenteric artery	May be occlusive or non-occlusive Splenic flexure and descending colon usual site	Tends to be limited in extent Usually single segment Bloody diarrhoea Some peritonism Bacterial invasion common Perforation relatively uncommon Most patients spontaneously recover Subsequent strictures may occur
Mesenteric vein thrombosis	Usually with co-existent portal or splenic venous thrombosis No underlying cause in 50% Others – cirrhosis, hepatoma, portal sepsis, trauma, prothrombotic states	Causes 5% of bowel 'infarcts' Similar presentation to arterial disease Difficult to diagnose preoperatively Thrombectomy usually unhelpful Resection of affected bowel Subsequent anticoagulation

Fig. 3.24 *Colonic ischaemia.*

Clinical features

Patients presenting with an acutely ischaemic bowel may present as an 'acute abdomen', particularly if the affected intestine has become gangrenous or has perforated due to full-thickness infarction (**Fig. 3.25**). The assessment of such patients should obviously include a search for evidence of vascular disease elsewhere or precipitants of hypotension and hypoperfusion. In the case of 'non-occlusive' ischaemia, a combination of chronically poor atheromatous circulation with an acute lowering of systemic blood pressure, such as an episode of cardiac failure, is often sufficient to precipitate infarction.

Patients may complain of acute severe abdominal pain or give a history of previous episodes of postprandial pain suggestive of intestinal 'angina'. Ischaemic colitis often results in bloody diarrhoea or, if necrosis is severe (in SMA occlusion, for example), frank rectal bleeding.

Investigation and treatment

Plain radiography may give some clues (**Fig. 3.26**), such as dilated loops of bowel, submucosal oedema and 'thumbprinting' of the mucosa. If an IMA lesion has caused distal colonic infarction, then this may be visible with a sigmoidoscope (see **Fig. 3.20**), but it is rare for significant rectal involvement to occur in view of the factors mentioned earlier.

Visceral angiography is extremely useful in identifying the precise location of an occluded vessel and can help the surgeon plan resection. In more chronic cases, it is possible to perform mesenteric angioplasty or stent insertion to relieve narrowed vessels.

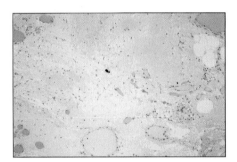

Fig. 3.25 *Colonic necrosis due to mesenteric infarction. Haematoxylin and eosin-stained view showing extensive necrosis of the ascending colon, resected from a patient with a superior mesenteric artery thrombosis.*

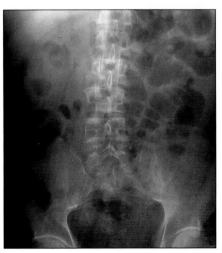

Fig. 3.26 *Acute superior mesenteric artery occlusion. This 35-year-old man presented with acute severe abdominal pain, and had a history of previous hyperlipidaemia and coronary artery disease. His plain abdominal film shows numerous loops of non-specifically dilated small bowel in the left side of the abdomen. At laparotomy, he had a complete occlusion of the SMA and required jejunal, ileal and ascending colonic resections. He was subsequently dependent on parenteral nutrition.*

On the other hand, where the clinical diagnosis of SMA occlusion is already made and the patient is dangerously ill, then laparotomy should not be delayed. The type of surgery will obviously depend on the site and extent of the infarction, but the surgeon will need to be prepared not only to resect non-viable bowel, but also to reconstitute the SMA circulation. This may require embolectomy or a bypass procedure for more proximal occlusions. Almost inevitably, extensive small bowel resections are required and patients may be left with the 'short gut syndrome' or chronic intestinal failure.

Ischaemic colitis due to an IMA lesion runs a less florid course. Arterial reconstruction and bowel resections are usually not necessary, although late stricturing may occur and subsequently require surgical intervention. Perforation of the ischaemic left colon is fortunately uncommon, but can occur and should obviously prompt a laparotomy. Otherwise, treatment is mainly supportive with intravenous fluids, antibiotics, restriction of oral intake and continued observation.

CHRONIC INFLAMMATORY BOWEL DISEASE

UC and Crohn's disease have much in common – both are chronic, relapsing inflammatory disorders of unknown aetiology – but there are important differences, such that inflammatory bowel disease (IBD) can be assigned to either aetiology in about 90% of cases. The remainder are termed 'indeterminate' colitis, although a definitive diagnosis may become apparent later.

The aetiology and pathogenesis of IBD are complex and continue to be intensively investigated. What seems apparent is that both Crohn's and UC may be the result of an environmental trigger affecting a genetically predisposed individual (**Figs 3.24** and **3.25**). The genetic component has been suggested by the increased incidence of IBD in first-degree relatives of affected individuals and the greater concordance rates among monozygotic than dizygotic twins, although this seems stronger for Crohn's than UC. Having an affected relative with UC or Crohn's will also put the individual at a higher risk of developing *either* disease.

The genetics of IBD are too complicated to be explained by simple Mendelian inheritance of a single gene. In about 10% of affected families with UC an autosomal dominant transmission has been described, but for the majority of individuals it seems that there are numerous interactions between different genes, with multiple loci acting independently, together with an undoubted environmental contribution. Possible mechanisms in the pathogenesis of IBD are listed in **Fig. 3.27**. Genetic influences may be summarised as follows:

- Genetic factors are more influential in Crohn's disease than UC
- Overall risk of IBD in first-degree relatives is 5–15%
- Within families, greater concordance in disease phenotype (e.g. fistulating versus non-fistulating Crohn's)
- Risk greater in relatives of patients affected at young ages
- Anticipation of Crohn's disease (occurring earlier in each generation)
- Candidate genes may lie on chromosomes 3, 7, 12 and 16

Epidemiological studies have identified cigarette smoking as a possible influence on the development of IBD. While smoking is a risk factor for developing Crohn's disease, it seems that non-smokers and ex-smokers are at greatest risk of developing ulcerative colitis. Some trials have even shown some clinical benefit from transdermal nicotine patches, but the basis of this epidemiological association still remains to be explained.

Possible mechanisms in the pathogenesis of inflammatory bowel disease

Factor	Evidence
Genetic component	Epidemiology; twin studies; IBD families Linkage to chromosomes by microsatellite screening Rare associations with other genetic disorders (such as Turner's syndrome and glycogen storage disease)
Inflammatory response	Various human and animal studies (including transgenic 'knockout' models) suggest roles for cytokines, neuropeptides, free radical injury, prostaglandins, leukotrienes and cell-adhesion molecules
Abnormal colonic mucus	Seems more relevant to UC than Crohn's Mucin chains show reduced sulphation, increased sialylation and shorter oligosaccharide components May affect mucosal 'barrier' function of mucins Mucus production influenced by cigarette smoking
Intraluminal microflora	Various bacteria implicated at one time or other (e.g. *Bacteroides, Listeria, Mycobacteria, E. coli*) Luminal antigens may act as 'trigger' Trials of antituberculous drugs have shown no effect Recent suggested role for *Mycobacterium paratuberculosis* in Crohn's (small studies showing good response to courses of clarithromycin)
Dietary factors	More evidence for a role in Crohn's than UC Crohn's can improve with 'bowel rest' or elemental diet (but no evidence that this alters luminal microflora)

Fig. 3.27 *Possible mechanisms in the pathogenesis of inflammatory bowel disease.*

ULCERATIVE COLITIS

Natural history

UC has a peak age of onset between the years of 15 and 30 but can occur at any stage in life. In Europe and the USA, prevalence is about 150 per 100 000. The incidence is approximately the same in both sexes.

The hallmark of UC is an inflammation of the large intestine extending proximally and contiguously from the rectum. The clinical manifestations depend largely on the severity (or depth) of the inflammation, its extent (whether a pancolitis or local proctitis) and the development of subsequent complications.

The disease tends to follow one of four patterns. Most individuals (about 70%) will have a chronic relapsing/remitting illness with intervening periods of good health. A second group will have progressive chronic disease without remission (10%), although their symptoms may vary with time. Thirdly, around 10% of patients will present with an acute fulminant colitis that requires colectomy. Finally, a few patients will suffer a single self-limiting attack of colitis and have no progression to chronicity.

Clinical features

Acute 'fulminant' colitis has already been discussed. Less severe flare-ups of chronic UC tend to cause similar symptoms, albeit less florid.

123

Proctitis leads to tenesmus, faecal urgency and the passage of bowel motions accompanied by pus, blood or mucus. Rectal bleeding or abdominal pain may also occur and episodes of left-sided colitis are often followed by right-sided 'proximal constipation' that may be visible on a plain abdominal film.

On examination, the features of acute colitis should be sought (see pp. 113–114) along with the presence of extra-intestinal manifestations (see chapter 6). The diagnosis of UC, however, rests mainly on the sigmoidoscopic appearances together with rectal histology and radiological imaging.

Investigations

At sigmoidoscopy, the colorectal mucosa in UC can adopt a spectrum of changes, ranging from non-specific increases in vascularity, through oedema and inflammation, to severe ulceration and a haemorrhagic, friable mucosa. In acute disease, a combination of inflammation and oedema can cause a pseudopolypoid appearance (**Fig. 3.28**).

Histological biopsy specimens (**Fig. 3.29**) should always be taken and stool sent for culture to exclude the other causes of colitis mentioned earlier.

The pathological features of UC are compared with those of Crohn's disease in **Fig. 3.30**.

Routine laboratory tests may give some support to a diagnosis of inflammatory bowel disease but are seldom diagnostic. Haematological indices may show leucocytosis, thrombocytosis, anaemia (iron deficiency or the anaemia of chronic disease) and raised ESR. The levels of acute-phase proteins such as CRP and ferritin may be elevated and the albumin level correspondingly decreased. With UC in remission, all of the indices may be normal.

A barium enema may reveal many of the sequelae of chronic UC, such as loss of haustral patterns, shortening of the colon and an increased sacrorectal space on lateral views should be avoided in acute colitis for the reasons mentioned earlier, but if acute changes are present, ulceration and pseudopolyps may be seen. In the longer term, a raised mucosal lesion may suggest a carcinoma.

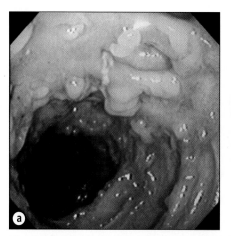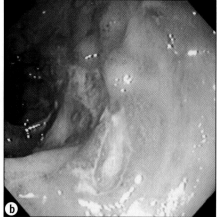

Fig. 3.28 *Colonic 'pseudopolyps' in active inflammatory bowel disease. In acute colitis the inflamed mucosa may develop a polypoid appearance, as (a) in this patient with a pancolitis due to UC. (b) Pseudopolyps may also occur in Crohn's disease, accompanied in this case by deep and superficial ulceration of the sigmoid colon.*

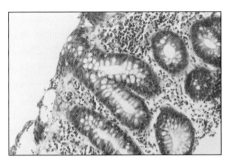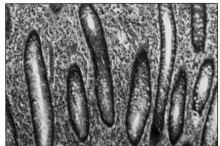

Fig. 3.29 *Histopathology of ulcerative colitis and Crohn's colitis. (a) Colonic biopsy specimen from a patient with UC, demonstrating a marked inflammatory cell infiltrate, with surface ulceration and crypt abscesses. (b) Histological specimen from a patient with severe Crohn's colitis, illustrating granuloma formation and chronic inflammatory changes.*

The pathology of inflammatory bowel disease: ulcerative colitis versus Crohn's colitis

Ulcerative colitis	Crohn's colitis
Rectum always involved	Rectum involved in only about 50% of cases
Anal lesions uncommon	Anal lesions in 75%
Terminal ileitis only if pancolitis (10%)	Terminal ileitis in at least 30% of colitics
Continuous proximal extension	Skip lesions
Deep fissuring uncommon	Frequent fissures, 'cobblestone' appearance
Colon shortened by muscle changes	Colon distorted by fibrous stricturing
Fistulation rare	Fistulae in 10% of cases
Inflammation limited to mucosa and submucosa	Transmural inflammation
Crypt abscesses common	Crypt abscesses rare
Mucosal goblet cell depletion	Normal goblet cell numbers
Granulomas absent	Granulomas in 75%

Fig. 3.30 *The pathology of inflammatory bowel disease: ulcerative colitis versus Crohn's colitis.*

Labelled white cell scanning can give a useful assessment of disease severity and extent during acute flare-ups (**Fig. 3.31**), but is of limited use once disease activity has settled.

A sigmoidoscopy with biopsy is usually sufficient to diagnose UC. However, much valuable information may be gained by a subsequent elective colonoscopy. In particular, this allows the opportunity to take biopsies from around the whole colon, in an effort to detect microscopic evidence of colitis. The true extent of disease has a bearing on the subsequent development of dysplasia and the need for regular surveillance. For patients with a diagnosis of uncomplicated proctosigmoiditis due to UC, assuming that a sigmoidoscopic and histological diagnosis has been made, the factors listed below should prompt a full colonoscopy, particularly if there is doubt cast on the diagnosis. Patients with the usual indications for a colonoscopy, listed on page 105, should obviously be investigated in any case:

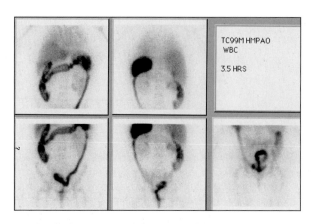

TC99M HMPAO
WBC

3.5 HRS

Fig. 3.31 *Labelled white blood cell scintigraphy in pancolitis. This patient with known UC was admitted to hospital with increasing bloody diarrhoea and tenesmus. These gamma camera images, taken 3.5 hours after an intravenous injection of labelled white blood cells, show significant accumulation of leucocytes along the entire colon.*

- If clinical features suggest ileal disease
  Steatorrhoea
  Nutritional deficiencies
  Low vitamin B_{12} level
  Chronic right iliac fossa pain
  Abdominal mass suggestive of terminal ileal origin
- Prior to elective surgery, especially if an ileoanal pouch is to be constructed
- At 8–10 years after onset of UC, in order to plan surveillance requirements

Medical treatment

Unlike those with severe acute colitis, the vast majority of patients with chronic UC can be managed on an outpatient basis. Careful explanation of the natural history of UC is essential. Patients need to be aware that most interventions (bar surgery) are not curative and some degree of maintenance treatment is usually necessary. Patient support groups are established in most countries, such as the National Association for Crohn's and Colitis in the UK. These organisations can be particularly helpful for patients with complicated disease or those faced with surgical stomas.

In general, the drug treatment of UC comprises steroids (local or systemic), 5-ASAs (again, locally or systemically) and in some cases the use of 'steroid-sparing' agents such as azathioprine on its metabolite 6-mercaptopurine. Disease activity and extent can be assessed by the methods mentioned earlier.

Patients with proctitis can be treated with a twice-daily rectal steroid, either prednisolone or hydrocortisone in the form of a foam enema or suppository. Many different proprietary formulations are available and patients will often have their own preference. The corticosteroid should be continued for 2 weeks after bleeding has stopped. Patients are usually started off on a 5-ASA preparation orally to maintain remission (see below). Rectal 5-ASA preparations can be helpful in some refractory cases but are relatively more expensive than their steroid counterparts.

Mild to moderate left-sided colitis can frequently be managed in a similar way to proctitis if not severe. Rectal steroids and an oral 5-ASA may be sufficient, but patients often require a course of oral prednisolone at a dose of 20–40 mg a day for 2 or 3 weeks before tapering the dose by about 5 mg every week.

The 5-ASA preparations are the cornerstone of maintenance treatment for UC, systemic steroids having no place in view of their well-known side-effects. Their precise mode of

Different types of 5-ASA preparation used in inflammatory bowel disease

Drug	Presentation	Site of activity
Sulphasalazine	5-ASA-sulphapyridine	Colon
Mesalazine	5-ASA alone	
a. Delayed release*	Resin-coated to release at pH > 6 or 7	Ileum and colon
b. Slow release**	Cellulose-coated microspheres	Ileum and colon
Olsalazine	5-ASA-5-ASA	Colon
Balsalazide	5-ASA-aminobenzoylalanine	Colon

*Proprietary examples include 'Salofalk', released at a luminal pH above 6, and 'Asacol', released at a pH above 7.
**An example is 'Pentasa', with cellulose-coated microgranules dispersed in the stomach and 5-ASA released throughout the small bowel.

Fig. 3.32 *Different types of 5-ASA preparation used in inflammatory bowel disease.*

action is still disputed, but *in vitro* studies have shown that they lead to inhibition of neutrophil chemotaxis, diminished platelet-activating factor release and some restraint of lymphocyte function.

Sulphasalazine, the longest-used of the drugs, consists of a 5-aminosalicylic acid molecule bound to sulphapyridine by a diazo bond. The drug is very poorly absorbed by the small intestine and so almost all of an oral dose reaches the colon, where the bond is lysed by bacteria and the 5-ASA is released. Unfortunately, the sulphonamide component can lead to a number of side-effects, including oligospermia, urinary discolouration, haemolysis, folate deficiency, methaemoglobinaemia and toxic dermal necrolysis. Sulphasalazine is well tolerated, however, in over 80% of patients and costs around a third of the price of newer 5-ASA preparations. None the less, its effects on fertility mean it should be avoided in young men.

A number of pharmacokinetic strategies have been devised to deliver oral 5-ASAs to the colon (**Fig. 3.32**). These agents are generally better tolerated than sulphasalazine, although adverse effects occur in about 10% of patients. Examples include blood dyscrasias, diarrhoea, nausea, pancreatitis and interstitial nephritis.

Overall, the 5-ASA drugs reduce the annual relapse rate in UC from about 70% to 30% of patients. Some, however, are unable to tolerate 5-ASAs or may suffer repeated relapses despite maintenance treatment and can require frequent courses of steroids. In these circumstances, consideration should be given to a 'steroid-sparing' maintenance drug such as azathioprine (at a dose of 2 mg/kg/day orally) or 6-mercaptopurine (1.5 mg/kg/day). These drugs can be very beneficial, although it may be 3 or 4 months before they exert an effect and they need to be continued for at least 2 years. Adverse reactions occur in some 10% of patients and include pancreatitis, myelosuppression and hepatitis. Close supervision is therefore required; patients will need a full blood count and liver function tests before starting treatment and then repeat measurements every couple of weeks in the first 3 months of therapy.

In the future, increases in our knowledge of the pathogenesis of inflammatory bowel disease may lead to better targeting of anti-inflammatory and immunosuppressive drugs. Current research is looking at ways of exploiting the cytokine network, including the use of cytokines such as interleukin-10 that have their own activity in down-regulating the inflammatory response. Other techniques may include the use of receptor antagonists to proinflammatory cytokines, such as tumour necrosis factor, or directing monoclonal antibodies against these agents and other targets, including cell adhesion molecules.

Surgical management

Emergency surgery, in the form of colectomy for fulminant colitis, has already been discussed, but patients with UC may benefit from surgical intervention in a number of other circumstances.

Colectomy offers the possibility of a cure for UC (although not for the extra-intestinal manifestations mentioned below, that are not related to colitic activity) and should be actively considered for those patients with chronic UC who are failing to improve with medical therapy. Other indications include the development of a carcinoma or persistent dysplasia on colonic biopsies, stricture formation or the rescue of patients who are intolerant of steroids or maintenance drugs.

As well as the introduction of steroid therapy, the other main factor in reducing UC mortality has been the improvement in surgical care. In particular, elective operations, carried out on patients who are generally in relatively good health, have altered management from simply being one of colectomy with ileostomy to that of reconstructive operations designed to maintain continence without stoma formation.

The 'classical' UC operation is that of proctocolectomy (designed to remove all the diseased bowel) with Brooke ileostomy formation. This operation has relatively low complication rates and the stoma is relatively easy to manage. Its simplicity means that it remains the operation of choice in acute severe colitis. Unfortunately there are significant adverse effects on the patient's quality of life as a result of the stoma. In one large follow-up study, over 30% of patients had restricted sexual activity, along with limitations on sporting, occupational and recreational activities.

As a result, surgeons have developed a number of alternatives to stoma formation. One option is that of abdominal colectomy with an ileorectal anastomosis. Whilst this does remove *most* of the colitic bowel, there is still the potential for further proctitis and subsequent complications. Indeed, subsequent proctectomy is necessary in up to 40% of patients and there remains a significant risk of rectal carcinoma.

Much more popular is the option of panproctocolectomy with subsequent formation of an ileal 'pouch'. This operation offers the potential of not only removing all the affected bowel, but also retaining continence without a long-term ileostomy. There are a number of variants on the procedure, but essentially it is a two-stage operation. At the first laparotomy, the colon and rectum are excised and a diverting ileostomy is formed. During this procedure, a reservoir or 'pouch' is constructed by mobilising a loop of distal ileum, doubling it back on itself in a 'J' shape and then using a surgical stapling device to create the pouch. The distal end of the pouch is anastomosed to the anus, with preservation of the sphincter mechanism. Two to three months later, a second operation is performed to close the protecting ileostomy. The end result is a successful restoration of faecal continence in most patients. Complications do occur, however, and include pelvic infection, strictures, fistulae, sexual dysfunction (in about 10%) and the subsequent development of 'pouchitis'. This latter condition occurs in about 20–30% of pouch recipients. Its pathogenesis is the subject of some controversy and there are even disagreements about its definition. There is some deterioration of pouch function with diarrhoea and usually some evidence of inflammation or ulceration.

Pouch dysfunction may be due to:

- The small intestine proximal to the pouch – e.g. excessive motility or bacterial overgrowth causing diarrhoea
- The pouch itself (most commonly) – pouchitis, scarring, infection
- The pouch outlet – anastomotic stenosis, fistulae (< 5%), irritation of perianal skin

Treatments are largely empirical and some cases respond to antibiotics while others are more successfully treated with topical steroids or immunosuppressive agents. The possibility should always be borne in mind that the original underlying disease may have been Crohn's disease after all.

Prognosis and long-term complications

Many of the complications of UC have already been mentioned. There are many extra-intestinal manifestations, particularly affecting the skin, eyes and joints, that are discussed in more detail in chapter 6. Primary sclerosing cholangitis occurs in 2–10% of patients with UC and this condition is outlined in chapter 4.

In patients who have had UC for many years, the colon is often shortened and there is a generalised loss of the normal haustral markings, a change often referred to as 'hosepipe colon' because of its smooth appearance (**Fig. 3.33**).

Moreover, patients with long-standing UC are at risk of developing dysplastic epithelial changes and even colonic adenocarcinoma. The risk is greatest amongst those patients with extensive disease and particularly with pancolitis. Overall, the cumulative risk of developing colon cancer is 3% after 15 years of disease, 5% at 20 years and 9% at 25 years.

As a result, regular colonoscopies in patients who have had UC for many years may detect dysplasia or early, treatable, carcinoma. There are variations amongst centres in terms of when to start surveillance and how long the intervals between screens should be. Data suggest that the initial screening colonoscopy should be at 8 years after the onset of disease in patients with pancolitis and at 12 years in those with UC known to be limited to the left side of the colon.

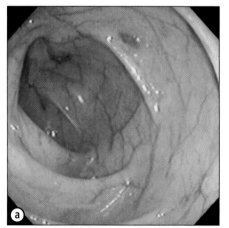 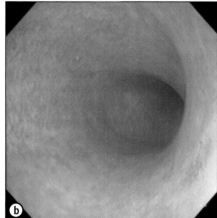

Fig. 3.33 *Normal colon. (a) This colonoscopic image shows the normal haustral markings of the colon. (b) This patient has had UC for many years. The haustral folds have been lost, giving rise to the smooth 'hosepipe' appearance.*

Histological biopsies should be taken from each region of the colon and, obviously, from any visibly abnormal mucosa. Care should be taken, however, to perform surveillance only when the UC is quiescent as inflammatory changes can mimic those of dysplasia on biopsy specimens.

Most centres would suggest screening colonoscopies every 2–3 years, assuming the previous surveillance biopsies showed no dysplasia. As mentioned earlier, colonoscopy itself is not without risk and informed consent is of vital importance.

CROHN'S COLITIS AND PERIANAL LESIONS

Clinical features

Crohn's disease can affect the gastrointestinal tract anywhere from the mouth to the anus. In descending order of frequency, the most commonly affected sites are the ileocaecal region, the colon, ileum alone, small bowel (diffuse), the stomach and the oesophagus. Small intestinal manifestations have been described in chapter 2 and the important pathological features of colonic Crohn's were mentioned earlier in this chapter (**Fig. 3.29(b)** and **Fig. 3.30**). An example of the colonoscopic appearance of acute Crohn's colitis is shown in **Fig. 3.28(b)**.

Treatment

The treatment of colonic Crohn's is similar to that of UC. Topical steroids or 5-ASA preparations are useful in treating anorectal disease and, unlike UC, Crohn's often responds to treatment with the antibiotic metronidazole, although courses should not exceed 3 months in view of the risk of peripheral neuropathy.

As with UC, moderate to severe disease will require systemic steroid therapy and some patients require azathioprine as a longer-term steroid-sparing drug. Oral 5-ASA preparations have been shown to have some effect in maintaining remission, although the benefit is much smaller than that seen in UC. Stopping cigarette smoking has been shown to reduce the relapse rate of Crohn's disease.

Unlike UC, dietary therapy may be beneficial in Crohn's disease, particularly for ileocaecal disease, where an elemental diet has been shown to be as effective as corticosteroid therapy.

Complications

In the long term, Crohn's disease can lead to stricturing of the colon (**Fig. 3.34**) or to fistula formation. The latter phenomenon, defined as an abnormal connection between two epithelial surfaces, may develop between the colon and the small bowel, external skin, vagina or bladder (**Fig. 3.35**). Fistulation can be particularly distressing for the patient. These lesions may discharge pus or faecal material into the urogenital tract or out on to the skin. Entero-enteric fistulae encourage bacterial overgrowth.

Patients with long-standing Crohn's colitis have a higher risk of developing colon cancer than the normal population. The increased risk is not as high as that associated with UC and the risk of cancer development does not seem to be related to the extent of colonic involvement in Crohn's (unlike UC). The role of colonoscopic surveillance in patients with Crohn's disease remains controversial.

Anal and perianal lesions are important elements of Crohn's disease and occur in 30–80% of patients, being more common in those with colonic disease than purely small intestinal involvement. Manifestations include perianal skin tags (which are quite common in the 'normal' population), fistulae, fissures, abscesses and sinuses. As with Crohn's disease elsewhere, the aetiology of perianal Crohn's remains obscure. In some ways, anal fissures and abscesses can be considered to be a local site of primary inflammatory activity

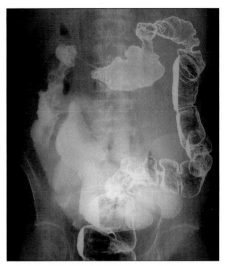

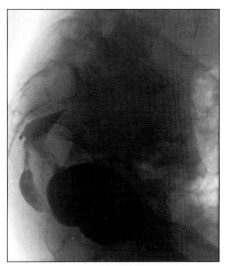

Fig. 3.34 *Stricturing in colonic Crohn's disease. This man with long-standing Crohn's colitis developed chronic colicky abdominal pains. The barium enema demonstrates marked stricturing of the colon. The most severe stricture in the proximal transverse colon (top left), has a shouldered margin and 'apple-core' appearance that is difficult to distinguish from a colonic carcinoma. Fortunately, at laparotomy, the strictures were found to be non-neoplastic.*

Fig. 3.35 *Rectovesical fistula. This woman with a history of severe Crohn's colitis developed recurrent urinary tract infections and complained of pneumaturia. A micturating cystogram was performed which, on this lateral view, shows the bladder anteriorly, with the contrast agent tracking posteriorly through a fistulous track to outline part of the rectum.*

like that seen in other parts of the gastrointestinal tract. Some authors have suggested that these external lesions are related to cutaneous manifestations of Crohn's disease and others have proposed that chronic diarrhoea of more proximal origin induces secondary changes in the anal region.

Some of these lesions may be asymptomatic and do not require intervention. On the other hand, the occurrence of anal pain should prompt careful assessment to exclude an abscess. This may necessitate examination under general anaesthesia, although recent evidence suggests a potentially useful role for endoanal MRI.

Patients with perianal disease are generally managed conservatively, as over-aggressive surgical intervention may lead to an outcome worse than the condition itself. Fluctuant abscesses are usually treated with simple surgical drainage, requiring little or no deroofing. The use of an antibiotic, such as metronidazole or ciprofloxacin, may be an effective treatment for a fistula, although persistent fistulae may be improved by the insertion of a loose 'Seton' suture to allow continued drainage.

Where perianal disease is thought to result from more proximal disease activity with subsequent diarrhoea, a defunctioning stoma is sometimes tried. Opinions on this technique are divided, but it may allow time for improvements in perianal sepsis in some patients.

Overall, some 75–85% of patients with Crohn's disease will require surgery at some stage. The usual indications are strictures with obstructive symptoms, failure of medical therapy to control activity, and local complications such as fistulae. Surgery for Crohn's disease is rarely 'curative' and, after a resection, about 50% of patients will relapse within 10 years, with around half of these requiring further surgery.

To summarise:

- Where possible, resections should be minimised to guard against eventual short-bowel syndrome
- Bypass procedures are generally avoided, as they carry a high risk of subsequent bacterial overgrowth and malabsorption
- Colonic isolation by split ileostomy may be useful in 'defunctioning' severely inflamed colon or resting severe perianal disease, before subsequently restoring continuity
- Surgery is usually performed under corticosteroid cover

COLLAGENOUS COLITIS

The growing use of colonoscopy and biopsies in the investigation of patients with diarrhoea has led to an increased recognition of collagenous colitis as a cause of disease. It is characterised by two elements, one clinical (chronic, watery diarrhoea with or without abdominal pain) and one histopathological (subepithelial deposition of collagen and chronic inflammatory changes on colorectal biopsy). Most patients are women (90%), with the majority presenting in the sixth or seventh decade of life. Collagenous colitis is estimated to account for up to 5% of adult cases of chronic diarrhoea.

Symptomatically, patients usually have watery diarrhoea, occurring 5–10 times a day. Some individuals may have crampy abdominal pains and sufferers are often misdiagnosed as having the irritable bowel syndrome. Usually, there is little to find on clinical examination.

Routine blood tests are usually normal (although the ESR can occasionally be raised). Stool microscopy and cultures are within normal limits and faecal osmolality measurement suggests a secretory-type diarrhoea which is further exacerbated by feeding. Radiological imaging and macroscopic inspection of the bowel at colonoscopy are both normal. The diagnosis relies on taking a histological biopsy specimen and demonstrating the pathognomonic subepithelial collagen deposition with an infiltrate of chronic inflammatory cells.

Treatment of collagenous colitis is difficult, not least because the natural history is variable, with many patients remitting spontaneously and others adopting a more chronic course. General measures are often helpful. Dietary secretagogues such as caffeine should be eliminated and many patients respond to a lactose-free diet. NSAIDs should be avoided as these may exacerbate the condition. Some studies have supported the use of stool bulking agents or antidiarrhoeal drugs including loperamide and codeine phosphate. Successful treatment has also been reported with 5-ASAs corticosteroids and courses of metronidazole.

LYMPHOCYTIC COLITIS

Like collagenous colitis, this is a recently recognised cause of chronic diarrhoea which also results in a watery diarrhoea with occasional abdominal cramping pains. Most patients are middle-aged, with a mean age of 53 years at diagnosis. Lymphocytic colitis is, however, equally common in both men and women.

Blood tests, faecal culture, radiology and colonoscopic inspection are all usually normal and the condition is diagnosed on the histological appearance of colorectal biopsies. The findings are those of an increased number of intraepithelial lymphocytes together with some epithelial surface damage and chronic inflammation in the lamina propria. Subepithelial collagen deposition is not present.

The same treatment methods used in collagenous colitis have been applied, with some success using anti-inflammatory drugs such as sulphasalazine or prednisolone.

COLONIC DIVERTICULOSIS

The term *diverticulosis* refers to the presence of diverticula (defined below), whereas *diverticulitis* is the clinical syndrome of inflamed diverticula which may perforate or lead to a local pericolitis. *Diverticular disease* is a general term encompassing this as well as the other complications of the condition.

Colonic diverticula are called 'pulsion' diverticula, referring to how the bowel mucosa is extruded through gaps in the colonic musculature, usually at vulnerable points where the blood vessels penetrate to the submucosa (**Fig. 3.36**).

Epidemiology

Diverticula are very common, particularly in the elderly. Post-mortem studies have shown a prevalence of about 9% in 50-year-olds, rising to 50% of those aged 70 or over. In most cases, the condition is merely an incidental finding, with only about 10% becoming symptomatic and less than a tenth of these requiring surgery.

Epidemiological studies suggest that diverticulosis is a consequence of the 20th-century westernised diet, with low fibre intake the main factor. It is rare in developing nations, less common amongst vegetarians than omnivores, and more common in women than men.

Aetiology

Pulsion diverticula are thought to arise as a result of chronically high intraluminal pressure exceeding the tensile strength of the bowel wall. Low-volume stools, resulting in a smaller colonic calibre, mean that the colonic musculature has to contract much harder in order to keep the stool moving. Consequently, these local increases in pressure may cause the mucosa to herniate through weak points in the circular muscle.

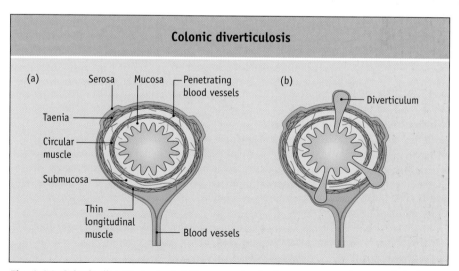

Fig. 3.36 *Colonic diverticulosis. (a) The normal colonic mucosa may be extruded along weak points in the musculature, particularly where the blood vessels pass through. (b) The resulting mucosal pocket is known as a diverticulum.*

133

Colonic diverticulosis: presentations and complications	
Asymptomatic	Most common
Chronic abdominal pain	With or without alteration in bowel habit
Acute diverticulitis	Pericolic inflammation Left iliac fossa pain, pyrexia, tachycardia May have local signs of peritonism
Pericolic abscess	Presentation can often be similar to diverticulitis Persistent pain, tenderness, incomplete obstruction May present as 'pyrexia of unknown origin' Abscess may drain into bowel – purulent diarrhoea
Diverticular perforation	Presentation depends on size of perforation Ranges from local peritonism to severe peritonitis Acute abdomen Subphrenic air on chest X-ray
Fistula formation	May occur into neighbouring viscera Vesico-colic, colo-vaginal, colo-enteric More common cause of fistulae than Crohn's Usually requires surgery
Rectal haemorrhage	Diverticular abscess may erode local artery Amount of blood lost is variable Most bleeds stop spontaneously
Intestinal obstruction	Usually chronic, intermittent May present with acute colonic obstruction Due to spasm, inflammation, stricture, abscess Rarely, adherent small bowel may be obstructed

Fig. 3.37 *Colonic diverticulosis: presentations and complications.*

With age, degeneration of mural collagen layers further reduces tensile strength. These changes are most pronounced in the sigmoid colon, an area which also usually develops the highest intraluminal pressures. Hence, the sigmoid is the most commonly involved site (95% of cases). Occasionally, the entire colon may be affected.

Clinical features and diagnosis

Diverticular disease may present in a number of ways (**Fig. 3.37**), although the most common presentations are related to the functional abnormalities of the colon: in other words, a change in bowel habit or the development of lower abdominal pain, much like that seen in the irritable bowel syndrome. Other cases may present with the complications listed. These vary in severity. Bleeding, for example, may be occasional and intermittent or acute and life-threatening.

Diverticulosis is usually diagnosed by a combination of sigmoidoscopy (**Fig. 3.38**) and barium enema. It is important to remember that diverticula are often an incidental finding and a coexisting colonic carcinoma should always be excluded (**Fig. 3.39**). The presence of severe diverticular disease and the subsequently tortuous sigmoid can make colonoscopy more difficult, with the additional hazard of perforating a diverticulum with the endoscope.

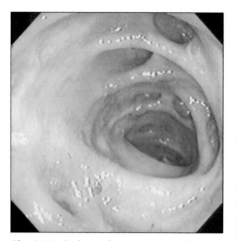

Fig. 3.38 *Endoscopic appearance of colonic diverticulosis. Multiple sigmoid colonic diverticula. The endoscopist needs to be extremely careful, as the inadvertent intubation of a diverticulum may perforate the colon.*

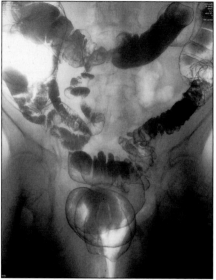

Fig. 3.39 *Colonic diverticula as incidental pathology. This elderly lady had a history of chronic lower abdominal pain, altered bowel habit and anaemia. The barium enema shows extensive sigmoid diverticula, together with a few small left-sided polyps. The mid-transverse colon has an 'apple-core' stricutre, in this case due to an adenocarcinoma.*

Treatment

The management of 'uncomplicated' diverticulosis is largely dietary. Patients should be encouraged to eat a high-fibre diet including wholewheat cereals, wholemeal bread and daily fresh fruit and vegetables. Some patients may require supplementation with bran or ispaghula husk. Other patients may respond to treatment with lactulose, although this is relatively expensive. Abdominal pain may be treated with an antispasmodic agent such as mebeverine.

Patients who present with an acute diverticulitis or an abscess should be treated as inpatients, kept nil-by-mouth in order to rest the bowel and given intravenous fluids. Suitable intravenous antibiotics should be given, after taking blood cultures, such as cefuroxime 750 mg and metronidazole 500 mg at 8-hourly intervals.

Some abscesses may settle on this regimen but some form of intervention is usually required. An abdominal CT scan is useful in demonstrating the abscess cavity and a drain can sometimes be placed. Surgical drainage may be performed by direct incision; a resection of the affected portion of bowel is often required.

Patients may present with an acute abdomen due to perforation, faecal peritonitis and septicaemia. Emergency resuscitation and prompt institution of antibiotic treatment are required preoperatively. The most widely used operation is a Hartmann's procedure, where the diseased colon is removed, the proximal colon brought out as an end colostomy and the distal colon oversewn. Surgery is hazardous in these circumstances, but the mortality of faecal peritonitis is approximately 50%.

Histological classification of colorectal polyps

Neoplastic (adenomatous)*	Non-neoplastic	Submucosal
Benign	Hyperplastic (metaplastic)	Lymphoid
Mild dysplasia	Mucosal (mechanical)	Lipoma
Moderate dysplasia	Hamartomatous	
Severe dysplasia		
Malignant		
Adenocarcinoma		

Adenomatous polyps are commonly described according to their appearance as tubular, tubulovillous or villous adenomas. The tubular, pedunculated type are most common (80%). The more sessile villous adenomas and intermediate tubulovillous variety account for 5–10% and 10–15% respectively.

Fig. 3.40 *Histological classification of colorectal polyps.*

Elective surgery can be planned for those with recurrent diverticulitis, fistula formation or recurrent subacute obstruction, or where endoscopic and radiological findings suggest a colonic carcinoma.

COLORECTAL POLYPS

The term 'polyp', derived from the Latin *polypus* ('many-footed'), is simply a descriptive term for any tissue that protrudes from the mucosal surface of the bowel. Importantly, polyps are not only very common, particularly in older people, but may be benign, premalignant or cancerous depending on their histological appearance. A basic classification is shown in **Fig. 3.40**. The main distinction is between neoplastic (such as benign, but potentially malignant adenomas) and non-neoplastic types (which include hamartomas, metaplastic polyps and inflammatory lesions).

Aetiology

The vast majority of polyps occur sporadically but they may also be part of a polyposis syndrome (**Fig. 3.41**), in which the affected bowel may be carpeted with a multitude of polyps (**Fig. 3.42**). Some of these syndromes have a clear inheritance pattern, such as the autosomal dominant transmission of familial adenomatous polyposis (FAP). Research carried out by the American National Polyp Study has shown that even 'sporadic' polyps may have an inherited component, as individuals who have a first-degree relative with an adenomatous polyp before the age of 60 years are themselves at higher risk of developing a similar lesion.

The architecture of an adenomatous polyp is important. Although most are tubular adenomas, the villous type carries a higher incidence of dysplasia and malignant transformation. Tubular adenomas are found to be malignant in just 5% of cases, compared to 40% of villous polyps.

Size, too, is relevant as the larger the polyp, the more likely it is to be villous and the more likely it is to transform. Studies at St Mark's Hospital (UK) showed that while only 1% of polyps smaller than 1 cm in diameter were found to be malignant, nearly 50% of those larger than 2 cm contained an adenocarcinoma. As a result, the concept of an adenoma-adenocarcinoma (or polyp-cancer) sequence is now widely accepted:

Polyposis syndromes

Familial adenomatous polyposis (FAP)	• Hundreds to thousands of colorectal adenomas
	• Autosomal dominant inheritance usually
	• 25% have no previous family history
	• Germline mutation in APC gene on chromosome 5
	• Adenomas begin to occur in second decade of life
	• Colorectal cancer by third or fourth decade
	• Hyperplastic gastric polyps in 50%
	• Duodenal adenomas in 80% (malignant potential)
	• Annual screening colonoscopy from age of 12 years
	• If multiple adenomas found, refer for colectomy
	• Screening duodenoscopy for other polyps
	• Sulindac (NSAID) may decrease FAP colonic polyps
	• APC mutation analysis allows screening of relatives
	• Variant forms noted:
	    Osteomas, epidermoid cysts (Gardner's syndrome)
	    Desmoid tumours (occur in 10% of FAP)
	    Congenital hypertrophy of retinal pigment epithelium

Turcot's syndrome	• May be a variant of FAP (controversial) • Colorectal adenomas occur in lower numbers than FAP • May be autosomal recessive • Associated astrocytomas, medulloblastomas
Cronkhite–Canada syndrome	• Probably not inherited • Polyps in stomach, colon, duodenum, small bowel • Non-neoplastic, but carcinomatous change described • Protein-losing enteropathy • Mean age of onset is 60 years • Associated alopecia, nail atrophy, hyperpigmentation
Peutz–Jeghers syndrome	• Autosomal dominant, high penetrance • Multiple hamartomatous polyps • Anywhere in gastrointestinal tract, small bowel most common • Total number of polyps usually below 100 • Mucocutaneous pigmentation (mouth, hands) • Usually presents in second or third decade of life • May develop intussusception or anaemia • Increased risk of gastrointestinal malignancies
Juvenile polyposis	• Multiple gastrointestinal polyps • Usually hamartomatous, some adenomas may occur • Familial in 25% of cases • Usually presents in childhood – bleeding, obstruction • Increased risk of cancer, especially if adenomatous

Fig. 3.41 *Polyposis syndromes.*

• Geographical prevalence rates of adenomas correlate with incidence of cancers
• Risk of developing an adenoma and risk of cancer both increase with age
• Both adenomas and cancers are more common on the left side of the colon

- Synchronous adenomatous polyps are commonly found in patients with colon cancer
- Risk of cancer rises with increasing size of adenoma
- Colonoscopic removal of adenomas reduces subsequent cancer incidence
- Follow-up studies of unresected adenomas support an average time of 5–10 years for progression to adenocarcinoma*

*The time for this sequence, however, can be accelerated in the hereditary non-polyposis colorectal cancer syndrome (HNPCC). A study utilising barium enema or colonoscopic screening of individuals with HNPCC noted a surprisingly high incidence of colorectal cancers occurring within 3.5 years of a normal investigation, suggesting that HNPCC patients may have an accelerated adenoma-cancer progression.

Detection, treatment and surveillance

The detection of colonic polyps is often purely coincidental. Owing to their relatively high prevalence, particularly in older age groups, adenomas are frequently found during endoscopic or radiological imaging of the colon in patients with gastrointestinal symptoms.

If a small polyp (< 1 cm diameter) is discovered at sigmoidoscopy, the lesion should be biopsied and the histology reviewed. The need for a full colonoscopy depends on the nature of the polyp. If it is found to be hyperplastic in nature, then further colonoscopy is unnecessary (although it should be noted, particularly with larger polyps, that adenomas and even carcinomas may have a hyperplastic component). If the lesion is adenomatous, then a full colonoscopy will be necessary to detect synchronous polyps more proximally.

If a larger polyp (> 1 cm) is found at sigmoidoscopy, a biopsy is unnecessary, as the patient should be referred for a full colonoscopy with diathermy snare removal of the polyp (see **Figs. 3.18** and **Fig. 3.43**) and retrieval for histological examination (**Fig. 3.44**). Polypectomy is a relatively safe procedure in trained hands, with a perforation rate of around 0.1%.

Approximately a third of individuals with a distal adenoma detected at sigmoidoscopy will have a synchronous polyp more proximally, which may be cancerous in some cases. If the distal adenoma is less than 1 cm in size (and shows nothing worse than mild to moderate dysplasia on histology), then data from the St Mark's Hospital studies suggest that a follow-up colonoscopy may not be necessary, as the risk of carcinoma is no greater than the general population.

After removal of a colonic adenoma, surveillance colonoscopies are recommended to reduce the risk of subsequent neoplasia. The US National Polyp Study found that after

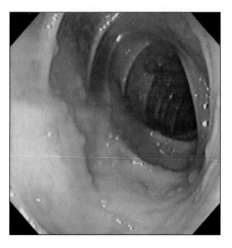

Fig. 3.42 Familial adenomatous polyposis (FAP). Colonoscopic view showing multiple polyps in a patient with FAP. This young woman was one of the 25% of FAP cases without a preceding family history and unfortunately presented with a metastatic adenocarcinoma of the colon.

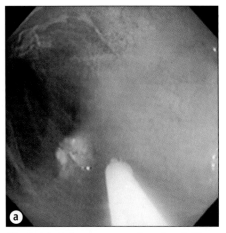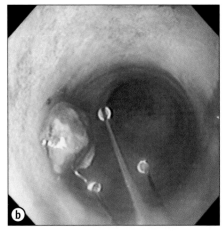

Fig. 3.43 *Polypectomy and retrieval. The endoscopist ensnares the polyp with the diathermy loop, which is placed around the stalk of the polyp. (a) The snare is tightened and heated by an electrical current, simultaneously cutting through the polyp and coagulating the blood vessels to leave a cauterised base. Wisps of smoke can also be seen in the lumen. If the polyp has a long, thick stalk (more than 1 cm in diameter), then the injection of adrenaline and/or a sclerosant into the base will help to minimise any potential bleeding. (b) The polyp itself is retrieved using a tripod device passed through the biopsy channel of the endoscope. Excised polyps should always be sent for histopathological analysis.*

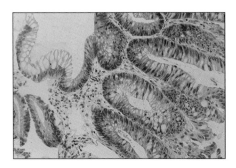

Fig. 3.44 *Colonic polyp histology. This high-power view of a tubular adenoma demonstrates the glandular epithelium with evidence of moderate dysplasia.*

complete removal of all colorectal adenomas it is safe to defer the next colonoscopy for 3 years. This interval should be shorter if there are doubts about the polyps being completely excised (if bowel preparation was poor, for example) or if large sessile polyps were found. The management of polyps found to contain malignant cells is discussed below.

COLORECTAL CANCER

Adenocarcinomas account for almost all colorectal malignancies, with lymphomas and carcinoids being responsible for less than 0.1%. Anal cancers such as squamous cell carcinomas or melanomas may occasionally invade the rectum.

The terms 'colorectal cancer' and 'adenocarcinoma' are used synonymously here.

Epidemiology

Colorectal cancer is the second commonest cause of cancer death, after bronchial carcinoma, in the USA and UK. Each year, over 130 000 new cases are reported in the

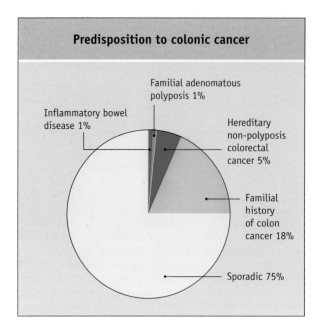

Fig. 3.45 *Predisposition to colonic cancer. Despite the high incidence of colon cancer in certain at-risk groups, it is still the 'sporadic' cases that make up the largest proportion of cancers.*

USA, and some 25 000 in the UK. The lifetime risk of developing colon cancer for an average, asymptomatic individual is about 5%. The incidence rises linearly with age between 30 and 70 years. Colonic cancer is approximately equal in men and women, although rectal lesions are slightly commoner in men.

There are a number of different conditions which may predispose to the development of colonic adenocarcinoma, but it is the sporadic tumours in 'average-risk' individuals that account for the majority of cases (**Fig. 3.45**).

The relative risks in Europe and North America can be ten times as high as those in the developing nations. There are also considerable variations within each population, those living in urban areas having a higher incidence than their rural counterparts. Immigrants adopt the risk of their new country within approximately two to three decades, reflecting an undoubted environmental influence.

Most interest has centred on finding proposed intraluminal carcinogens, including dietary factors. A high intake of dietary fibre was first suggested almost 30 years ago as offering some protection against colonic cancer, reducing the risk by as much as 35%. This was thought to be a result of decreased colonic transit time minimising the period of epithelial exposure to carcinogenic material, although other theories have suggested that bacterial fermentation of fibre may lead to protective substances being formed. Conversely, a diet rich in red meat and animal fats is associated with an increased incidence of cancer development.

Insights into the pathogenesis of colorectal cancer have been offered by studies of 'chemoprevention', the use of specific chemicals that may prevent or reverse carcinogenesis. Suggested examples include the dietary factors mentioned above and, more recently, the surprise finding that certain NSAIDs may reduce the development of colorectal cancer. Evidence has largely been based on some animal models of carcinogen-induced colorectal cancers along with an epidemiological association between NSAID use and a lower incidence of malignancy. More recent clinical trials have shown that patients with FAP who took the NSAID sulindac had a reduction in both the number and size of adenomas.

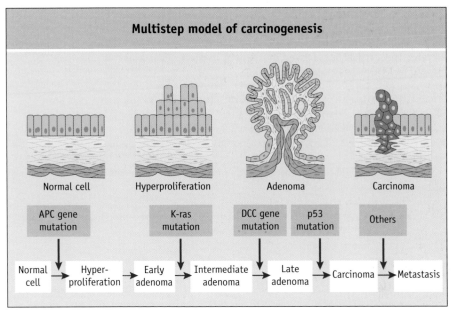

Fig. 3.46 *Multistep model of carcinogenesis. The stepwise genetic alterations that lead to colorectal cancer.*

Genetics and molecular biology

As we have seen, familial genetic factors are responsible for approximately 25% of colonic cancers and environmental influences on individuals with a more subtle genetic predisposition may account for many more cases. Interestingly, the genes involved in the inherited forms of colon cancer are generally the same ones that become abnormal in the sporadic types.

Genetic research into colorectal cancer has been aided by the presence of premalignant lesions that may undergo a stepwise progression into malignancy. Scientific data have supported the adenoma-carcinoma sequence and have led to the theory of multistep carcinogenesis, whereby a sequence of separate genetic alterations leads to an adenocarcinoma (**Fig. 3.46**). The relevant genes are closely involved in the normal control of cell growth and either the loss of tumour-suppressor genes or the promotion of oncogene products may lead to carcinogenesis. Tumour-suppressor genes encode proteins that restrain cell growth, maintain the differentiated phenotype or initiate programmed cell death (apoptosis). An example of this is the familial adenomatous polyposis APC gene, which is defective from the beginning of life in those with FAP and is somatically inactivated in most cases of sporadic colorectal neoplasia.

Oncogenes give rise to proteins involved in signal transduction (usually from the plasma membrane to the nucleus) and the regulation of expression of other genes involved in cellular proliferation. One example of this is the *RAS* oncogene family, which includes genes that encode GTPase enzymes, mutation of which may lead to an uncontrollable mitogenic stimulus. Indeed, *RAS* mutations are frequently found in large adenomas and colorectal cancers.

An alternative to the model of multistep carcinogenesis has been developed from observations of the system of DNA mismatch repair genes. These encode for a complex group of enzymes concerned with the identification and correction of the mispairing of nucleotides during DNA synthesis. If this system is defective then the cell becomes much more sensitive to mutagenic stimuli and neoplastic transformation. Hence, this mechanism of carcinogenesis has been termed the mutator pathway, and seems to be the basis of tumour development in cases of HNPCC.

Hereditary non-polyposis colorectal cancer (HNPCC)

This syndrome is responsible for about 5% of colorectal cancer cases. Despite its name, patients with this condition may develop small numbers of polyps, but more significantly these individuals have a strong predisposition to developing carcinomas, particularly in the proximal colon.

HNPCC usually follows an autosomal dominant pattern, although non-penetrance may be observed in some gene carriers.

The diagnostic criteria for HNPCC families are:

1. Three or more relatives with colorectal carcinoma, one being a first-degree relative of the other two.
2. At least two family generations affected.
3. One or more family members affected below the age of 50 years.

As mentioned earlier, HNPCC tumours are thought to arise from genetic instability, the result of defective DNA mismatch repair systems. Four abnormal human genes have been identified (**Fig. 3.47**) in HNPCC and patients typically have an inactivating mutation in each of the DNA mismatch repair genes. Significantly, the presence of these mutations in colorectal cancer may increase their resistance to chemotherapeutic agents.

Patients with a family history that meets the HNPCC criteria outlined above require colonoscopic screening. Individuals at risk should be offered a screening colonoscopy at 2-year intervals from the age of 20–25 years which should be continued up to the age of 40, when screening should be increased to an annual basis.

Anatomical sites of colorectal cancers

The distribution of carcinomas in the colon is shown in **Fig. 3.48**. Half of all cancers occur in the rectum (**Fig. 3.49**), with a further 25% in the sigmoid colon (**Fig. 3.50**). If we assume that a flexible sigmoidoscope will reach the proximal descending colon, then up to 80% of colonic cancers will be within reach – a fact of some significance with regard to potential screening of the general population (see below).

Patients with HNPCC buck this trend and are more likely to develop tumours in the right side of the colon. Furthermore, recent epidemiological studies have suggested that as the general population increases in age, so are right-sided lesions becoming more common.

Candidate gene mutations described in HNPCC		
Gene	**Location**	**Found in**
hMSH2	Chromosome 2p	Found in 40% of HNPCC families
hMLH1	Chromosome 3p	Found in 30% of HNPCC families
hPMS2	Chromosome 7q	Two families
hPMS1	Chromosome 2q	One family

Fig. 3.47 *Candidate gene mutations described in HNPCC.*

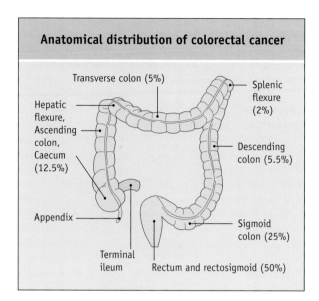

Anatomical distribution of colorectal cancer

Transverse colon (5%)

Splenic flexure (2%)

Hepatic flexure,
Ascending colon,
Caecum (12.5%)

Descending colon (5.5%)

Appendix

Sigmoid colon (25%)

Terminal ileum

Rectum and rectosigmoid (50%)

Fig. 3.48 *Anatomical distribution of colorectal cancer.*

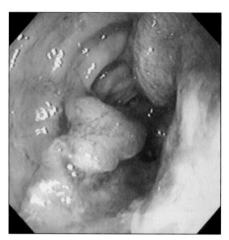

Fig. 3.49 *Adenocarcinoma of the rectum. This patient complained of tenesmus and rectal bleeding. The sigmoidoscopic view shows an exophytic adenocarcinoma in the proximal rectum.*

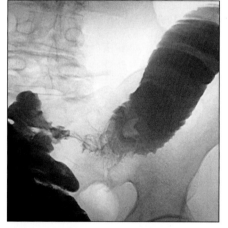

Fig. 3.50 *Sigmoid colonic cancer. This close-up view of a barium enema demonstrates a tight, irregular 7 cm 'apple-core' stricture in the sigmoid colon, with dilatation of the proximal bowel. Sigmoidoscopy and biopsy confirmed the diagnosis of an adenocarcinoma.*

Importantly, colonic cancers may arise at more than one site in the same individual. Approximately 5% of patients with adenocarcinoma will have two or more synchronous tumours and 30% will have an adenomatous polyp elsewhere in the colon. It is vital that patients with large bowel cancer have their entire colon examined by barium enema or, ideally, colonoscopy.

Symptomatology of colorectal cancer.		
Symptom	**Prevalence in right colon lesions**	**Prevalence in rectal or left colon lesions**
Rectal bleeding	5% Usually altered blood May present with anaemia	50% of left colonic tumours 70–90% of rectal carcinomas
Abdominal pain	50–60%	50–60%
Altered bowel habit*	20%	60–70%
Tenesmus	Very rare	50–60% of rectal tumours
Symptomatic bowel obstruction	20%	20% left colon 6% rectal

*May be constipation or diarrhoea, occurring in roughly equal proportions.

Fig. 3.51 *Symptomatology of colorectal cancer.*

Clinical features

The clinical diagnosis of colorectal cancer can be very difficult. Not only are the symptoms (**Fig. 3.51**) and signs frequently vague, but there is also considerable overlap with many other conditions such as diverticulosis, inflammatory bowel disease and functional disorders. Alterations in bowel habit, rectal bleeding, anaemia, abdominal pain and weight loss should always prompt consideration of an underlying neoplasm. Colorectal cancer is by no means a disease confined to the elderly and some 3% of cases arise before the age of 35. Generally, right-sided lesions tend to present more insidiously, often with constitutional symptoms such as malaise, weight loss, anorexia or anaemia.

Complications of colonic cancer may be the presenting feature. About 20% of patients present with an episode of obstruction and some 10–15% with perforation. Intussusception and fistulation are recognised, though rare, presentations. Acute life-threatening rectal bleeding is uncommon and more likely to be the result of coexisting diverticular disease or angiodysplasia.

Clinical examination of the patient is often unremarkable. Attention, however, should be paid to the patient's general appearance, looking for signs of anaemia, cachexia or rare systemic manifestations such as thrombophlebitis, acanthosis nigricans or dermatomyositis. Abdominal palpation may reveal a liver enlarged with secondary deposits, the presence of ascites or a palpable primary tumour. About half of patients with right-sided or transverse colonic tumours will have a palpable mass, but this is felt in only 5–10% of left-sided tumours. Digital rectal examination may reveal a low rectal cancer and should be performed in all patients.

Investigations

General investigations in patients with the above symptoms and signs may detect some evidence of an underlying neoplasm. Blood sent for routine haematology and biochemistry tests may show iron deficiency anaemia or, depending on the relevant metastases, deranged liver function or hypercalcaemia.

Levels of the tumour marker carcinoembryonic antigen (CEA) can be assayed in peripheral blood. Limitations on its sensitivity and specificity mean that CEA has little or no place in the primary diagnosis of colorectal cancer but it can be of great use

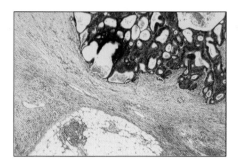

Fig. 3.52 *Histology of colonic adenocarcinoma. Haematoxylin and eosin-stained transverse colonic biopsy from the patient shown in Fig. 3.39. There is an adenocarcinoma invading transmurally through the colonic musculature.*

postoperatively, where serial measurements in the same patient may detect a rising CEA level associated with disease recurrence.

Plain radiography is similarly of limited use in diagnosing colorectal cancer. An abdominal film may show dilated bowel loops in cases presenting with obstruction, but is usually normal in the uncomplicated patient.

Definitive imaging of the carcinoma requires either colonoscopy or contrast radiography. The criteria for selecting patients for these investigations have been discussed earlier in this chapter.

Contrast radiography can be extremely valuable and cancer detection rates have been estimated to be as high as 95–8% in some studies. In cases of suspected obstruction or possible perforation, a water-soluble contrast enema should be used (e.g. 'gastrograffin'), but in other circumstances a double-contrast barium enema with adequate bowel preparation is the procedure of choice. The classical appearance of a colonic cancer is an annular 'apple-core' stricture with shouldered margins (see **Fig. 3.39** or **Fig. 3.50**) but similar appearances may result from IBD (**Fig. 3.32**). The main disadvantages of contrast radiography are the lack of histological confirmation and poor visualisation of certain areas, particularly the rectosigmoid junction, which means it should usually be combined with flexible sigmoidoscopy.

Colonoscopic examination offers the ability to biopsy affected areas, remove polyps and take photographs of lesions, as well as looking for synchronous cancers or adenomas. Some of the pros and cons of colonoscopy are shown in **Fig. 3.8**. At colonoscopy, the adenocarcinoma may be seen as a stricture, an exophytic growth (**Fig. 3.49**) or a polyp. Similar appearances, however, can occur in other conditions – diverticular disease, IBD or adenomatous polyps, for instance. The final arbiter is usually the histopathologist's assessment of biopsied material (**Fig. 3.52**). However, endoscopic biopsies can be subject to sampling error and it must be kept in mind that biopsies from cancerous regions may just show evidence of inflammation or 'benign' changes such as adenoma or hyperplasia. If the clinical suspicion of carcinoma is high, then affected areas should be rebiopsied or excised as appropriate.

Some of the imaging modalities discussed earlier (CT, MRI, ultrasound) have their uses, particularly in preoperative staging and the detection of metastatic disease. The proponents of fine-cut, CT scanning 'virtual colonoscopy' support its role in the diagnosis of colonic tumours, but the requirement for tissue biopsy still remains.

Histologically, colonic adenocarcinomas tend to form a recognisable glandular epithelium with variable amounts of mucin secretion. The glandular architecture is usually still present in the poorly differentiated tumours, albeit less easily recognised. Mucin may be demonstrated microscopically by using the periodic acid-Schiff (PAS) staining technique. So-called 'signet-ring' cells, where the cytoplasm is almost completely occupied by mucin, may be found, although these are associated with a poorer prognosis.

145

Tumour staging

The prognosis for an individual patient with colorectal cancer depends on many variables:

- Deep local invasion of bowel wall*
- Involvement of draining lymph nodes (especially if multiple nodes involved)*
- Metastases in liver, bone or lung*
- Poorly differentiated tumour histology
- Signet-ring cells on histology
- Aneuploidy of tumour cells
- Genetic deletions (particularly DCC and p53)
- Evidence of perineural or venous infiltration
- Extremes of patient age (both very young and very old)
- Clinical presentation with 'complicated' tumour (obstruction or perforation)
- High preoperative carcinoembryonic antigen (CEA) level
- Medical comorbidity

*Most important.

The Dukes' staging system (**Fig. 3.53**) is used throughout the world and allows an accurate assessment of disease severity and prognosis. However, it is based on the pathologist's view of invasion and takes no account of clinical features, such as the degree of tumour fixation found at laparotomy or (in the original unmodified Dukes' system) the presence of distant metastases. Consequently, many clinicians utilise the TNM (tumour, nodes, metastases) staging system.

Whichever system is used, it is obvious that patients with the least advanced stage will have the best prognosis. Unfortunately, early presentation of colorectal cancer is still the exception rather than the rule. Dukes' A tumours are found in only 5–10% of patients, whereas about 25% of colorectal adenocarcinomas will already have established hepatic metastases at the time of diagnosis.

Treatment

Surgery remains the mainstay of colorectal cancer treatment, although adjuvant therapies are becoming more important (**Fig. 3.54**). It is still the only therapy that can be said to be potentially 'curative', although sadly this is not always possible.

The surgeon needs to be sure that there are no synchronous cancers or polyps elsewhere in the colon and some form of colonic imaging is necessary, as mentioned earlier. The type of resection performed for a colonic adenocarcinoma (**Fig. 3.55**) depends on several factors. Along with the primary tumour, a wide 'resection margin' of adjacent bowel is removed (usually at least 5 cm from each side) together with the relevant draining lymph

Modified Dukes' staging system for colorectal cancer		
Stage	**Features**	**5-year survival**
A	Tumour confined to the mucosa	90–5%
B1	Tumour growth into muscularis propria	75–80%
B2	Tumour growth through muscularis propria and serosa (full thickness)	60%
C1	Tumour spread to 1–4 regional lymph nodes	25–30%
C2	Tumour spread to more than 4 regional lymph nodes	
D	Distant metastases (liver, lung, bones)	<1%

Fig. 3.53 *Modified Dukes' staging system for colorectal cancer.*

Treatment of colorectal cancer	
Surgery	'Curative' or 'palliative' En-bloc resection of tumour and draining lymph nodes Relieves or prevents complications (e.g. obstruction) Staging accuracy improved by inspection of tumour Resection of liver metastases in certain circumstances

Chemotherapy	1. In *advanced* disease (e.g. distant metastases):
	   20% response rate to 5FU alone
	   Improves short-term survival
	   No further survival benefit with combination chemotherapy
	2. As *adjuvant* to surgery:
	   Delays tumour recurrence
	   Improves survival in patients with Dukes' C tumours
	   Controversial in cases of Dukes' B

Radiotherapy	Most useful for rectal cancers Reduced recurrence rate for Dukes' B2 and C Can be pre- or postoperative (or both) May cause radiation enteritis in adjacent bowel
Endoscopic palliation	Useful for obstructing rectal cancers if poor surgical candidate Nd YAG laser obliteration of tumour Argon-beam coagulation Usually short-term benefit; frequent applications required
Possible future therapies	?Immunomodulation ?Tumour DNA vaccination ?Gene therapy (e.g. insertion of 'suicide' prodrug activating enzymes)

Fig. 3.54 *Treatment of colorectal cancer.*

nodes. Surgery is further influenced by consideration of the arterial blood supply to the affected bowel.

Even where the advanced stage of the tumour makes curative intent impossible, surgery is still performed in the majority of patients. A palliative resection and anastomosis should delay, if not prevent, the development of obstruction or perforation.

Rectal carcinomas usually require a different surgical approach, depending on the precise location of the primary tumour. For high rectal or rectosigmoid lesions it is usually possible to perform an anterior (abdominal) resection with a primary anastomosis. Low rectal tumours, however, have traditionally required an abdominoperineal excision, with complete removal of the rectum and anus, necessitating a permanent colostomy. Recent developments in surgical technique, principally the use of end-to-end anastomotic staplers, have allowed sphincter-saving resections to become commonplace, as long as it is possible to leave a 2 cm resection margin. Without this, or if there is extensive local disease or invasion, an abdominoperineal excision remains necessary.

After a 'curative' surgical resection, it is possible to identify those patients at high risk of disease recurrence. Examples include primary tumours that have penetrated the bowel wall to its serosal surface or those that have already involved the lymph nodes. In these circumstances, the use of adjuvant chemotherapy may reduce the recurrence rate, particularly if given in the early postoperative phase whilst tumour burden is low.

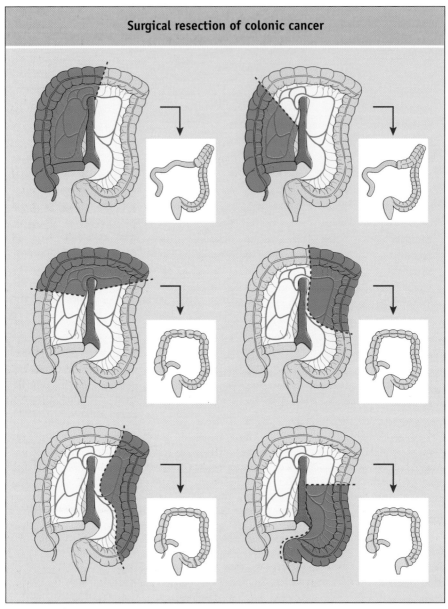

Fig. 3.55 *Surgical resection of colonic cancer. The extent of bowel resected is shown for a given tumour, depending on its location, the draining lymph nodes and its blood supply. The anastomoses are demonstrated in the insets.*

This is a controversial field and long-term prospective studies are continuing. The currently available data support the use of postoperative chemotherapy for patients with Dukes' C disease. Combination therapy regimes, comprising either 6 months of

5-fluorouracil (5FU) and leucovorin or 12 months of 5FU and levamisole, appear equally effective. The survival benefits seen with these drugs in patients with Dukes' C lesions have not been proven in those with Dukes' B carcinomas.

Patients with advanced metastatic or unresectable disease clearly have a poor prognosis. Systemic chemotherapy has been studied in this group and trials do show some short-term improvement in survival for approximately 20% of patients treated with 5FU. More intensive combination drug treatments have not shown any further survival benefit and are associated with greater toxicity.

Radiotherapy has been shown to reduce the local recurrence rate (usually 45–50%) of rectal cancers of stage B2 or C, if given pre- or postoperatively. The main side-effect is the development of radiation enteritis affecting adjacent bowel (see **Fig. 2.40**).

Finally, surgery may be utilised for those individuals with distant metastatic spread. The commonest site of metastasis is the liver, involved in up to 25% of patients at the time of diagnosis. The 5-year survival for patients with liver metastases, if left alone, is extremely low. As a result, some surgeons have developed the approach of resecting hepatic metastases in certain circumstances. Essentially, the primary tumour should be excised with curative intent, there should be no other non-hepatic metastases and hepatic disease should be 'resectable'. The definition of this term varies between authors, but usually means solitary lesions or up to four metastases confined to one lobe (although others will resect focal disease in multiple lobes). Five-year survival rates have been reported to be as high as 30% after such surgery.

In the future, attention seems likely to switch to developing novel anti-tumour strategies that could eradicate micrometastatic disease. Speculative therapies might include the use of 'gene therapy' techniques, using tumour oncogene proteins to increase the immunogenicity of cancer cells or inserting so-called 'suicide' genes that encode for chemotherapy prodrug activating enzymes into malignant cells. Until these or any other theories become a reality, the emphasis will continue to be on improving the screening and early diagnosis of colorectal cancer.

Management of the malignant polyp

Approximately 5% of apparently 'adenomatous' colonic polyps are found to contain a cancer. These lesions are an important subdivision of colorectal adenocarcinoma, not least because they may be potentially 'cured' endoscopically and cause something of a dilemma for the gastroenterologist.

The difficulty lies in judging whether a colonoscopically removed polyp, found to contain malignancy, can be safely considered to have been 'cured' in the way that is readily accepted for adenomatous lesions. Follow-up studies have shown that the risk of tumour recurrence or spread to lymph nodes in these circumstances is approximately 10%. The key features that identify those lesions that are likely to spread or recur after excision are the presence of poor histological differentiation, venous or lymphatic invasion, involvement of the polyp resection margin or invasion of the bowel wall submucosa.

If any of these factors is present, surgical resection of the affected area of colon should be considered. Clearly, the risk-benefit ratio of an operation may be influenced by other factors such as the patient's general health and fitness for surgery and so decisions will need to be tailored to the individual's circumstances.

Screening for colorectal cancer

There is now a considerable body of evidence to show that screening programmes can reduce colorectal cancer mortality. Not only is the disease relatively common, but there is also a well-defined premalignant stage (the adenoma) with a long latency. Furthermore, the presenting stage of a colorectal cancer shows a strong inverse association with patient survival. Given that there are readily available treatments for both the 'benign' polyp and early carcinoma, the detection of these lesions assumes even greater importance.

In these circumstances, a proposed screening method would have to be accurate, safe, acceptable to patients and cost-effective. These factors have to be balanced against one another. For instance, performing an annual colonoscopy on the general population would obviously detect many polyps and early cancers, but such a scheme would be extremely costly and labour-intensive and would expose patients to unnecessary discomfort and the risk of colonoscopic complications.

The different methods of screening for colon cancer are:
- Faecal occult blood testing
- Flexible sigmoidoscopy ('one off' or at regular intervals)
- Colonoscopy
- Barium enema
- Possibly 'virtual colonoscopy' in the future

The key distinction to be made is that of identifying 'average-risk' individuals as opposed to those who have another condition (family history, IBD, previous polyps or carcinoma) that makes them a higher risk for the development of a cancer. This has an important influence on both the method and frequency of screening used.

Some studies have used either double-contrast barium enema or colonoscopy as the screening method, but these are probably not suitable for surveillance of the general 'average-risk' population, where compliance, cost and complications become even more relevant. Therefore, attention has been most centred on methods that detect faecal occult blood (FOB) or involve flexible sigmoidoscopy (**Fig. 3.56**).

Faecal occult blood testing. FOB testing relies on the fact that most colorectal cancers and adenomatous polyps will bleed, at least intermittently. This, however, seems more true for cancers than polyps and FOB testing is probably better at detecting early-stage cancers than their benign precursors. If the FOB test is positive, then the patient should undergo a full evaluation with a colonscopy.

The most widely used FOB tests involve the patient applying a sample of their faeces to paper that is impregnated with chemical reagents. The 'guaiac' reaction utilises the pseudoperoxidase activity of haemoglobin to facilitate a change in the colour of an indicator dye and this forms the basis of the Haemoccult II® test that has been used in the largest screening trials. There is some evidence that the sensitivity of FOB testing can be improved by combining the guaiac-based method with a monoclonal antibody against haemoglobin, although this does increase the cost. As it is, the pseudoperoxidase reaction can be affected by a number of variables that reduce reliability. Most importantly, sensitivity improves with the number of samples taken and so patients should take two samples from each of three consecutive stools. A false-positive result is more likely with rehydration of the sample, a non-colorectal blood source (gastric, duodenal or nosebleed) and if there is peroxidase activity in foods (red meat, broccoli or turnips). A false-negative result may be obtained if there is bacterial degradation of haemoglobin (an old sample), in the presence of ascorbic acid, or with reduced or absent bleeding (more likely in a left-sided lesion).

Three large, randomised, population-based screening trials have now been reported – from Minnesota (USA), Nottingham (UK) and Funen (Denmark).

The American study used an annual, rehydrated (to increase sensitivity) FOB test and found that the subsequent mortality from colorectal cancer was cut by about a third in the 46 000 patients studied. The two European studies, which between them enrolled over 200 000 patients with an 8–10-year follow-up, used a slightly different methodology, with

Comparison of various screening tests for colorectal neoplasia

	Faecal occult blood	Flexible Sigmoidoscopy (60 cm)	Double-contrast barium enema	Colonoscopy
Detection rate for polyps and cancers	50%	55%	90%	95%
False-negative rate	50%*	10%**	10%	5%
False-positive rate	2–5%	Negligible	2–4%	Negligible
Relative cost per single examination***	$	$$$$$$$$$$$$	$$$$$$$$$$$$$$$$ $$$$$$$$$$	$$$$$$$$$$$$$$$$ $$$$$$$$$$$$$$$$ $$$$$$$$$$$$$$$$ $$$$$

*The detection rate improves with the number of tests performed and so the false-negative rate falls as more stools are screened.
**Percentage of polyps or cancers that are missed within range of the sigmoidoscope, not the entire colon (which would be even higher).
***Costs directly involved in performing the test. The true indirect costs will often be greater – for example, the cost of investigating a false-positive FOB test or the additional costs of nursing care involved in colonoscopy.

Fig. 3.56 *Comparison of various screening tests for colorectal neoplasia.*

biennial non-rehydrated tests. The reduction in colorectal cancer mortality was 15 and 18% in these two studies. The difference between the studies probably reflected the closer screening interval and rehydrated methods used in the USA. As a positive FOB test would be investigated with a colonoscopy, it may just be differences in the resulting colonoscopy rates that are most important (3% colonoscopy rate in the European studies versus 28% in the USA).

The second major finding of these trials was a 'down-staging' of colorectal cancer, so that about 75% of the tumours detected in the FOB screening groups were Dukes' A or B, compared with just 50% of those that developed in 'controls'.

On the face of it, these are impressive results, but debate continues about the practicalities of introducing such a screening test into the general, asymptomatic population. Even in the closely monitored conditions of the trials, patient acceptability seemed a problem – only 60–7% of individuals selected agreed to have at least one examination, with about a third of these patients not complying with their subsequent biennial tests. When outside the setting of a clinical trial, compliance rates are as low as 25%.

Furthermore, the relatively 'cheap' costs of the FOB tests must be weighed against the economics of subsequently investigating positive results, many of which will turn out to have been false. If rehydrated FOB specimens are used, about fifty people with a positive

test need to be investigated in order to diagnose one cancer. It has been estimated that the introduction of annual testing of all Americans over the age of 50 years would generate up to 5 million extra colonoscopies each year, at a potential cost of several billion dollars.
Flexible sigmoidoscopy. Flexible sigmoidoscopy, either at regular intervals (approximately every 5 years) or as a 'one-off' investigation at the age of 50 years, has also been proposed as a suitable screening technique for the 'average-risk' population. There is already some data from case-control studies that have shown a 60% reduction in mortality from rectosigmoid cancers. Large population-based trials of screening with 60 cm flexible sigmoidoscopy are currently progressing in Europe and North America.
Who, when and how often? It is easier to make screening guidelines for those groups that can be identified as 'high-risk' for colorectal cancer (**Fig. 3.57**) than for the general population. It is difficult to say which is the optimum screening method – and equally difficult to make firm guidelines about screening intervals. The reductions in mortality seem to support annual or biennial FOB screening from the age of 50 years, possibly coupled with a flexible sigmoidoscopy which may then be repeated at 5-year intervals.

ANGIODYSPLASIA

Angiodysplasia, also known as colonic vascular ectasia, is a common cause of recurrent lower gastrointestinal bleeding in the elderly. The condition is comprised of degenerative ectatic blood vessels which are usually identifiable at colonoscopy (**Fig. 3.58**) or angiography (see **Fig. 3.16**), while remaining difficult to demonstrate at laparotomy or in routine pathological specimens.

Angiodysplastic areas are most commonly found in the caecum and ascending colon, although careful visceral angiography in these patients may demonstrate associated small intestinal lesions. Bleeding commonly occurs, usually in a low-grade, recurrent form, and the condition often presents as an idiopathic iron deficiency anaemia. Massive haemorrhage is relatively uncommon, but well recognised.

Screening for colorectal cancer in 'high-risk' groups	
Previous colorectal cancer	Colonoscopy at 1 year after 'curative' resection If clear, further screening at 3-yearly intervals
Previous adenomatous polyp	Colonoscopy at 3-yearly intervals
Colonic Crohn's or ulcerative colitis	Screening colonoscopy, with biopsies, after 8 years If known distal colitis only, screen after 15 years Repeat procedure every 1–2 years Consider colectomy if dysplasia found
Familial adenomatous polyposis	Genetic testing and counselling Screen at-risk relatives (first- and second-degree) Annual flexi-sigmoidoscopy from age 12 Reduce interval to 3-yearly after age 40
HNPCC	Genetic testing and counselling Colonoscopy 2-yearly from age 20 Increase to annual intervals after age 40

Fig. 3.57 *Screening for colorectal cancer in 'high-risk' groups.*

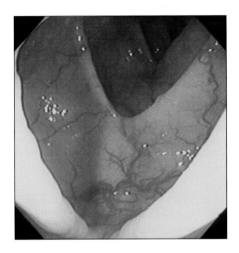

Fig. 3.58 *Colonic angiodysplasia. Colonoscopic view demonstrating a cluster of ectatic blood vessels in a patient with recurrent iron-deficiency anaemia.*

Debate has raged about whether or not colonic angiodysplasia is associated with valvular heart disease. Up to 25% of patients with angiodysplasia have aortic stenosis, but a number of prospective and retrospective studies have failed to confirm that this is indeed a true association.

The management of angiodysplasia depends upon the circumstances. Ectatic areas found incidentally at colonscopy should be managed conservatively if there has been no bleeding, as the absolute risk of significant bleeding is quite small. On the other hand, patients with active haemorrhage clearly require haemostasis and this can be achieved by interventional angiography (with coil embolisation), colonoscopic ablation (laser, electrocoagulation or heater probe) or surgical resection. Medical treatments aimed at reducing the number of bleeding episodes, using oestrogenic drugs, have been tried but the results of clinical trials have been conflicting.

THE IRRITABLE BOWEL SYNDROME

This constellation of functional intestinal disorders constitutes a major part of the workload of gastroenterologists in Europe and North America. The irritable bowel syndrome (IBS) is the result of complex interactions between psychosocial factors, disordered bowel motility and altered intestinal sensation. For many years it was difficult to offer a definition of IBS, but formal diagnostic criteria have now been developed, most notably the 'Rome criteria'. These dictate continuous or recurrent symptoms of:

1. Abdominal pain or discomfort
- Relieved by defaecation
- and/or associated with change in stool frequency
- and/or associated with change in stool consistency
2. Two or more of the following
- Altered stool frequency (> 3/day or < 3/week)
- Altered stool consistency (hard, soft or loose)
- Passing mucus per rectum
- Sensation of abdominal bloating or distension

The Rome criteria have been criticised, particularly for not recognising the important subgroup of IBS patients who have an abnormally high gastrocolic reflex (increased urge to defaecate postprandially) and for the need to have both abdominal pain and altered bowel habit present in order to fit the diagnosis.

Epidemiology

The symptoms of IBS are extremely common in the general population. Surveys suggest that at any one time, 20% of Americans and Europeans meet the diagnostic criteria and yet only about 10% of these individuals will seek medical advice. The factors that single out this subgroup are still not clearly defined. Those who present to physicians have variously been reported as showing a subjectively poor 'quality of life', having more absenteeism from work and a greater number of consultations for gastrointestinal and non-gastrointestinal illnesses alike. Despite the sexes being approximately equal in the prevalence of symptoms, Caucasian women are much more likely to present than their male equivalents, whilst in Asian societies this ratio is reversed.

IBS is more common in the age group 30–64 years than 65–93. However, this may reflect the traditional view that IBS is more difficult to diagnose confidently in older patients (because of the possibility of colorectal cancer, for example) and the tendency to identify other disorders such as diverticulosis as a cause of symptoms.

While the prevalence of IBS symptoms in the population remains steady, there is an equilibrium of patients 'dropping in' and 'dropping out'. Often patients will develop IBS for 2–3 years and then symptoms will gradually subside; others pursue a more chronic course.

Pathophysiology

The development of IBS involves contributions from cerebral psychosocial factors, the brain–gut axis of the autonomic nervous system and a combination of altered bowel motility and luminal sensation. Possible aetiological factors in the development of IBS include:
- Psychological – increased incidence of affective disorders, somatisation, phobias compared to controls
- Abnormal motility
- Altered patterns of visceral sensation (hyperalgesia)
- Intraluminal factors – e.g. dietary intolerance, changes in fibre intake (high or low), bile acids, altered bowel flora
- Inflammation – some evidence for subtle increase in mast cell numbers in mucosa and muscularis propria
- Infection – up to 30% of IBS cases develop post-infection; mechanism possibly due to changes in microbial flora or increased motility

IBS patients commonly demonstrate psychological symptoms including anxiety states, somatisation disorders and neurotic traits. Some studies have even suggested that about 50% of IBS patients meet the diagnostic criteria for a psychiatric illness. Certainly, many patients report exacerbations of symptoms around the times of occupational or domestic crises and the influence of these factors on the autonomic nervous system is well recognised.

Many abnormalities of gut motility have been described in IBS. Patients with diarrhoea have been shown to have increased jejunal contractions (particularly postprandially), accelerated whole-gut transit times and a correlation between proximal colonic motility and the degree of diarrhoea. Conversely, patients with colicky pain and constipation can be seen to have intense clusters of colonic contractions during periods of colicky pain.

The prevalence of distensive symptoms such as a 'bloating' sensation in the abdomen has led to the realisation that many IBS patients have abnormal visceral sensation. This can be quantified experimentally by balloon distension studies (**Fig. 3.59**). These have demonstrated a lower threshold for the sensation of 'urgency', with increased reflex motor contractions when the rectum is distended (in those with diarrhoeal symptoms) or a lower threshold for pain in those with discomfort as a predominant symptom.

154

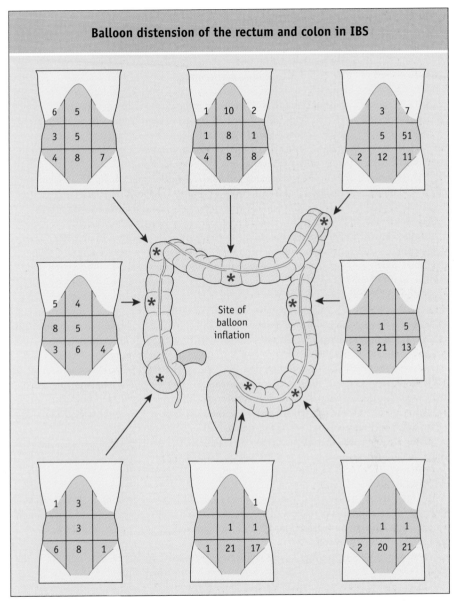

Balloon distension of the rectum and colon in IBS

Fig. 3.59 *Balloon distension of the rectum and colon in IBS. The sites and relative intensities of pain experienced by IBS sufferers when a balloon was inflated at different points in the large bowel.*

Other authors have searched for possible intraluminal factors that may 'irritate' the bowel. These may just be precipitants of symptoms in IBS rather than truly aetiological factors and candidates have included malabsorbed sugars (fructose, sorbitol, lactose), dietary allergens, fatty acids and bile salts. There have even been reports of IBS symptoms amongst heavy users of sorbitol-containing chewing gums and mints.

Clinical features and diagnosis

Essentially, the symptoms are those already mentioned above. To some extent it is possible to subclassify patients according to their main complaint and identify diarrhoea-predominant, constipation-predominant and pain-predominant (or pain-gas-bloat) individuals and to tailor treatment methods accordingly.

Accuracy of the history is all-important. For instance, a truly liquid large-volume diarrhoea is not a feature of IBS and is more likely to be due to other pathology. 'Diarrhoea' in IBS relates more to increased stool frequency and feelings of urgency.

Specific enquiry should be made about symptoms suggestive of 'organic' disease, particularly rectal bleeding, bloody diarrhoea, steatorrhoea and weight loss. These should prompt referral for the necessary investigations.

There is often a degree of overlap with functional disorders elsewhere. This includes other gastrointestinal disorders such as non-ulcer dyspepsia, globus hystericus and sphincter of Oddi dysmotility. IBS patients are more likely to have fibromyalgia, chronic fatigue syndrome, migraines or an 'irritable bladder'.

Routine physical examination should be within normal limits; signs of anaemia, vitamin deficiencies, cachexia or endocrine abnormalities should lead to a reconsideration of the diagnosis. Many patients have some colonic tenderness, but examination of the abdomen and rectum is usually unremarkable.

The main clinical dilemma in IBS is knowing how far to investigate patients. After taking a detailed history and performing a full physical examination, it is reasonable to undertake a limited series of investigations. This will serve the dual purpose of excluding other conditions and reassuring the patient, but over-investigation may prolong the patient's anxiety. A reasonable compromise is to take blood for routine biochemistry, full blood count, haematinics, thyroid function tests and inflammatory markers such as ESR or CRP. Stool should be sent for microbiological analysis and a sigmoidoscopy performed in those with diarrhoea. The insufflation of air during this latter test often provokes a reproduction of the patient's pain. Those over the age of 40 years should have the remaining colon imaged with a barium enema.

Many clinicians use therapeutic trials, with some of the drugs mentioned below, as part of the diagnostic process.

Management

Many IBS patients are worried about a possible sinister cause underlying their symptoms. They require a careful explanation of the features of IBS and reassurance about its 'benign' nature. Exacerbating factors such as lifestyle, stresses and dietary factors should be minimised.

In those whose dietary fibre intake is low, it is reasonable to increase the amount in the diet. However, many patients will have unsuccessfully tried high-fibre diets already. Those who consume excessive caffeine or alcohol should reduce their usage and exclusion diets (in those with diarrhoea) may be tried if the patient is supervised by a dietician. A particular example is that of lactose intolerance which may show a dramatic response to an exclusion diet or can be diagnosed using a lactose-hydrogen breath test (see chapter 2).

Drug treatments should be used cautiously in IBS. As the condition is not life-threatening it is difficult to justify long-term treatment with drugs that may have significant side-effects (**Fig. 3.60**). Some can be beneficial, depending on the predominant symptom, but there is frequently a high placebo response.

Antispasmodic drugs, such as mebeverine, peppermint oil or dicyclomine, can be used to control the pains of a 'spastic' colon by reducing muscular contraction. Simple antidiarrhoeal drugs, such as loperamide, may help reduce stool frequency in diarrhoea predominance.

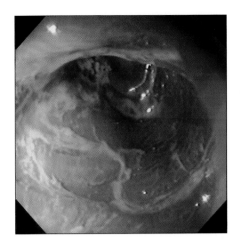

Fig. 3.60 Melanosis coli. *Long-term use of laxatives, as in this patient with constipation-predominant IBS, can lead to melanosis coli. At colonoscopy the large bowel mucosa is heavily pigmented with a purple-black discolouration.*

Soluble-fibre bulking agents such as ispaghula husk are commonly used and can have beneficial effects on both constipation and diarrhoea. If constipation fails to respond to the usual methods of increasing fibre, exercise and fluid intake, then an osmotic laxative or faecal softener may be useful, but stimulant laxatives should be avoided.

Many gastrointestinal units have developed psychological approaches including the use of hypnotherapy, biofeedback and formal psychotherapy. Some patients may respond to treatment with antidepressant drugs where appropriate.

Future developments may include the use of agents that reduce visceral sensation or inhibit gastrocolic reflexes. Putative agents under investigation include selective M3 muscarinic antagonists, somatostatin analogues, $5HT_3$ antagonists and tachykinin receptor blockers. For the moment, though, physicians need to be able to recognise the symptoms of IBS, differentiate it from more sinister intestinal disease and offer general supportive care based on symptomatology and backed by the therapeutic approaches outlined above.

chapter 4

The Liver and Biliary Tree

STRUCTURE AND FUNCTION

EMBRYOLOGY

The embryological origins of the liver, bile ducts and pancreas are closely related (**Fig. 4.1**). In particular, the vascular and biliary connections between the liver and the rest of the gastrointestinal tract are essential for its normal functioning. Embryological abnormalities of these systems can therefore result in potentially life-threatening conditions that may present to paediatricians or gastroenterologists. Similarly, the symbiotic relationship between these organs means that disease processes affecting one will often affect the other.

Some of the important embryological defects that may occur are listed in **Fig. 4.2**. The reader is referred to one of the standard textbooks of paediatric gastroenterology for further details.

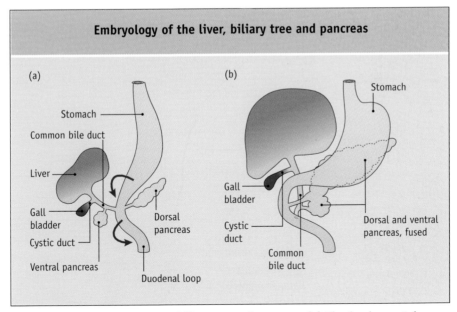

Embryology of the liver, biliary tree and pancreas

Fig. 4.1 *Embryology of the liver, biliary tree and pancreas. (a) The developmental anatomy of the biliary tree at 5 weeks of gestation. (b) After fusion of the dorsal and ventral pancreatic ducts, at 7 weeks.*

Developmental abnormalities and variations of the liver and biliary tree and pancreas

Abnormality	Significance
Liver	
Riedel's lobe	Elongated right lobe May be mistaken for true hepatomegaly Can extend below umbilicus Normal liver function Ultrasound diagnostic
Portal vein anomalies	Persistent ductus venosus Atresia or agenesis rare
Arterial anomalies	May arise from superior mesenteric or left gastric rather than coeliac artery Rarely of significance
Biliary tree	
Alagille's syndrome	Some cases familial, others spontaneous mutations Deficiency of intrahepatic interlobular bile ducts Chronic cholestasis Congenital abnormalities common in other organs Infrequent progress to cirrhosis, hepatoma or liver failure Survival often limited by associated cardiac abnormalities
Extrahepatic biliary atresia	1 in 10 000 live births Destruction or absence of extrahepatic bile ducts Poor prognosis without surgery (Kasai hepatoportoenterostomy) or liver transplant
Bile duct variations	Accessory bile ducts (from individual liver segments) Duplication of common bile duct Agenesis or duplication of cystic duct

Choledochal cysts	1 in 15 000 live births
	Cystic dilatation of intra- or extrahepatic bile ducts
	Cholestatic jaundice
	Long-term risks:
	   Secondary biliary cirrhosis
	   Episodic cholangitis
	   Cyst wall carcinoma
	Treatment: surgical excision with choledochojejunostomy

Caroli's syndrome	Cystic dilatations of bile ducts, associated with congenital hepatic fibrosis May occur with polycystic renal disease
Double gall bladder	Rare (1 in 10 000) May be associated with extrahepatic biliary atresia
Floating gall bladder	Abnormally mobile Vulnerable to torsion

Fig. 4.2 *Developmental abnormalities and variations of the liver and biliary tree and pancreas.*

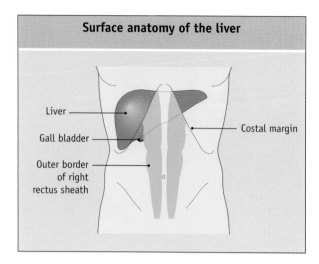

Surface anatomy of the liver

Liver

Gall bladder

Outer border of right rectus sheath

Costal margin

Fig. 4.3 *Surface anatomy of the liver. The liver descends by up to 3 cm during inspiration and is just about palpable below the costal margin in normal adults.*

ANATOMY

The liver

The liver is the largest of the internal organs, weighing between 1.2 and 1.8 kg, and occupies most of the right upper quadrant of the abdomen. The surface anatomy of the liver (**Fig. 4.3**) corresponds to an anterior upper border roughly parallel with the fifth right intercostal space and a lower border that runs obliquely upward from the right ninth to the left eighth costal cartilage. The fundus of the gall bladder usually lies beneath the junction of the right rectus sheath and the ninth costal cartilage. The posterior surface of the liver is concave and bears a 5 cm long transverse cleft, the porta hepatis. The lesser omentum descends from the margins of the porta and contains the hepatic artery, portal vein and common bile duct. The porta lies just in front of the vena cava and behind the gall bladder.

The convex anterior surface of the liver is divided by the attachment of the falciform ligament into two lobes, the right being approximately twice the size of the left. The area of right lobe between the falciform ligament and gall bladder is sometimes termed the quadrate lobe, and an area known as the caudate lobe can be delineated by the inferior vena cava and ligamentum venosum on the posterior surface. These subdivisions of the liver are not of any functional significance and are of little relevance when considering surgical resections, for example. A more useful anatomical description is based on the distribution of blood vessels and bile ducts within the liver (**Fig. 4.4**). The liver can thus be divided into eight functionally distinct segments. Principally, Cantlie's line extends from the vena cava to the gall bladder, divides the liver into two functional lobes and represents a relatively bloodless field sometimes used as a resection margin. The further subdivision into eight segments is based on each having its own pedicle of blood vessels and bile ducts.

The liver is made up of a wide range of cell types. About 60% are hepatocytes, but there are also significant numbers of biliary epithelial cells and 'non-parenchymal' cells including endothelium, Kupffer cells and stellate cells.

The microscopic architecture of the liver is vitally important for its successful function. The hepatocytes lie in plates separated by blood-filled sinusoids that are arranged radially around a central efferent hepatic vein (**Fig. 4.5**) with peripheral portal tract areas that contain distal branches of the hepatic artery, portal vein and bile duct. This histological 'lobule' is perhaps the best anatomical description of the liver microarchitecture, while a

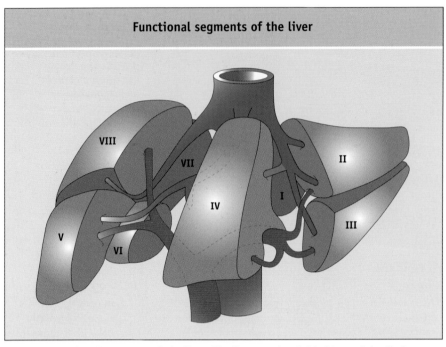

Functional segments of the liver

Fig. 4.4 *Functional segments of the liver. The liver can be divided into eight distinct segments based on blood supply and biliary drainage.*

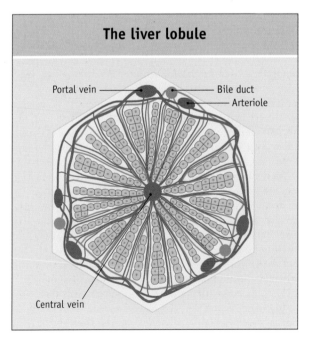

The liver lobule

Fig. 4.5 *The liver lobule. Blood from the hepatic artery and hepatic portal vein flows from the portal tracts toward the central vein, which in turn drains into the hepatic vein. The portal tracts also contain branches of the bile ducts and lymphatics.*

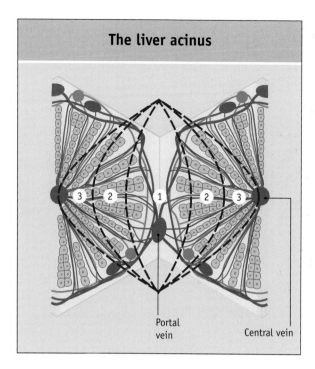

The liver acinus

Portal
vein

Central vein

Fig. 4.6 *The liver acinus. According to this model, the central vein is taken to be at the periphery of the functional unit. The branches of the portal vein and hepatic artery are at its centre and a gradient of relative hypoxia develops as blood flows towards the central vein (with oxygen tensions being highest in-zone-1 and lowest in zone-3).*

functional model is better represented by the 'acinus' (**Fig. 4.6**). As blood flows into the liver via the hepatic artery and portal vein and towards the central vein there is a progressive reduction in oxygenation. Consequently, there are important variations in susceptibility to tissue injury at different sites within the acinus.

The hepatic sinusoids are lined with fenestrated endothelial cells which are separated from the hepatocytes by the space of Disse (or perisinusoidal space) containing extracellular matrix proteins. Other cells present in the sinusoidal walls are the phagocytic Kupffer cells, which are a vital part of the reticuloendothelial system, and the hepatic stellate cells (also known as Ito cells, lipocytes or pericytes). The latter have some myofibroblast activity which may help regulate sinusoidal blood flow and are now recognised as important agents in the repair of hepatic injury; increased stellate cell activation appears to be a key factor in the development of liver fibrosis. The hepatocytes themselves display marked polarity in their structure. The hepatocyte membrane directly facing the sinusoid has numerous microvilli, some of which extend through the endothelial fenestrations, reflecting the extensive number of receptors and transport mechanisms in this area of the cell. Microvilli are also seen on the opposite side of the cell, which borders the bile canaliculus formed between adjacent hepatocyte plates and which represents the initial site of bile secretion. The hepatocyte's lateral surface has numerous gap junctions and desmosomes that anchor it to its neighbours.

After secretion into the canalicular spaces, bile is collected in the smallest intrahepatic bile ductules which gradually coalesce to form bigger and bigger ducts. The smaller ducts have a cuboidal epithelium which becomes progressively more columnar as the ducts increase in size.

163

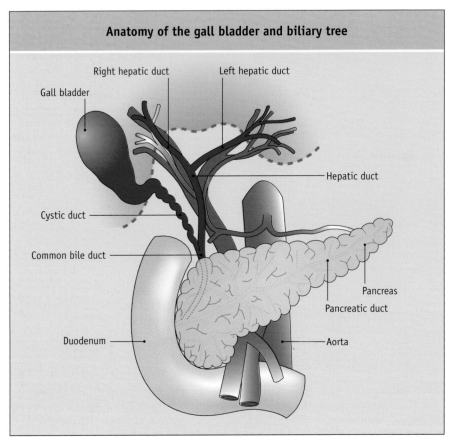

Anatomy of the gall bladder and biliary tree

Fig. 4.7 *Anatomy of the gall bladder and biliary tree.*

The biliary tree and gall bladder

The intrahepatic bile ductules gradually merge to form larger ducts that drain the eight
functional liver segments. Within the right hemiliver, the union of these branches creates an
anterior and a posterior sectoral duct that in turn merge to form the right hepatic duct. In
most individuals, the right hepatic duct extends outside the liver for just 1 cm. Ducts
draining the three segments of the left hemi-liver form the left hepatic duct which runs a
longer course than the right, before joining with it to create the common hepatic duct
(**Fig. 4.7**). After merging with the cystic duct from the gall bladder, the common hepatic
duct becomes the common bile duct (CBD), which initially lies within the lesser omentum
close to the portal vein and hepatic artery. To some extent, the wall of the CBD becomes
thicker, and its lumen narrower, as it progresses towards the ampulla. Usually, the CBD is
approximately 7 cm long and its diameter ranges from 4 to 12 mm. The larger bile ducts
receive their blood supply from a plexus of vessels derived from branches of the right
hepatic artery.

The gall bladder is a purse-like sac that stores approximately 50 ml of bile. It measures
8–10 cm in length and can be divided into a fundus, body and neck. It has a muscular wall
and is lined by columnar epithelium. The lining mucosa forms a small recess close to the
neck, known as Hartmann's pouch, which can be the site for gallstone impaction.

164

Anomalies of the cystic duct are relatively common and it may join the right hepatic duct or occasionally the more distal portion of the CBD.

PHYSIOLOGY

The liver

The complex physiology of the liver has been one of the factors that have delayed the development of artificial liver support devices. Whereas the heart can be considered as a pump or the kidneys as filters, the liver performs a wide variety of important functions (**Fig. 4.8**). Its central role in carbohydrate, protein and fatty acid metabolism reflects the territory of the portal venous circulation, drawing blood from the gut and pancreas. This same blood can also become a conduit for gut-derived pathogens, potential antigens and orally administered drugs, and so hepatic physiology is further geared to their handling

The functions of the liver	
Metabolic	Carbohydrate metabolism Apolipoproteins Fatty acid metabolism Transamination and deamination of amino acids Storage of fat-soluble vitamins Drug metabolism and conjugation
Synthetic	Urea Albumin Clotting factors Complement C3 and C4 Ferritin Transferrin C-reactive protein (CRP) Haptoglobin α_1-antitrypsin α-fetoprotein α_2-macroglobulin Caeruloplasmin
Excretory	Bile synthesis Excretion of drug metabolites
Endocrine	Breakdown of hormones and cytokines 25-hydroxylation of vitamin D
Immunological	Fetal development of B lymphocytes Removal of circulating immune complexes Removal of activated CD8 T lymphocytes Phagocytosis and presentation of antigens Probable role in developing oral tolerance Production of lipopolysaccharide-binding protein Cytokine release – e.g. TNF-α, interferons Transport of immunoglobulin A
Miscellaneous	Capacity for liver regeneration Regulation of angiogenesis

Fig. 4.8 *The functions of the liver.*

and disposal. The portal venous blood contributes some 75% of the acinar supply, with the remaining 25% derived from the hepatic artery. There is evidence of differential metabolism within the acinus – the better-oxygenated zone 1 hepatocytes perform more gluconeogenesis and glutathione synthesis than their zone 3 equivalents. These latter centri-acinar cells contain more glycolytic enzymes and more cytochrome p450 metabolic capacity and have a mechanism of bile formation that is less dependent on the presence of bile salts.

Changes in blood levels of glucose, plasma proteins, clotting factors and lipids are important features of many liver diseases.

Liver regeneration. Unlike most of the other solid organs, the adult liver maintains a capacity for self-regeneration When the ability of hepatocytes to replenish the liver is limited, a population of pluripotent 'oval' cells derived from tiny bile ductules can proliferate and repopulate the liver with hepatocytes and biliary cells. Oval cells themselves may originate in the bone marrow.

The liver's ability to regenerate after tissue injury or surgical resection is striking. From animal studies of sequential partial hepatectomies, we know that it is possible to remove two-thirds of the liver on 12 successive occasions. Mathematical models suggest that a single rat hepatocyte can undergo approximately 34 cell divisions, producing enough cells to form about 50 rat livers. In the light of this, it is fair to say that despite their highly specialised functions, hepatocytes are not terminally differentiated cells.

Immunological functions. The liver is a central component of the immune system. The phagocytic Kupffer cells, which make up 15% of the liver cell mass and comprise some 80% of the body's total macrophage population, are vitally important scavengers of foreign antigens and present them to lymphocytes. The hepatic lymphocyte population is highly specialised, with B lymphocytes making up less than 5% of the total. The vast majority are T cells which show a higher preponderance of CD8 cells over CD4 (the opposite to what is seen in the circulation), as well as a recently described population of lymphocytes known as 'NK-T' cells. Representing only 5% of circulating lymphocytes, these NK-T cells make up 40% of the intrahepatic population and, as their name would suggest, have some features in common with 'natural killer' cells.

Abnormal immunological responses are a feature of many types of hepatic illness.

Bile secretion, the biliary tree and the gall bladder

Bile. Bile is an important aid to the alimentary tract, augmenting the digestion and absorption of fats. It is also an important route for the excretion of hepatic metabolites and waste products such as cholesterol, bilirubin and heavy metals. Secretion requires the activity of both hepatocytes, the source of 'primary' bile, and the cholangiocytes that line the bile ductules. This biliary epithelium is far from being just a passive physical barrier and is instead accountable for secreting about 40% of the 600 ml volume of bile produced each day, as well as largely determining its fluidity and pH.

The main constituents of bile are shown in **Fig. 4.9**. The bile acids are formed within hepatocytes from cholesterol, largely by hydroxylation of the ringed structure, and are then made more water-soluble by conjugation with glycine, taurine or sulphate. They have detergent-like properties and form micellar aggregates that help emulsify dietary fats, assist with the action of pancreatic and brush-border lipases and essentially solubilise the intraluminal fat. The conjugated bile salts are subsequently reabsorbed by specific active transport in the terminal ileum, although about 20% of intestinal bile is deconjugated by ileal bacteria. The unabsorbed bile undergoes further bacterial metabolism in the colon, with conversion to so-called 'secondary' bile acids, and about 50% of these are reabsorbed in turn. The enterohepatic circulation of bile salts is normally very efficient, 80–5% of

Composition of bile

Constituent	Comments

Bile acids
  Cholic acid
  Chenodeoxycholic acid
  Deoxycholic acid
  Ursodeoxycholic acid (trace only)
	Conjugated to taurine, glycine or sulphate
	Highly efficient enterohepatic circulation
	Synthesis balances faecal losses

Bilirubin	Largely conjugated to glucuronide
Cholesterol	One-third reabsorbed in intestine
Trace metals	Iron, manganese, zinc, copper, lead
Drug metabolites	Tend to be higher molecular weights than those excreted in urine Polar molecules usually unaltered Lipophilic metabolites usually conjugated

Fig. 4.9 *Composition of bile.*

circulating conjugates being taken up by the liver on a single pass through the portal venous route.

Owing to their detergent-like actions, bile salts are cytotoxic if concentrations are high enough, but the cell membranes of the biliary tree and intestine are protected both by the presence of other intraluminal lipids (phosphatidylcholine in the biliary tree or fatty acids in the intestine) and by their own plasmalemma content of cholesterol and glycolipids.

Bilirubin is derived from the breakdown of red blood cells (75%), the catabolism of other haem proteins (22%) and ineffective bone marrow erythropoiesis (3%). It is a yellow pigment with a tetrapyrrole structure and is insoluble in water. As a result, unconjugated bilirubin is transported in the circulation as a complex with albumin, although a tiny amount may circulate in isolation (**Fig. 4.10**). The lipid-soluble bilirubin is made water-soluble by the liver in a series of steps comprising specific uptake, conjugation and excretion (**Fig. 4.11**). These three stages are very closely integrated in the hepatocyte, which maintains a constant downward gradient from blood to cytoplasm by excretion of bilirubin into the canaliculus.

Virtually no conjugated bilirubin is reabsorbed from the biliary tree or intestines. However, luminal bacteria in the terminal ileum and colon are capable of deconjugating bilirubin and converting it to a water-soluble tetrapyrrole known as urobilinogen. About a fifth of the urobilinogen is reabsorbed and excreted by the kidney, while further amounts appear in the stool as stercobilinogen.

Role of the biliary tree. Once bile has been secreted by the hepatocytes it undergoes considerable modification as it passes down the biliary tree. Water is drawn into the bile through paracellular junctions by osmosis. Glutathione is split into its constituent amino acids which are reabsorbed, as are luminal glucose and some organic acids. Bicarbonate and chloride ions are actively secreted into bile by a mechanism largely dependent on the cystic fibrosis transmembrane regulator (CFTR). Cholangiocytes also contribute IgA by exocytosis.

The gall bladder. Given the important role of bile in fat digestion, it seems appropriate that the body has mechanisms to store and release bile in large quantities after meals. The gall bladder acts in such a capacity, holding around 50 ml of bile that can be released in response

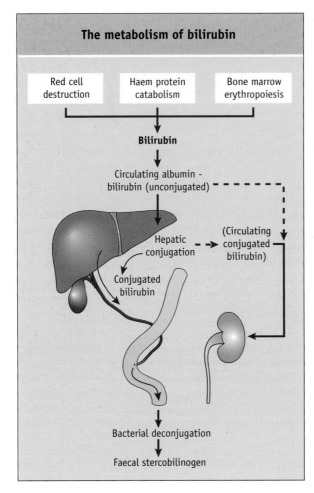

The metabolism of bilirubin

| Red cell destruction | Haem protein catabolism | Bone marrow erythropoiesis |

Bilirubin

Circulating albumin - bilirubin (unconjugated)

Hepatic conjugation → (Circulating conjugated bilirubin)

Conjugated bilirubin

Bacterial deconjugation

Faecal stercobilinogen

Fig. 4.10 *The metabolism of bilirubin. Once bile is taken up and conjugated by the liver, some leakage of bilirubin mono- and diglucuronides does occur, but these normally account for less than 5% of circulating bilirubin. In bile, more than 80% is conjugated as the diglucuronide form.*

to the ingestion of food. It is, however, not essential to human digestion (as testified by the experience of individuals who have had a cholecystectomy). In the fasting state, about half of the bile continuously flowing down the hepatic duct is directed to the gall bladder for storage, dependent on the relative pressures in the vessels. During its time in the gall bladder, bile is concentrated by the net reabsorption of sodium, calcium, chloride and bicarbonate ions followed by diffusion of water and there is a lowering of the intracystic pH. The gall bladder is capable of reducing the volume of its stored bile by 80–90%.

Control of biliary motility and secretion. The gall bladder, extrahepatic bile ducts and sphincter of Oddi are motile structures and the efficient flow of bile depends on maintaining an adequate pressure gradient. The hormone cholecystokinin (CCK) is the most potent physiological stimulus to gall bladder contraction but there is also an autonomic nervous component, with parasympathetic fibres causing contraction and sympathetic fibres causing relaxation of the gall bladder. CCK levels rise highest in response to dietary long-chain fatty acids, amino acids and carbohydrates (in decreasing order of potency) but gall bladder contraction occurs in response to any meal and even after drinking water. The main hepatobiliary effect of the hormone secretin is to increase the secretion of fluid and electrolytes by the biliary epithelium.

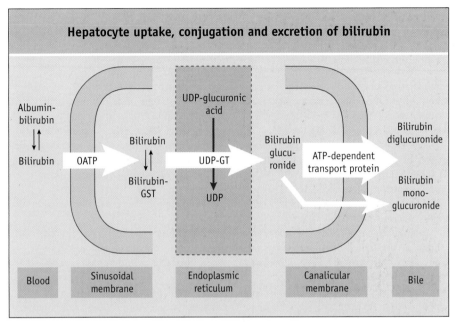

Fig. 4.11 *Hepatocyte uptake, conjugation and excretion of bilirubin. The uptake of circulating bilirubin across the sinusoidal membrane can be competitively inhibited by some organic anions such as bromosulphthalein and indocyanine green and has been termed the organic ion-transporting polypeptide (OATP). Bilirubin GST effectively acts as a reservoir, storing bilirubin prior to conjugation and thereby helping to maintain a downward gradient from the sinusoid. Other abbreviations: UDP-GT = uridine diphosphate glucuronyl transferase, GST = glutathione S-transferase, ATP = adenosine triphosphate.*

SYMPTOMS AND SIGNS

In many instances, diseases of the liver, biliary tract or pancreas can present with similar patterns of symptoms to other parts of the digestive system – with abdominal pain, weight loss, diarrhoea or bleeding. However, in many cases, owing to the well-hidden retroperitoneal location of the pancreas, for example, or the variety of metabolic functions performed by the liver, conditions can present in a less well-defined, more insidious manner. Liver disease is frequently an incidental finding, discovered on 'routine' laboratory tests or on the screening of blood donations. As part of the assessment of all patients, a full history should be taken and a complete physical examination performed.

Abdominal pain

Pain due to inflammation of the gall bladder or pancreas can be among the most severe of abdominal symptoms. Parenchymal liver diseases are less common causes of pain, but its occurrence can give a significant clue to the presence of worsening pathology.

Conditions that stretch the liver capsule may result in upper abdominal pain, felt most obviously on the right side. Causes include acute hepatitis, venous obstruction (due to right heart failure or the Budd–Chiari syndrome, for example) or the presence of rapidly enlarging intrahepatic mass lesions. While cirrhosis itself is painless, the development of right upper quadrant pain in such a patient may be a presenting symptom of a hepatocellular carcinoma, a venous thrombotic episode or perhaps an associated peptic ulcer.

Non-specific abdominal pain in patients with ascites may be an indicator of spontaneous bacterial peritonitis (see below), although patients are more likely to present with encephalopathy or other evidence of hepatic decompensation. Gallstones are usually asymptomatic but where stones give rise to biliary colic, attacks of pain can be quite severe with a typical colicky pattern lasting for at least half an hour. Pain that persists for more than 6 hours is more likely to represent acute cholecystitis. Classically, the pain of biliary colic is worst postprandially but can occur at any time. Most episodes of true biliary colic represent periods when the cystic duct is intermittently blocked by stones. As visceral pain, it is often poorly localised to the upper abdomen and the differential diagnosis includes peptic ulceration, non-ulcer dyspepsia, gastro-oesophageal reflux disease, pancreatitis, renal stones and colonic disorders. It is more commonly felt in the epigastrium than the right upper quadrant and radiates to the right shoulder in about half of cases.

Pain due to acute cholecystitis may initially be generalised over the upper and central abdomen, becoming more localised as the surrounding peritoneum is inflamed. It most commonly presents as an uncharacteristically severe attack of pain in a patient with previous episodes of biliary colic, although may of course occur *de novo*. The pain may sometimes radiate through to the back and, because of the presence of significant inflammation, fever and rigors may occur. The presence of jaundice should suggest either a hepatic infection or ascending cholangitis. Pancreatic pain is classically located across the upper or central abdomen and radiates through to the back. In the case of acute pancreatitis it can be overwhelmingly severe and the multiple exacerbations seen in cases of chronic pancreatitis can be similarly agonising. Chronic abdominal pain is one of the presenting features in more than 50% of cases of pancreatic cancer.

Jaundice

Jaundice (also known as icterus) can be considered as both a symptom and a sign. Mild jaundice may not be noticed by the patient and may only be detected by an alert physician, but most jaundiced individuals or their relatives will spot the yellow discolouration of sclerae, skin or mucous membranes. In normal individuals, the serum bilirubin is below 18 μmol/l, with less than 5% present in the conjugated form. Jaundice is not usually clinically detectable until levels have risen above at least 30 μmol/l (**Fig. 4.12**).

The key to finding the cause of jaundice is to consider whether the hyperbilirubinaemia is of unconjugated or conjugated type as this significantly narrows the differential diagnosis (although many liver diseases lead to a combination of the two) (**Fig. 4.13**). This can be done biochemically but important clues can also be gained from a thorough history and examination.

Conjugated bilirubin is water-soluble and specific enquiry should be made for symptoms suggesting 'cholestatic jaundice' – dark urine, pale stools and pruritus. Patients

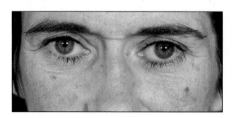

Fig. 4.12 *Jaundice. This patient with alcoholic cirrhosis demonstrates the yellow sclerae seen with hyperbilirubinaemia. She also has multiple facial telangiectasia.*

Differential diagnosis of jaundice, based on the nature of the hyperbilirubinaemia

Specific abnormalities of bilirubin metabolism

Unconjugated hyperbilirubinaemia	Haemolysis
	Gilbert's syndrome
	Crigler–Najjar syndrome types I and II
Mixed or predominantly conjugated hyperbilirubinaemia	Rotor's syndrome
	Dubin–Johnson syndrome

Parenchymal liver disease

Hepatocellular dysfunction	Viral hepatitis
	Toxins (e.g. alcohol, paracetamol, *Amanita phalloides*)
	Autoimmune hepatitis
	Metabolic disorders
	Pregnancy-associated disorders
	Drug reactions
	Ischaemia
	Budd–Chiari syndrome
Intrahepatic cholestasis	Inflammation or destruction of bile ductules
	Primary biliary cirrhosis
	Primary sclerosing cholangitis
	Ductopenic drug reactions
	Graft versus host disease
	Transplant rejection
	Infiltrative conditions
	Malignant neoplasms
	Sarcoidosis
	Tuberculosis
	Amyloidosis
	Granulomatous drug reactions
	Benign recurrent intrahepatic cholestasis
	Postoperative cholestasis
	Cholestatic drug reactions
	Total parenteral nutrition

Bile duct obstruction

Choledocholithiasis	
Bile duct strictures	Neoplastic
	Primary sclerosing cholangitis
	Surgical injury
	Acquired immunodeficiency syndrome (AIDS) cholangiopathy
	Post-choledocholithiasis
	Post-transplantation
Extrinsic compression	Lymphadenopathy
	Neoplasia
	Pancreatitis
	Aneurysms

Fig. 4.13 *Differential diagnosis of jaundice, based on the nature of the hyperbilirubinaemia.*

Important aspects of history-taking in patients with jaundice or suspected liver disease

Subject	Relevance
Duration of jaundice Abdominal pain Associated symptoms – anorexia, lethargy, weight loss, pale stools, dark urine, pruritus	May help to discriminate patients with 'hepatocellular' jaundice from those with posthepatic (or 'surgical') jaundice
Disorientation, memory loss, clumsiness, difficulty in performing complex tasks, dysarthria	Neurological sequelae of chronic alcohol abuse Hepatic encephalopathy Hepatolenticular degeneration (Wilson's disease)
Easy bruising or bleeding Ankle swelling Abdominal distension (ascites)	Together with encephalopathy, suggestive of hepatic decompensation
Alcohol intake (past and present)	Alcoholic liver disease Pancreatitis
Drugs and medications (including prescribed drugs, over-the-counter medicines, herbal remedies, recreational drugs and, particularly, history of intravenous drug abuse)	Drug reactions Paracetamol overdosage Ecstasy-induced hepatitis Risk of viral hepatitis and human immunodeficiency virus (HIV)
Previous episodes of jaundice	Viral hepatitis Gallstone disease
Blood transfusions and previous surgery	Many patients are unaware of having received transfusions during previous surgery Risk factor for viral hepatitis Post-surgical biliary strictures Retained stones after cholecystectomy Halothane hepatitis
Family history of jaundice or liver disease	Isolated hyperbilirubinaemias Haemolytic anaemias Familial contacts with viral hepatitis Inherited metabolic liver diseases
Sexual history	Pregnancy-associated liver disorders Jaundiced contacts Risk of viral hepatitis or AIDS
Country of origin or history of foreign travel	Viral hepatitis Schistosomiasis Liver fluke infection Amoebiasis
Occupation	Health-care workers (hepatitis viruses) Farmers/animal workers (hydatid) Sewage workers (leptospirosis) Exposure to industrial toxins Alcoholic drinking patterns
Sports and recreation	Water sports (leptospirosis) Anabolic steroid misuse Wild mushroom-picking

Fig. 4.14 *Important aspects of history-taking in patients with jaundice or suspected liver disease.*

should also be asked about episodes of abdominal pain, distension, easy bruising, weight loss, anorexia and lethargy. Where parenchymal liver disease is suspected, attention should be paid to the presence of risk factors (**Fig. 4.14**) that may point to the likely aetiology.

An algorithm for the diagnostic approach to the jaundiced patient is shown in **Fig. 4.15**.

Steatorrhoea

Patients may develop fat malabsorption in cases of exocrine pancreatic insufficiency and also in severe cases of obstructive jaundice. This may present as obvious steatorrhoea or with complications such as deficiencies of fat-soluble vitamins. The diagnosis and management of malabsorption are discussed in chapter 2, while the intestinal sequelae of pancreatic insufficiency are described later in this chapter.

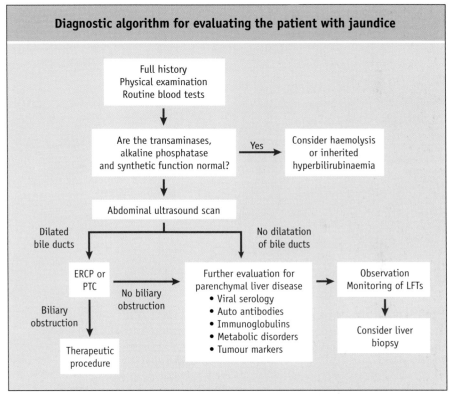

Fig. 4.15 *Diagnostic algorithm for evaluating the patient with jaundice. 'Routine blood tests' should always include clotting studies as a measurement of synthetic liver function (and, together with the platelet count, they should be used to assess the risk of bleeding if invasive tests are considered). Most automated laboratories will measure albumin, bilirubin, at least one transaminase, alkaline phosphatase and γ-glutamyl transpeptidase as part of the 'liver function tests'. Depending on local availability and expertise, a CT scan or MRI cholangiography would be reasonable alternatives to an ultrasound scan. A rapid presentation of jaundice with coagulopathy and encephalopathy is more suggestive of acute hepatocellular failure (ERCP = endoscopic retrograde cholangiopancreatography, PTC = percutaneous transhepatic cholangiography, LFTs = liver function tests).*

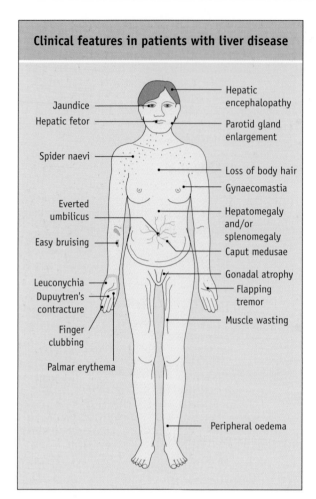

Clinical features in patients with liver disease

Jaundice

Hepatic fetor

Spider naevi

Everted umbilicus

Easy bruising

Leuconychia

Dupuytren's contracture

Finger clubbing

Palmar erythema

Hepatic encephalopathy

Parotid gland enlargement

Loss of body hair

Gynaecomastia

Hepatomegaly and/or splenomegaly

Caput medusae

Gonadal atrophy

Flapping tremor

Muscle wasting

Peripheral oedema

Fig. 4.16 *Clinical features in patients with liver disease.*

PHYSICAL SIGNS OF CHRONIC LIVER DISEASE

The physician may detect a wide range of physical signs in patients with liver disease (**Fig. 4.16**). In many instances, these are manifestations of cirrhosis or chronic hepatitis, but evidence may also be found of complications such as portal hypertension or ascites and patients may display evidence of risk factors (such as injection marks in an intravenous drug abuser) or of extrahepatic damage from aetiological agents such as alcoholic neuropathy or cardiomyopathy.

Some signs are more reliable than others. Combinations of signs such as jaundice, a flapping tremor, multiple spider naevi (**Fig. 4.17**), gynaecomastia, ascites (**Fig. 4.18**) and oedema are reliable indicators of chronic liver disease. Traditionally, the presence of tattoos (**Fig. 4.19**) or body-piercing has been suggested as indicating a higher risk of viral hepatitis, although some authors have argued that these individuals are no more likely to carry such viruses once the influences of other lifestyle activities (intravenous drug abuse or sexual promiscuity, for example) are excluded.

The physical examination of a patient with liver disease should begin with the history. Is the patient disorientated, confused or dysarthric, for example? Is there an alcoholic

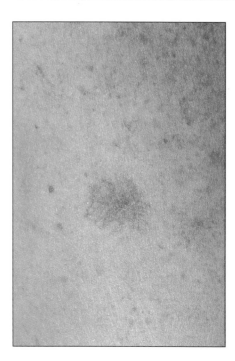

Fig. 4.17 *Cutaneous spider naevi. These telangiectatic lesions are comprised of a central spiral arteriole with multiple radiating precapillary vessels. Pressure on the central arteriole causes the whole lesion to blanch. They occur almost exclusively on the upper half of the body and two or three may be found in normal individuals.*

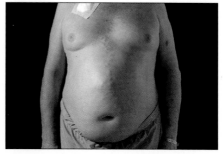

Fig. 4.18 *Physical signs in alcoholic cirrhosis. This patient has a distended abdomen due to ascites, together with a caput medusae pattern of engorged abdominal wall veins flowing away from the umbilicus. He also has bilateral gynaecomastia. The sticking plaster covers the site of a recently removed central venous catheter inserted following a variceal haemorrhage. See also Fig. 4.28 (b).*

fetor? Many alcohol-dependent patients seek to disguise this by using mints or chewing gum. A general inspection should reveal any obvious jaundice, muscle wasting, abdominal distension or malnutrition.

The patient should be asked to extend his or her arms, to allow inspection of the hands (**Fig. 4.20**) and also to demonstrate a tremor. This is best achieved with the elbows fully extended and the palms hyperextended backwards, as if trying to stop traffic. The fingers should be kept extended and spaced slightly apart. The fine tremor of alcohol withdrawal is easily distinguished from the more coarse 'flap' of hepatic encephalopathy. This can sometimes be made more obvious by gently hyperextending the patient's palm against the observer's; the flap may then be felt as a gentle beating as the extensor and flexor muscles attempt to remain in balance. This same neuromuscular sign can be demonstrated in many patients with hepatic encephalopathy as the so-called 'milkmaid's grip' – when asked to squeeze the examiner's fingers at a constant pressure, the patient is unable to maintain a tonic contraction and instead 'milks' the gripped fingers with subtle clonic contractions and relaxations. Many patients with hepatic encephalopathy have a fetor hepaticus – musty, sweet-smelling breath, probably due to high levels of mercaptans in the circulation. More formal techniques for demonstrating the presence or severity of hepatic encephalopathy are discussed later in this chapter.

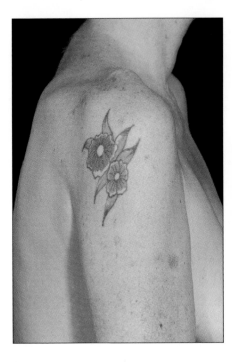

Fig. 4.19 *Tattoos and spider naevi. Tattooing in a patient with chronic hepatitis C infection. A more likely route of acquiring the virus was the patient's previous history of intravenous drug abuse. This picture also demonstrates multiple spider naevi.*

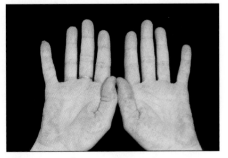

Fig. 4.20 *Palmar erythema. A common sign in cirrhosis, particularly that of alcoholic origin, erythema can also be found in thyrotoxicosis, rheumatoid disease, pregnancy and sometimes as a variation of normal.*

Abdominal palpation may uncover a range of physical signs in patients with liver disease. The liver may be palpable and should be checked for tenderness (as in venous congestion or acute hepatitis), pulsatility (in tricuspid regurgitation, for example) or an irregular outline (which may suggest metastatic disease). The size of the liver in cirrhosis varies, some patients having a small shrunken organ whilst others have a more easily palpable or obviously enlarged liver. Splenomegaly may be present if there is portal hypertension.

Depending on whether ascites (see pp. 263–265) is tense, moderate or mild, the intra-abdominal fluid may be detected by demonstrating a fluid thrill, shifting dullness or a positive ascitic 'puddle' sign. In this latter manoeuvre, smaller amounts of peritoneal fluid manifest as peri-umbilical dullness when the patient adopts a position on all fours.

INVESTIGATIONS

BLOOD BIOCHEMISTRY

Measurements of serum bilirubin, aminotransferases, alkaline phosphatase, gamma-glutamyl transpeptidase (γGT) and albumin are popularly referred to as 'liver function tests' or LFTs (Fig. 4.21). In many cases, such tests may detect asymptomatic liver and biliary diseases prior to clinical presentation.

The tests can be grouped into three main categories. Elevations in the aminotransferase enzymes (also known as transaminases), alanine aminotransferase (ALT) and aspartate aminotransferase (AST) usually reflect some degree of hepatocellular injury or inflammation. On the other hand, pathology affecting the intra- or extrahepatic biliary tree

Biochemical liver function tests

Marker	Normal Range	Significance
Bilirubin	5–18 μmol/l	Non-specifically raised in liver disease, but also in haemolysis and biliary obstruction. In isolation, may suggest inherited hyperbilirubinaemia
AST ALT	5–40 iu/l 5–35 iu/l	Raised following inflammation or necrosis of hepatocytes. Usually not necessary to measure both. However, AST:ALT ratio of >2 suggestive of alcoholic hepatitis
Alkaline phosphatase γGT	30–130 iu/l 5–50 iu/l	Usually raised together in cholestasis, biliary obstruction or hepatic infiltration. Alkaline phosphatase also produced by bone, intestine and placenta
Albumin	35–45 g/l	Reflects synthetic function of liver. However, levels also fall with malabsorption, protein-losing enteropathy, critical illnesses ('reverse' acute-phase protein), burns and nephrotic syndrome
Lactate dehydrogenase	240–524 iu/l	Low sensitivity and specificity for liver disease. May be highest in ischaemic hepatitis. Levels also raised after muscle damage or haemolysis

Fig. 4.21 Biochemical liver function tests. Abbreviations are explained in the text. As normal values can vary between laboratories, readers are advised to check with their local clinical chemistry department.

leads to elevations in the alkaline phosphatase or γGT. The third group can be said to represent the synthetic function of the liver and includes the production of albumin, urea and clotting factors (see below). In the setting of acute liver failure, the blood glucose and arterial pH can also be considered as surrogate markers of hepatic functional reserve. Bilirubin can be raised in most types of hepatobiliary pathology.

These 'rules' are frequently broken, however, and there is often considerable overlap between hepatitic and cholestatic patterns. For example, extrahepatic biliary obstruction will cause a raised bilirubin, alkaline phosphatase and γGT, but there is almost invariably some irritation and secondary inflammation of the hepatocytes caused by the biliary obstruction. Consequently, there will usually be at least a mild rise in serum transaminases. The converse is also frequently true. Most significant forms of hepatitis often lead to a variable degree of cholestasis and there may be a consequent rise in alkaline phosphatase and γGT. Hence, most clinicians work on the basis of pattern recognition, picking out what seems to be the 'dominant' distribution of raised enzymes.

As highlighted in **Fig. 4.22**, these biochemical measurements can give rise to occasional diagnostic pitfalls. It is important to remember the possibilities of extrahepatic disease, particularly where the pattern of abnormal LFTs seems unusual or if there is just one abnormal value. It would be unusual, for example, to have a serum AST value twenty

Diagnostic pitfalls and unusual patterns of abnormal liver function tests	
Situation	**Possible explanation**
Isolated raised transaminase	Consider non-hepatic source, e.g. myositis, myocardial infarction, haemolysis
Isolated raised γGT	Consider alcohol excess, but may also be raised with enzyme-inducing drugs, early hepatic infiltration and fatty liver (hepatic steatosis)
Isolated raised alkaline phosphatase with normal γGT	Consider extrahepatic source. In practice, this is usually of bony origin and the levels of calcium, phosphate, parathyroid hormone and vitamin D should be checked. Most laboratories can measure alkaline phosphatase isoenzymes
Isolated hyperbilirubinaemia	Exclude haemolysis and Gilbert's syndrome

Fig. 4.22 *Diagnostic pitfalls and unusual patterns of abnormal liver function tests.*

times the normal upper limit with otherwise completely normal LFTs – a non-hepatic source should also be considered, such as muscle, and there is always the remote possibility of laboratory error.

Haemostasis and the liver

Haemostatic abnormalities and liver disease often go hand in hand (**Fig. 4.23**). This reflects not just the liver's role as the source of plasma proteins and clotting factors, but also its production of the proteins that normally inhibit coagulation, control fibrinolysis or cause activation of fibrinolysis. Many patients with liver disease have thrombocytopenia and deficiencies of vitamin K or vitamin C. The prothrombin time (or its international normalised ratio, INR) is the parameter that is most widely used for prognostic purposes, such as in the Child–Pugh score (see p. 254). Similarly, prolongation of the prothrombin time is one of the criteria used to determine the need for liver transplantation in acute liver failure. The prothrombin time is particularly sensitive to deficiencies in clotting factors V, VII and X. Vitamin K is required for the synthesis of factors II, VII, IX and X, acting as a cofactor for the γ-carboxylation of their glutamate residues. Each time this reaction occurs, an epoxide of vitamin K is formed. The enzyme that converts it back to the active form, vitamin K epoxide reductase, is the therapeutic target of warfarin.

A deficiency of active vitamin K, whether due to anticoagulation, dietary deficiency or malabsorption, will have the net effect of prolonging the prothrombin time. Since hepatic stores of the vitamin are limited, a deficiency state can result within 4 weeks of dietary withdrawal. The accuracy of the prolonged prothrombin time in assessing the liver's synthetic capacity is best confirmed by excluding vitamin K deficiency with an intravenous injection of 10 mg of the vitamin at least 12 hours prior to repeating the test.

Immunological tests

Measurement of autoantibodies can be very useful in the diagnosis of liver and biliary disease and is discussed on pages 213, 238–242. A positive anti-smooth muscle antibody

Haemostatic abnormalities in liver disease

Reduced clotting factor synthesis	Hepatocellular dysfunction Vitamin K deficiency (dietary or due to malabsorption)
Reduced production of coagulation inhibitors	Antithrombin III Protein C Protein S
Increased fibrinolysis	Diminished production of tissue plasminogen activator inhibitor (TPA-I)
Qualitatively abnormal clotting factors	Dysfibrinogenaemia (excessive sialysation of fibrinogen molecule) may cause prolonged thrombin time
Disseminated intravascular coagulation (DIC)	Low-grade DIC often present in cirrhosis May reflect endotoxaemia and poor clearance of activated clotting factors
Thrombocytopenia	Hypersplenism Chronic hepatitis C infection
Capillary fragility	Vitamin C deficiency
Increased thrombotic risk	Antiphospholipid antibodies (anticardiolipin antibodies, lupus anticoagulant) more common in chronic hepatitis C

Fig. 4.23 *Haemostatic abnormalities in liver disease.*

may suggest autoimmune chronic active hepatitis, anti-mitochondrial antibodies are found in primary biliary cirrhosis and a pANCA (perinuclear anti-neutrophil cytoplasmic antibody) is often found in primary sclerosing cholangitis. A number of autoantibodies, particularly against the thyroid gland, have been described in chronic hepatitis C. There is often a degree of overlap between these various autoantibodies and their disease associations.

Patients with autoimmune hepatitis may demonstrate a raised serum level of IgG, whilst IgM is often raised in primary biliary cirrhosis and IgA in alcoholic liver disease.

Markers of metabolic liver diseases

In α_1-antitrypsin deficiency the diagnosis is confirmed by measuring the serum level of the enzyme. With haemochromatosis and Wilson's disease, the tests are a little more complicated. As discussed later in this chapter, genetic haemochromatosis is characterised by iron overload affecting a whole range of organ systems. The serum iron and ferritin levels are usually elevated, but these can fluctuate in other disease states. Measurement of transferrin saturation is also helpful and there is now a genetic test that can be performed on peripheral blood. With Wilson's disease, the serum copper and caeruloplasmin are usually reduced but again these levels may fluctuate in other liver diseases too. As in haemochromatosis, a liver biopsy may be very valuable but another sensitive and specific test for Wilson's disease is the measurement of 24-hour urinary copper excretion, before and after a penicillamine challenge.

Tumour markers

The most widely applicable tumour marker in the context of liver disease is α-fetoprotein (AFP), which is raised in about 80% of cases of hepatocellular carcinoma. The protein is expressed by dividing hepatocytes and by peribiliary oval cells and so modest elevations are often seen in the context of liver regeneration or during chronic hepatitis. A series of progressive rises in the AFP level, however, should raise the suspicion of a developing carcinoma. The marker is also produced by some germ cell tumours.

Recently, a number of tumour markers based mostly on epithelial mucins have been described for adenocarcinomas of the biliary tract and pancreas. One example is CA19–9, produced by a wide range of gastrointestinal epithelia. Elevated serum levels are found in about 70% of bile duct cancers, 50% of hepatocellular carcinomas, 40% of gastric adenocarcinomas and 30% of colonic cancers. As with many tests, sensitivity and specificity depend on the chosen cut-off value, but the presence of a CA19–9 value above 40 iu/l is 75–90% sensitive and 80–95% specific for ductal pancreatic cancer. Importantly, the specificity of a raised CA19-9 deteriorates rapidly in the presence of jaundice, and many non-neoplastic conditions that 'irritate' the biliary tree (such as cholangitis or choledocholithiasis) or pancreas (such as chronic pancreatitis) may lead to elevated levels. A related marker, CAM17–1, is currently being evaluated in clinical studies and appears to be of potential use in the diagnosis of pancreatic cancer.

QUANTITATIVE TESTS OF LIVER FUNCTION

Although frequently of use to the researcher, most of the described methods of quantifying dynamic liver function (**Fig. 4.24**) have had little clinical impact. The Child–Pugh score and the blood tests listed above are more widely used.

Quantitative tests generally rely on the liver's ability to clear an administered substance from the blood. In the case of drugs with a high first-pass metabolism (such as lignocaine or indocyanine green) this can be heavily influenced by changes in the rate of liver blood flow. Those which assess clearance of substances with a low first-pass metabolism (such as antipyrine) give a more accurate reflection of hepatocyte function.

DIAGNOSTIC RADIOLOGY

Plain radiography

The plain abdominal X-ray is generally less valuable in hepatopancreaticobiliary disease than in other forms of digestive disease. There are, however, some important exceptions. Calcified tissue is easily demonstrated, whether this be chronic calcific pancreatitis, calcium-containing gallstones (10–20% of all gallstones are radio-opaque), the walls of hydatid liver cysts or the so-called porcelain gall bladder (**Fig. 4.25**). Gas may be visible in the biliary tree after damage to the ampulla of Vater caused by passing a gallstone, following an endoscopic sphincterotomy or after the formation of a choledochoenteric fistula.

Ultrasound scanning

Transcutaneous ultrasound. The ultrasound scan is generally the first-line imaging test for hepatobiliary and pancreatic disease. It is particularly suited for imaging focal liver lesions and the gall bladder (**Fig. 4.26**) and for determining the presence of biliary tract obstruction.

Focal liver lesions are usually detected when above 1 cm in diameter and the experienced ultrasonographer can distinguish cysts, abscesses, haemangiomas and malignant neoplasms. Subtle, diffuse hepatic changes can sometimes be difficult to identify although the hyperechogenicity of a fatty liver is usually detectable.

Quantitative tests of liver function

^{14}C Aminopyrine breath test	Taken by mouth, aminopyrine is demethylated by hepatic cytochrome p450, releasing $^{14}CO_2$. Overall results reflect functional hepatocyte mass.
Galactose elimination test	After i.v. injection, galactose eliminated by hepatic galactokinase. Useful measure of reserve, but may be affected by extrahepatic metabolism
Caffeine clearance	Demethylated by cytochrome p448. Easily affected by drug interactions and cigarette smoking
MEGX test	Lignocaine converted to MEGX metabolite by cytochrome p450. Correlates less well with hepatic function than aminopyrine or galactose tests
Asialoglycoprotein receptor assay	Uses ^{99}Tc-labelled asialoglycoprotein analogue to measure scintillation density of liver receptors. Normally, these receptors are ubiquitously expressed by hepatocytes and clear circulating asialoglycoproteins. Good correlation with functional hepatocyte mass
Indocyanine green clearance	Dye is taken up almost exclusively by hepatocytes and excreted unchanged in bile. Serial blood levels measured after i.v. injection. Good correlation with hepatocyte mass. Rare instances of anaphylaxis

Fig. 4.24 *Quantitative tests of liver function.*

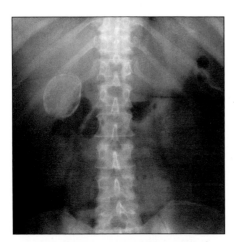

Fig. 4.25 *Porcelain gall bladder. This plain abdominal radiograph demonstrates the severe intramural calcification of the gall bladder which may be, but is not always, associated with chronic cholecystitis. Its main significance is the marked tendency to develop gall-bladder carcinoma (up to 20% of cases).*

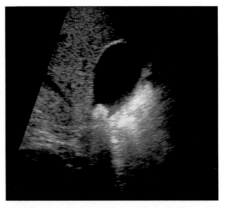

Fig. 4.26 *Ultrasound scanning of the gall bladder. The classical appearance of a gallstone. The gall bladder appears as the black, fluid-filled cystic space adjacent to the liver parenchyma and the gallstone is the bright focal lesion at its inferior edge. Projecting below the stone is a typical dark 'acoustic shadow'.*

The addition of real-time Doppler scanning increases the sensitivity and specificity of ultrasound scans and is also an excellent method of assessing vascular structures and blood flow. It is consequently very useful in detecting hepatic venous thrombosis, portal venous thrombosis and, particularly after liver transplantation, hepatic artery ischaemia or occlusion. Doppler affords the detection of reversed portal vein flow in portal hypertension and the development of collaterals (such as splenic 'varices') and can assess flow through portosystemic shunts.

Endoscopic and laparoscopic ultrasound. Imaging can be further refined by using endoscopic and laparoscopic probes to visualise the pancreas, biliary tree or liver. These images, however, can be difficult to interpret, require experienced operators and are relatively expensive. Even so, pancreaticobiliary imaging is likely to join the staging of oesophageal tumours as one of the areas in which endoscopic ultrasound may be useful.

Contrast enhancement. In order to increase the discrimination of focal liver lesions, a number of different intravenously injected ultrasound contrast agents are being developed. An example is the use of injected microbubbles of air or carbon dioxide; these oscillate rapidly in the presence of an ultrasound signal to give off a high-intensity signal. One such commercially available agent, known as Levovist (**Fig. 4.27**), shows promise in enhancing the appearance of liver tumours and may help to distinguish benign from malignant nodules in cirrhosis.

Computed tomography CT

This method of cross-sectional imaging displays the abdomen as a series of slices viewed as if looking from below. Conventional CT scans are now gradually being superseded by spiral CT. Spiral CT scans acquire their images much faster and the examination can be completed with just one breath-hold. Resolution is also increased so that small lesions are more easily identifiable.

Compared to ultrasound scanning, CT has the advantage of displaying all the abdominal organs on the same image plain and without major artefacts due to bowel gas or subcutaneous fat. The use of an intravenous contrast agent enhances the appearance of vascular lesions (**Fig. 4.28**); scans can clearly discriminate between different causes of abdominal masses (**Fig. 4.29**) and aid the staging of malignant disease (**Fig. 4.30**). The rapid acquisition of images, combined with the use of intravenous contrast, enables the

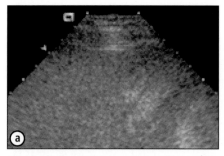 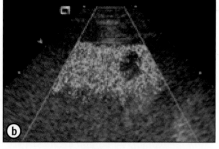

Fig. 4.27 *Levovist® scanning. A liver metastasis from a pancreatic adenocarcinoma. (a) Conventional grey-scale Doppler ultrasound (b) Colour Doppler mode 3 minutes after the injection of a microbubble contrast agent. The tumour is barely detectable on the grey-scale view, but is clearly defined with the Levovist® technique as an area of low-signal intensity. This is because metastases do not take up the microbubbles during the hepatic phase of scanning and so appear as defects on the colour images.*

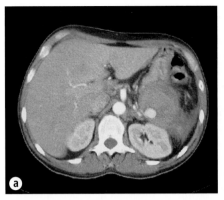 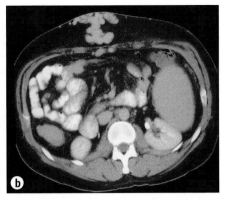

Fig. 4.28 *Computed tomography. (a) This intravenous contrast-enhanced abdominal CT scan shows a pseudoaneurysm of the splenic artery with a surrounding haematoma that has developed following pancreatitis. The pseudoaneurysm is visible as the large white spot just anterior to the patient's left kidney. (b) An incidental example of vascular enhancement, this abdominal CT scan shows the 'caput medusae', venous collaterals clearly visible on the anterior abdominal wall in a man with portal hypertension.*

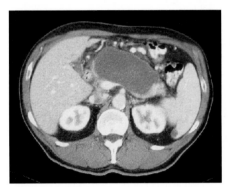 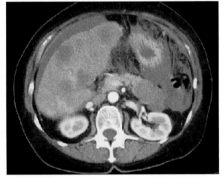

Fig. 4.29 *Pancreatic pseudocyst. The fluid-filled mass in the anterior abdomen is a large pseudocyst that has replaced much of the pancreas as a complication of acute pancreatitis.*

Fig. 4.30 *Staging of pancreatic adenocarcinoma. This contrast-enhanced scan shows a large low attenuation mass replacing the tail of the pancreas (visible just anterior to the patient's left kidney). There are also multiple liver metastases and ascites.*

radiologist to view the images at different vascular phases after the intravenous injection. This 'biphasic' scanning technique is very useful in assessing the vascularity of liver lesions such as haemangiomas.

CT arterioportography requires placement of a catheter in the coeliac axis or superior mesenteric artery, allowing a higher delivery of contrast that greatly increases the sensitivity for diagnosing small metastatic deposits in the liver.

Oral cholecystography

With the recent advances in biliary tract imaging, the oral cholecystogram is being used less and less. It involves taking an oral contrast agent, such as iopanoic acid or sodium iopodate, that is absorbed and then excreted in the bile. Radiographs are then taken in varying positions so that the biliary tract is free from overlying bowel gas.

Oral cholecystography has probably been of most use in the selection of patients for non-surgical treatment of gallstones. It is of little benefit in jaundiced patients as insufficient contrast enters the biliary tree and it is similarly inappropriate in extensive small bowel or pancreatic disease as not enough oral contrast is absorbed.

Percutaneous transhepatic cholangiography (PTC)

The development of improved catheters and guide-wire techniques in the 1970s led to the advent of fine-needle PTC as both an important diagnostic and therapeutic tool. Although much of its diagnostic role has been usurped by ERCP (see below) it remains a very valuable tool for diagnosing biliary tract disease, particularly where the bile ducts are occluded or ERCP has been unsuccessful.

PTC involves a long thin (0.7 mm diameter) needle advancing into the liver under aseptic conditions and radiography screening control. The bile ducts are punctured and the position is confirmed by intraductal injection of non-ionic contrast medium. In view of the hepatic puncture required, patients should be kept under close observation for 24 hours post-procedure for signs of haemorrhage or biliary peritonitis.

PTC also has an important therapeutic role, allowing percutaneous drainage and relief of jaundice due to malignant biliary obstruction in particular. Self-expanding metallic stents can also be inserted.

It is usually a very successful technique in experienced hands (biliary puncture rates of 95–100% if the system is dilated) and overall complication rates are between 5 and 10%. These complications can be serious, though, and include haemorrhage, biliary peritonitis, sepsis and death. Consequenctly, the main contraindication is coagulopathy and this should be reversed (for instance, by vitamin K or fresh frozen plasma if the prothrombin time is prolonged) prior to the procedure. Broad-spectrum antibiotics are also given to cover the procedure.

Endoscopic retrograde cholangiopancreatography (ERCP)

Diagnostic ERCP allows the inspection and cannulation of the ampulla of Vater, with the ability to inject contrast and visualise the pancreatic ductal system, biliary tree and gall bladder. Specimens can be obtained from suspected neoplastic lesions for cytopathological analysis and samples of bile or pancreatic juice can be aspirated. It is now possible to study biliary dysmotility with sphincter of Oddi manometry. Importantly, ERCP also offers therapeutic techniques such as the removal of impacted ductal stones, stenting of strictures and sphincterotomy.

After a 6-hour fast, the patient lies in the left lateral position and is sedated, usually using an intravenous combination of pethidine and a benzodiazepine. Prophylactic antibiotics are usually given and are essential in cases with suspected biliary obstruction, a history of cholangitis, pancreatic pseudocyst and in the elderly who are at greatest risk. Antibiotic policies differ between units, but oral ciprofloxacin is as effective as intravenous cefuroxime.

A special side-viewing endoscope is passed and the oesophagus, stomach and duodenum inspected before reaching the ampulla. Cannulation is then made slightly easier by limiting duodenal peristalsis with an injection of hyoscine or glucagon. As the cannula is introduced, small amounts of contrast agent (such as iopromide) are injected under X-ray screening control. By selecting the pancreatic or common bile ducts, the biliary tree and pancreas can be clearly demonstrated (**Fig. 4.31**) and radiographs taken of their appearance. Cannulation of the ampulla may be rendered difficult or impossible by previous surgery such as a Billroth II gastrojejunostomy or a Roux-en-Y choledochojejunostomy.

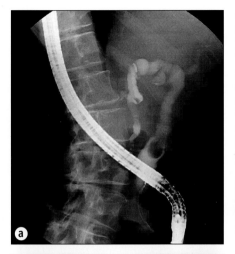

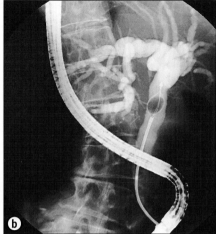

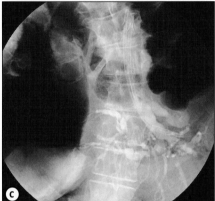

Fig. 4.31 *ERCP for impacted gallstones. (a) An impacted gallstone in the common bile duct. The stone itself is visible as the round black shadow within the contrast medium and there is obvious dilatation of the obstructed biliary system. The metallic shadow of the endoscope gives a useful comparison of size. (b) The endoscopist extracts the stone using a wire basket, having previously widened the ampulla with a sphincterotomy to permit its easy removal. (c) To facilitate the free drainage of bile and remaining stones, two biliary stents are inserted and left* in situ.

Depending on the pathology encountered, various therapeutic procedures may be performed. These include facilitating biliary drainage and stone extraction with a sphincterotomy, balloon dilatation of strictures, crushing of gallstones using a mechanical lithotripter, insertion of biliary or pancreatic stents (**Fig. 4.32**) and removal of stones using a balloon catheter sweep or wire basket.

ERCP can be extremely helpful in many situations (**Fig. 4.33**) but it is important to appreciate the risks of the procedure. In addition to the usual dangers of sedation and endoscopic intubation, the complications of ERCP (particularly following therapeutic procedures) include haemorrhage, intestinal perforation, acute pancreatitis and cholangitis. These serious adverse events occur in 2–5% of cases and overall the procedural mortality rate is 0.1–0.2%.

Magnetic resonance imaging (MRI)

Using MRI technology, it is possible to obtain high-quality cross-sectional images of the liver, biliary tree and pancreas. The ability to tailor the image acquisition process has the potential to make MRI the modality of choice for imaging focal liver lesions (**Fig. 4.34**). Tissue-specific contrast materials can be administered, such as manganese chelates that are taken up by hepatocytes (**Fig. 4.35**) or iron oxide particles that are absorbed by Kupffer

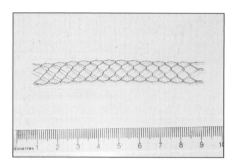

Fig. 4.32 *Self-expanding metallic ERCP stent. This device is inserted across a stricture by first passing a guide-wire and then 'railroading' the stent into position. Metallic stents have higher long-term patency rates, particularly in malignant strictures, but are more expensive than polyethylene ones.*

Indications for ERCP	
Diagnostic	
Suspected biliary tract disease	Investigation of jaundice, abnormal LFTs or bile duct dilatation on ultrasound scan
Suspected pancreatic disease	Possible neoplasm
	Assessment of chronic pancreatitis
Therapeutic	
Choledocholithiasis	Sphincterotomy or balloon dilatation of ampulla
	Lithotripsy (mechanical, extracorporeal shockwave or laser-induced)
	Stone extraction
	Biliary drainage (endoprosthetic stent or nasobiliary tube)
Acute cholangitis	Sphincterotomy
	Stone extraction
	Drainage
Pancreatic or bile duct strictures	Stent placement
	Balloon dilatation
Ampullary or bile duct dysmotility	Sphincterotomy
	Ampullary dilatation
Acute gallstone pancreatitis	Sphincterotomy
	Stone extraction
Chronic pancreatitis	Stone extraction (if applicable)
	Consider sphinecterotomy, stent insertion

Fig. 4.33 *Indications for ERCP.*

cells, in order to maximise resolution. By using specially adapted non-magnetic equipment, therapeutic procedures can be performed with MRI guidance. Thermal ablation of tumours can be more accurately targeted using heat-sensitive image sequences (**Fig. 4.36**) that give real-time feedback on the extent of tissue damage.

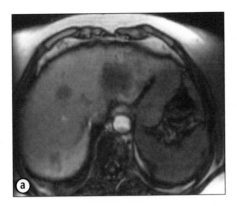

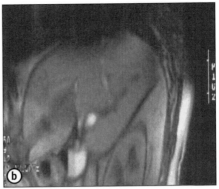

Fig. 4.34 *Magnetic resonance imaging of the liver. One useful aspect of MRI is the ability to acquire views in more than one plane. (a) An axial view, similar to that used for CT scanning, demonstrating multiple low-density liver metastases from a colonic adenocarcinoma. (b) In a different patient with liver metastases, similar low-density areas can be seen in the coronal plane. The diminished resolution is due to this scan being taken in an open-configuration 0.5 Tesla magnet used for interventional procedures, which has a lower resolution than the 'conventional' 1.5 Tesla magnet.*

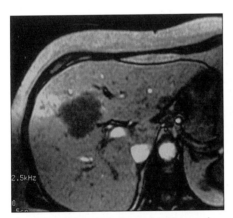

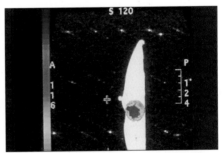

Fig. 4.35 *Contrast-enhanced MRI scanning of the liver. Using MnDpDp, a manganese chelate that is selectively taken up by normal hepatocytes, this scan shows a hepatocellular carcinoma as a clearly defined area of low intensity.*

Fig. 4.36 *Thermal-sensitive MRI. Special colourisation sequences allow a spectrum of appearances that represent different temperatures within a tissue. Here, a liver tumour is undergoing thermal ablation, with the red colour corresponding to a temperature above 60°C (and therefore causing necrosis). By monitoring the energy delivered in this way, the radiologist is able to deliver therapy in a more precise manner.*

187

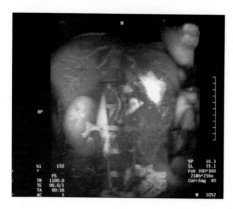

Fig. 4.37 *Magnetic resonance cholangiopancreatography (MRCP). An obvious obstruction of the common bile duct (arrowed), with consequent dilatation of the proximal biliary tree.*

Magnetic resonance cholangiopancreatography (MRCP)

MRCP is a relatively recent development that can produce high-quality images of the pancreas and biliary tract without requiring an endoscope, injection of contrast or exposure to radiation. The pictures obtained are strikingly similar to those gathered using ERCP (**Fig. 4.37**).

Magnetic resonance spectroscopy (MRS)

MRS is a non-invasive technique that allows the indirect measurement of various metabolites *in vivo* (**Fig. 4.38**). This can provide important localised information on hepatic biochemistry. An example of a hepatic phosphorus-31 spectrum is shown in (**Fig. 4.39**). This is still a research tool at present, but it has already been shown that certain pathological conditions have characteristic 'metabolic fingerprints' on MRS.

Radionuclide imaging

The reticuloendothelial elements of the liver cause it to be delineated on scintigraphic scans that use radiolabelled white cells or colloid, but these are relatively inefficient ways of studying its anatomy or function. Better information can be gained by using radiopharmaceuticals that are excreted in the bile and these can be particularly helpful in studying the actions of the gall bladder in suspected acute cholecystitis.

Technetium-labelled hepatic iminodiacetic acid (HIDA) is one such agent, being taken up by the liver within 5 minutes of an intravenous injection. Scanning over the next 30 minutes progressively reveals the gall bladder, common bile duct and duodenum. Failure of the gall bladder to be visualised within 30–40 minutes usually occurs in acute cholecystitis, as obstruction of the cystic duct is present in 95% of cases. A patchy distribution of HIDA excretion over the biliary tree is sometimes seen in cases of sclerosing cholangitis. Other uses for HIDA scanning include the detection of biliary leaks after laparoscopic cholecystectomy and the study of acalculous biliary pain. In this latter group, failure of the gall bladder to eject more than 40% of its volume after an infusion of CCK on HIDA scanning defines patients who might benefit from cholecystectomy despite normal ultrasound scanning.

The majority of neuroendocrine tumours that arise in the gastrointestinal tract express somatostatin receptors on their surface. By radiolabelling somatostatin analogues such as octreotide (**Fig. 4.40**), scintigraphy can be used in their localisation. False negatives occur

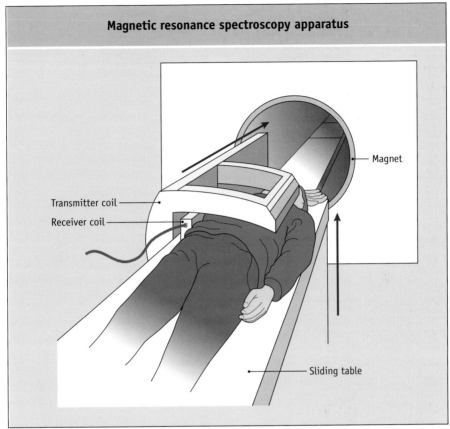

Magnetic resonance spectroscopy apparatus

Transmitter coil

Receiver coil

Magnet

Sliding table

Fig. 4.38 *Magnetic resonance spectroscopy apparatus. A patient is about to be placed in the MR scanner for a spectroscopic examination of the liver. The transmitter coil emits an MR pulse and the overlying receiver coil picks up the radiofrequency signal subsequently given off by the liver. This signal encodes the biochemical information that is the basis of MR spectroscopy.*

in about 10–20% of cases and, as splenic tissue usually actively binds the analogue, ectopic splenic tissue (such as a pancreatic splenunculus) can be a rare cause of a falsely positive 'hot spot'.

Vascular imaging

Angiographic assessment of tumours (**Fig. 4.41**) can be invaluable when planning surgery, and areas of vascular displacement, invasion or tumour 'blush' may be demonstrated. Arteriovenous malformations (AVMs) can also be revealed (see **Fig. 7.3**). Selective transcatheter arterial embolisation can be used to stop hepatic bleeding (following percutaneous liver biopsy, for example), to block AVMs or to cause necrosis of intrahepatic tumours (see chapter 6).

Venography is used extensively in the diagnosis of obstructed hepatic veins (Budd–Chiari syndrome, see below), but recent developments in interventional radiology have opened up a series of new uses for venous imaging in patients with liver disease.

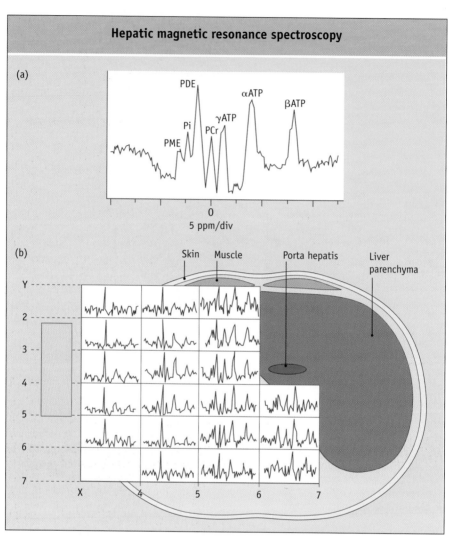

Fig. 4.39 *Hepatic magnetic resonance spectroscopy. (a) ^{31}P spectroscopy is a non-invasive source of information about the levels of important metabolites such as the three (α, β and γ) ATP signals in a characteristic 'spectrum' (b) These can be localised to different areas of the liver, giving valuable information about cell membrane turnover and hepatic gluconeogenesis. A typical phosphorus-31 MR spectrum of the liver in vivo contains six resonances: phosphomonoesters (PME) – cell membrane precursors and intermediates of carbohydrate metabolism; inorganic phosphate (Pi); phosphodiesters (PDE) – cell membrane degradation products, endoplasmic reticulum and intermediates of carbohydrate metabolism; and three resonances attributable to ATP. Phosphocreatine (PCr) is derived from overlying muscle.*

Intravascular pressure can be measured and, using balloon inflation 'wedge' techniques, the portal pressure can be determined. The pressure gradient between the portal and hepatic venous systems is generally an accurate guide to the degree of portal hypertension, but can underestimate the severity if there is a presinusoidal component.

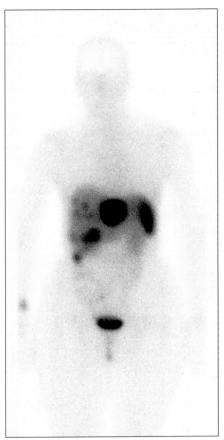

Fig. 4.40 *Octreotide scintigraphy. Radiolabelled somatostation analogues such as ^{123}I Tyr-octreotide can be used to localise the 80–90% of neuroendocrine tumours that express somatostatin receptors. In this example, there is an area of increased uptake in the head of the pancreas due to an islet cell tumour, with multiple liver metastases shown as 'hot spots'.*

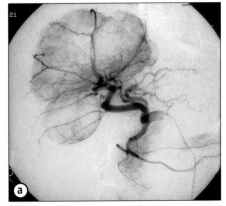

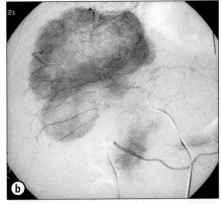

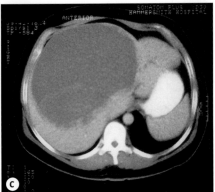

Fig. 4.41 *Hepatic arteriography. (a) Wide displacement of the normal arterial branches during the arterial phase. (b) This was followed by a tumour 'blush' of abnormal circulation in the venous phase, caused by a large cystic liver mass. Histology revealed this to be a non-functioning neuroendocrine tumour. (c) CT scan of the same patient.*

At the same time as the hepatic veins are cannulated, it is possible to take a sample of liver histology by advancing a needle into the hepatic parenchyma (a transjugular liver biopsy, as discussed below). This can be particularly helpful where coagulopathy precludes conventional percutaneous biopsy.

The jugular to hepatic venous route can also be used to create a small transjugular intrahepatic portosystemic shunt (TIPSS) to reduce portal pressure. The TIPSS procedure is described on page 261.

Pancreatic neuroendocrine tumours are frequently very small and hard to localise by cross-sectional imaging. Selective venous sampling at venography, although technically demanding, can detect the tumour site in over 80% of cases.

LIVER BIOPSY

The histological assessment of a biopsy specimen can be considered the 'gold standard' for the diagnosis and assessment of liver disease. However, a liver biopsy is not a procedure to be undertaken lightly and certainly not by the inexperienced. In the right hands, the risk of a complication occurring is relatively small, but is still appreciable and potentially life-threatening.

A liver biopsy is most commonly performed in the setting of known or suspected chronic liver disease, but is also carried out in some cases of acute liver dysfunction, particularly where routine serological tests have been unhelpful (by the transjugular route if there is coagulopathy), and is also extremely valuable in assessing the integrity of liver grafts post-transplant. The histological assessment may be necessary to clinch a diagnosis (for instance, whether or not cirrhosis is present) or to grade the severity of known pathology (such as chronic active hepatitis).

Methodology

Samples for histological assessment can be taken in a number of ways (**Fig. 4.42**), but the most widely used is that of percutaneous sampling using a Menghini or Tru-Cut needle.

Liver biopsy techniques	
Method	**Features**
Percutaneous biopsy	Most simple methodology Note contraindications (see Fig. 4.44) Use Menghini, Tru-Cut or spring-loaded device +/− Ultrasound guidance
Plugged biopsy	Similar to above Needle track plugged with gelatine sponge material if mild to moderate coagulopathy
Transjugular liver biopsy	Useful if significant coagulopathy Multiple biopsies can be taken Samples may be smaller or more fragmented
Laparoscopic liver biopsy	Useful in assessing malignancy Allows targeted biopsy of lesions and inspection of peritoneum

Fig. 4.42 *Liver biopsy techniques.*

The core of liver tissue is aspirated up into the Menghini needle using a vacuum syringe technique, whilst the Tru-Cut has a cutting sheath that slices a small streak of liver into the device.

The pathologist may be assisted by special staining techniques for iron (**Fig. 4.43**), fat collagen, viruses, α_1-antitrypsin or hepatotropic viruses. Samples can also be sent for biochemical analysis, to estimate the total hepatic iron or copper content.

Contraindications

There are some important contraindications to the procedure (**Fig. 4.44**) and thorough consideration should be given to the risk:benefit ratio before performing a liver biopsy in

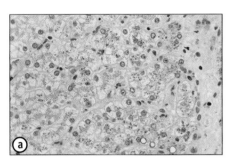 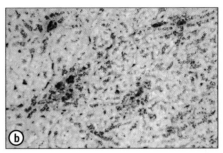

Fig. 4.43 Hepatic iron overload. High-power views of liver biopsy specimens taken from a young man with a history of multiple blood transfusions for thalassaemia. (a) The iron deposition is visible as brown granules in the haematoxylin and eosin (H&E) stain. (b) This is made much more obvious with Perl's stain, which colours the haemosiderin bright blue. In this case, the iron has been predominantly taken up by Kupffer cells, but there is also deposition within portal tract septae and the hepatocytes themselves. Hepatic iron deposition also occurs in alcoholic liver disease and primary haemochromatosis.

Contraindications to percutaneous liver biopsy	
Coagulopathy	Increased risk of bleeding Avoid if prothrombin time prolonged by > 3 secs or platelet count < 90×10^9/l
Uncooperative patient	Patient needs to be able to perform specific breath-hold during procedure May be impossible if encephalopathic, dyspnoeic or educationally subnormal
Significant ascites	More mobile, 'floating' liver Increases bleeding risk Consider performing procedure after ascites drained or use transjugular route
Extrahepatic biliary obstruction	Dilated biliary tree increases chances of bile duct or gall bladder injury If absolutely necessary, biopsy may be possible under imaging control

Fig. 4.44 Contraindications to percutaneous liver biopsy.

any patient. Because of the increased risk of haemorrhage, percutaneous biopsy should be avoided in patients with impaired clotting or low platelet counts. It is the author's practice to perform the procedure only if the prothrombin time is within 3 seconds of the upper limit of normal and the platelet count is above $90 \times 10^9/l$. Vitamin K (if there is sufficient time) or fresh frozen plasma can be given to correct mild to moderate clotting impairment, and thrombocytopenic patients can be given pooled platelet transfusions, ideally with measurement of the increment before biopsying. In many centres, 'plugged' biopsies are performed in cases of mild coagulopathy; a sterile gelfoam material is injected into the track as the biopsy is withdrawn. If a liver biopsy is really necessary in the setting of significant coagulopathy it should be carried out by the transjugular route.

Significant ascites results in a relatively more mobile liver that tends to increase the risk of intraperitoneal bleeding. The fluid should be drained prior to the procedure. In view of the liver's subdiaphragmatic location, patients need to hold their breath briefly in expiration as the biopsy is taken. Those unable to cooperate, whether due to confusion or dyspnoea, would be at much higher risk of liver trauma and percutaneous biopsy should be avoided.

Complications

Complications are uncommon but potentially life-threatening. The most obvious is haemorrhage, with bleeding occurring either into the liver itself (and subcapsular haematomas can be particularly painful), into the biliary tree (presenting as haemobilia) or into the peritoneum. For this reason, patients are kept on bed rest, usually for 6–7 hours post-procedure, with close monitoring of pulse and blood pressure.

Significant haemorrhage should be managed with the usual resuscitation and correction of clotting abnormalities; the bleeding source should be treated with selective embolisation at arteriography (if facilities are immediately available) or by laparotomy.

Surrounding structures may be damaged by a misdirected needle, with consequences such as pneumothorax, biliary peritonitis (due to gall bladder perforation) or penetration of adjacent bowel. Bacteraemia is well described, especially in the immunocompromised, and seeding of malignant cells may occur in the needle track after biopsying hepatic tumours. Based on a prospective audit carried out by the British Society of Gastroenterology, haemorrhage occurs in about 1–2% of cases, although only half of these require transfusion. The overall mortality risk in this audit was estimated at between 0.1 and 0.3%.

The most common 'complication' is that of pain, either at the biopsy site, radiating across the upper abdomen or occurring in the right shoulder tip. This can be minimised by carefully explaining the procedure (and its risks) to the patient beforehand, by using adequate local anaesthetic at the biopsy site and by making provision for parenteral analgesia (such as intramuscular pethidine) afterwards.

The risk of bleeding rises greatly if more than two 'passes' of the needle are made. If no adequate specimen is obtained after two attempts, the procedure should be abandoned and repeated at a later date (ideally under ultrasound guidance).

Opinion is divided as to whether all liver biopsies should be performed under ultrasound guidance. Some studies have suggested a lower rate of complications but others have failed to confirm this finding – and there are considerable cost implications for performing all biopsies under such guidance. At the very least, all patients should have had an ultrasound at some stage prior to the procedure, if only to exclude focal pathology such as tumours, cysts or vascular lesions and to rule out biliary obstruction in those with jaundice. Clearly, where a histological diagnosis of a focal tumour is required, the biopsy should be carried out under imaging control.

Technique

The practical method of how to perform a liver biopsy should be demonstrated and then closely supervised by a doctor experienced in the procedure. The actual technique will not be discussed in any further detail here.

DIFFERENTIAL DIAGNOSIS

GILBERT'S SYNDROME

Gilbert's syndrome is a harmless disorder of bilirubin metabolism and is the commonest of the inherited non-haemolytic hyperbilirubinaemias as well as being the one of most relevance to the non-paediatrician. Individuals with the syndrome have a normal life expectancy and suffer no long-term complications. The main significance of Gilbert's syndrome is that its early recognition should save the patient from unnecessary investigations.

The syndrome is often, but not always, familial and is characterised in most cases by diminished production of the enzyme bilirubin uridine diphosphate (UDP)-glucuronyl transferase, due to a mutation in the promoter region of the gene encoding the enzyme. The existence of other causative factors has been suggested by the occurrence of the promoter alteration in normal controls and one suggestion is that abnormally low hepatocyte uptake of organic anions may be responsible for establishing the phenotype in some individuals who are homozygotic for the gene mutation.

Clinical features

In most cases, the hyperbilirubinaemia of Gilbert's syndrome is detected incidentally on 'routine' blood biochemistry tests. However, it may manifest in late childhood or early adult life as an episode of jaundice. Certain circumstances can conspire to make the bilirubin level rise and suggested precipitant have included fasting, physical exertion, menstruation, psychological stress and febrile illnesses. The evidence is strongest for fasting and this phenomenon can even be exploited as a diagnostic test.

On examination, patients may be mildly icteric if the bilirubin level is high enough but there should otherwise be no physical signs of liver disease.

Diagnosis

The most important diagnostic issue is to exclude parenchymal liver disease and haemolysis. A diagnosis of Gilbert's syndrome can be made if the patient has had hyperbilirubinaemia either constantly or on at least two distinct occasions over a 6-month period. The other liver function tests – transaminases, alkaline phosphatase, γGT, albumin, prothrombin time – should all be normal. It seems reasonable also to send blood as part of a 'liver screen' for the viral, autoimmune and metabolic causes of hepatitis listed on pages 171, 197, 230, 233, 241 and 245, but these tests are unlikely to be positive with just an isolated hyperbilirubinaemia. The liver itself is histologically normal in Gilbert's syndrome but a biopsy is not necessary to make the diagnosis and should be reserved for cases where true parenchymal disease is suspected.

Haemolysis should be excluded with a blood film, a full blood count with reticulocyte quantification and measurement of serum haptoglobin. Radioisotope studies of red cell survival are not usually required, but about half of Gilbert's syndrome cases do have a demonstrable shortening in the red cell life span. This, however, is only mild and not sufficiently low to cause jaundice in itself. Some investigators have suggested the shortened red cell survival may be a metabolic consequence of the syndrome rather than its cause.

Where Gilbert's syndrome is suspected but the diagnosis is not certain, specific confirmatory tests can be employed. As mentioned earlier, fasting causes the hyperbilirubinaemia to increase (unlike in cases of 'true' chronic liver disease) and this can be achieved either by restricting the total daily calorific intake to less than 400 kcal for 3 days or by maintaining a carbohydrate-rich and virtually fat-free intake of less than 2500 kcal. Hyperbilirubinaemia can also be exacerbated (or even precipitated if normal in suspected Gilbert's) by giving a 30 mg dose of intravenous nicotinamide. A genetic test is available, but this should seldom be necessary and is relatively costly.

Treatment

The prognosis of Gilbert's syndrome is benign and treatment largely unnecessary. Phenobarbitone has been shown to reduce the icterus effectively if this is cosmetically troublesome (although its mechanism does not involve increasing the activity of UDP-glucuronyl transferase). However, due consideration needs to be given to the risk and benefits of this type of medication before embarking on prolonged courses of treatment.

VIRAL HEPATITIS

Hepatotropic viruses are a major worldwide cause of mortality and morbidity, infecting hundreds of millions of people. As well as their acute effects, infection with certain hepatitis viruses can result in long-term complications such as cirrhosis and primary liver cancer.

In addition to the true hepatotropic viruses, hepatitic illnesses can also be caused by other viral pathogens (**Fig. 4.45**). The patterns of illness caused by these agents vary widely, from asymptomatic subclinical infection to fulminant hepatitis with acute liver failure.

The known hepatitis viruses differ widely, but in some cases share certain characteristics (**Fig. 4.46**), such as the routes of transmission or the possibility of causing chronic disease.

Hepatitis A

Pathogenesis and epidemiology. Hepatitis A virus (HAV), a member of the picornaviridae family, is an RNA virus that is usually transmitted by the faeco-oral route, although it can occasionally be transferred by parenteral routes such as drug abuse if individuals are acutely infectious. It is particularly common in childhood and is associated with poor sanitation and low socioeconomic status. The majority of infections occur before the age of 5, with seroprevalence studies in westernised societies suggesting an exposure rate of between 40 and 70%. These rates seem to be falling in keeping with improved public health. One consequence of this may be that the normally subclinical childhood infection becomes less common, leaving non-exposed adults at risk of potentially more severe infection later in life.

The epidemiology in developing nations is rather different, with evidence of almost universal exposure to HAV in childhood. HAV-contaminated water and food supplies maintain an endemic level of infection in many developing countries and may infect the non-immune traveller.

Once acquired, HAV replicates within the hepatocyte, producing large quantities of virus that are released into both the bloodstream and the biliary tree, the latter transferring viral particles ultimately into the faeces.

Clinical features. There is an incubation period of between 2 and 6 weeks. During this time, the patient may develop a range of prodromal symptoms including anorexia, general malaise, nausea and fevers. Jaundice may then occur together with dark urine and pale stools. The icteric illness itself is usually fairly short-lived, rarely lasting beyond 6 weeks.

Viral causes of hepatitis	
Hepatitis A, B, C, D, E, G	See Fig. 4.44
Cytomegalovirus (CMV)	Neonatal infection occasionally severe Most adult disease self-limiting, anicteric Fulminant hepatitis rare, but recognised Reactivation common post-transplantation or if immunocompromised May be treated with ganciclovir
Epstein – Barr virus (EBV)	Hepatitis usually subclinical Jaundice in 10–15% only Hepatitis more severe with increasing age Fulminant hepatitis very rare
Human immunodeficiency virus (HIV)	May cause infectious mononucleosis-type illness like CMV or EBV Usually subclinical, rarely icteric
Herpes simplex virus	Very rare, but can be life-threatening in immunocompromised Elevated LFTs and fever common, but jaundice rare Only half of patients have evidence of active herpes infection elsewhere May be treated with aciclovir or famciclovir
Yellow fever	Transmitted by mosquitoes in Africa and South America May cause severe hepatic necrosis, together with viral infiltration of heart and kidneys Effective single-dose vaccine available (live, attenuated) for travellers
Measles	Hepatitis common but usually subclinical Abnormal LFTs in > 80% of cases May be more marked in adults Usually self-limiting
Varicella zoster virus	Abnormal LFTs common in childhood and adult infections Significant hepatic involvement tends to occur only as part of multisystem disease

Fig. 4.45 *Viral causes of hepatitis.*

Some individuals, despite resolving their acute hepatitis, develop a secondary cholestasis that may last up to 3 or 4 months. This seems to have an immunological basis and can be resolved even more quickly with a short course of corticosteroid therapy. HAV does not cause a chronic viral hepatitis. Some patients may have subsequent 'post viral' symptoms such as fatigue or lethargy.

Fulminant hepatitis is a life-threatening acute complication of HAV infection, but is fortunately rare, occurring in less than 0.3% of cases overall. As the risks of HAV infection rise with age, HAV acquisition has a mortality risk of almost 3% if infection occurs after the age of 50.

The hepatotropic viruses

Virus	Molecular biology	Route of transmission	Chronicity of infection	Possibility of causing acute liver failure?
Hepatitis A	RNA virus Non-enveloped Member of picornavirus family	Faeco-oral	Acute only	Yes, but rare (< 0.3%) More likely in older patients (> 50 yrs) or if pre-existing chronic liver disease
Hepatitis B	Member of hepadnavirus family Double-stranded DNA genome Uses reverse transcriptase	Parenteral	5–10% of adults and 95% of neonates develop chronic infection	Yes, but < 1%
Hepatitis C	Enveloped single-strand RNA virus Related to flaviviridae	Parenteral	Acute infection usually subclinical Chronicity in 50–80%	Controversial Extremely rare in western nations May occur in association with other viruses
Hepatitis D	Single-strand circular RNA virus Requires HBV in order to persist and be transmitted	Parenteral	Found in about 5% of HBV carriers May cause acute or chronic hepatitis	May cause fulminant hepatitis either as superadded infection with HBV or as naive coinfection
Hepatitis E	Non-enveloped single-strand RNA virus Member of caliciviridae family	Faeco-oral	Acute only	Rare Most likely in third trimester of pregnancy
Hepatitis G	Single-strand RNA virus Member of flaviviridae family	Parenteral	Persists in about 20% of cases	Almost certainly not (but may be acquired from blood products given during fulminant hepatitis)

Fig. 4.46 *The hepatotropic viruses.*

Diagnosis. Routine LFTs will show elevations, particularly in the serum transaminases (where levels into four figures are not unusual) and bilirubin levels, but there will usually also be some increase in 'cholestatic' markers such as alkaline phosphatase and γGT. In severe cases, there may be a coagulopathy and hypoalbuminaemia.

Specific diagnosis of HAV relies on the serological detection of an IgM antibody that persists for up to 6 months after an acute infection. Resolution of the acute infection is accompanied by a long-lasting IgG response that can be used to detect past exposure (and therefore immunity) to the virus (**Fig. 4.47**).

Treatment. There are no specific therapies for HAV infection and the vast majority of cases require nothing more than supportive care with bed rest, adequate fluid intake, antipyretic measures and avoidance of alcohol. Those most at risk of complications (particularly the older age groups and those with pre-existing chronic liver disease) should be monitored closely. It is clearly important to identify individuals with deteriorating LFTs or impaired synthetic liver function at an early stage. In the UK, HAV is a notifiable disease.

Prevention. Passive immunity can be transferred with specific anti-HAV immunoglobulin, but a more effective choice is one of the inactivated virion-based vaccines which give long-lasting immunity to HAV. Some proprietary formulations combine immunisation against HAV with protection against typhoid or hepatitis B.

Hepatitis B

Epidemiology. According to World Health Organisation estimates, hepatitis B virus (HBV) infects almost 400 million people worldwide. The diseases caused by the virus kill at least 1 million people each year.

The distribution of HBV is highly variable. Areas of high prevalence include China, south east Asia and Africa, with up to 60% of their populations infected at some stage in their lives and a chronic carrier rate of 8–10%. In these areas, the major route of infection

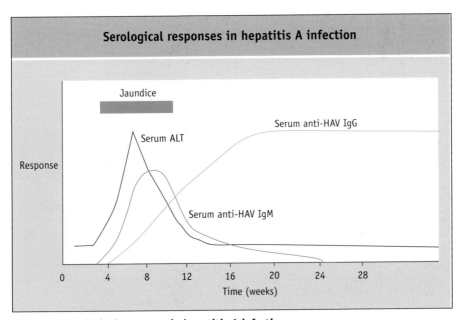

Fig. 4.47 *Serological responses in hepatitis A infection.*

199

Exposure-prone behaviour reported by patients with acute hepatitis B in the USA	
Risk factor	Proportion reporting (%)*
Heterosexual activity	39
Intravenous drug abuse	14
Homosexual activity	13
Familial/household contact	3
Occupational	1
None identified	29**

*Importantly, about 80% of those who denied an obvious risk factor had evidence of other high-risk behaviour (such as other sexually transmitted diseases, history of imprisonment or use of other illicit drugs).
**Figures based on studies carried out by Centers for Disease Control.

Fig. 4.48 *Exposure-prone behaviour reported by patients with acute hepatitis B in the USA.*

is vertical transmission from mother to offspring, with a slightly lesser role played by horizontal infection between siblings.

In areas with a relatively low prevalence, such as western Europe, North America, Australia and New Zealand, the rates of chronic HBV infection are between 0.5 and 1.5%. In the USA there are an estimated 1–1.25 million individuals chronically infected with HBV. Unlike the highly endemic areas, these countries experience mostly horizontal HBV transmission between young adults. In particular, certain 'at risk' groups can be defined that are based on the parenteral spread of the virus, such as intravenous drug abusers, the sexually promiscuous and certain occupational groups such as health-care workers (Fig. 4.48). However, the majority of adults at risk of exposure to HBV do not fit easily into 'high-risk' groups and preventative strategies should not be targeted exclusively away from the wider population.

One of the most important differences between areas of high and low endemicity is the effect of age of acquisition on the subsequent clinical course of HBV infection. HBV in immunocompetent adults is more likely to cause a symptomatic infection but is usually followed by resolution and a low rate of chronic carriage. The opposite is true in neonatal or early childhood infection where chronicity, albeit initially subclinical, is the rule. Acute HBV causes a clinically detectable illness in 30–50% of adults exposed, but in less than 10% of the under-5 age group. Similarly, subsequent chronic carriage rates can be over 90% for infants and neonates but only 2–10% for older children and adults. The significance of this is that 15–25% of those chronically infected will die prematurely as a result of chronic liver disease and its complications.

Virology. HBV is a member of the hepadnavirus family. Its genome consists of partially double-stranded circular DNA of about 3200 base pairs. The four most important regions of the genome are:

- S gene – encodes the viral surface or envelope proteins
- C gene – for the core region, encoding a nucleocapsid protein that holds the viral DNA
- X gene – encodes two proteins functioning as transcriptional activators which may have a role in HBV carcinogenesis
- P gene – for the viral DNA polymerase which also has some reverse transcriptase activity essential for HBV replication

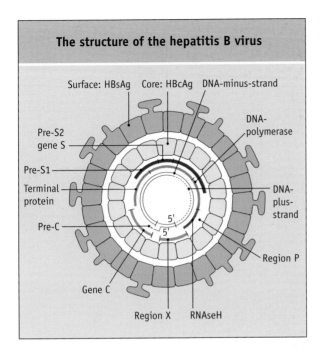

The structure of the hepatitis B virus

Surface: HBsAg   Core: HBcAg   DNA-minus-strand

Pre-S2 gene S

Pre-S1

Terminal protein

Pre-C

Gene C

Region X   RNAseH

DNA-polymerase

DNA-plus-strand

Region P

Fig. 4.49 *The structure of the hepatitis B virus.*

Both the S and C genes have upstream regions known as preS(1 + 2) and preC respectively. Different proteins can be produced depending on which site is the start of transcription. For instance, the S gene is able to produce three different envelope proteins, known as large, middle or small, by commencing transcription with preS1, preS2 or the S gene itself, respectively. The preS1 and preS2 regions are the most immunogenic portions of the surface antigen (or HBsAg) proteins. Recombinant HBsAg is now used for immunisation to create a protective defence against HBV.

In addition to the shedding of whole viral particles (**Fig. 4.49**) by infected hepatocytes, HBV envelope proteins may be released into the circulation without containing viral DNA. Consequently, serological tests (see below) may show HBsAg but not HBV DNA within the bloodstream.

The product of the C gene, known as core antigen or HBcAg, has an important role in the pathogenesis of HBV infection as peptide fragments of this protein can elicit a potent cellular immune response when expressed on the surface of hepatocytes. A modified protein product of this gene may find its way into the circulation after export from the hepatocyte and is known as e antigen or HBeAg. It has been suggested that e antigen may act as a 'tolerogen' for the related HBcAg, allowing replication to occur without a strong cytotoxic response. HBeAg in the serum is therefore a marker of active viral replication and relatively high infectivity, and patients with this marker will also have circulating HBV DNA.

Pathogenesis. The liver damage that occurs with HBV infection is related more to immunological injury than to any cytopathic effect of the virus. A more vigorous immune response, as seen in the immunocompetent adult, is also more effective at clearing the virus than the immature neonatal defences which allow a chronic infection to develop.

The cellular immune response is mainly against small epitopes of HBV proteins (particularly HBcAg) that are present on the surface of the hepatocyte and are recognised

201

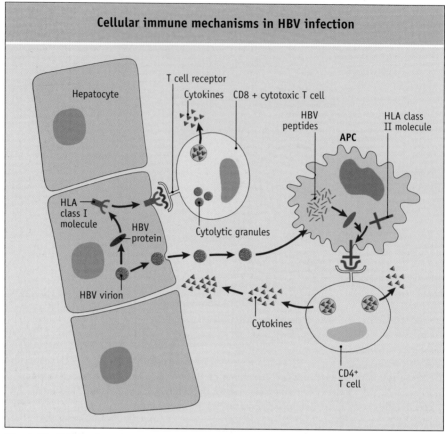

Cellular immune mechanisms in HBV infection

Fig. 4.50 *Cellular immune mechanisms in HBV infection. HBV core proteins are processed within the cytoplasm and presented on the hepatocyte surface in association with the peptide-binding groove on HLA class I molecules. This peptide-HLA complex is recognised by the appropriate clone of CD8+ T cell. Extracellular HBV virion particles are also taken up, processed and presented to helper T lymphocytes by antigen-presenting cells (APCs). The character of the immune response to these presented proteins is heavily influenced by the individual's T cell receptor repertoire and HLA polymorphisms. (HBcAg = hepatitis B core antigen; HBsAg = hepatitis B surface antigen)*

by human leucocyte antigen (HLA) class I- restricted CD8+ cytotoxic T lymphocytes (Fig. 4.50). Fragments of released viral proteins are also taken up by antigen-presenting cells and displayed to class II-restricted CD4+ lymphocytes. This leads to the release of cytokines and stimulation of cytotoxic T cell clones as well as encouraging B cell antibody responses. The net result of these events is an inhibition of viral replication, the destruction of infected hepatocytes and the production of circulating antibodies to diminish the likelihood of hepatocyte reinfection. Recent studies have shown that cytotoxic T cells are capable of inhibiting viral replication directly without destroying the hepatocytes and this may further influence the course and severity of liver damage.

Researchers have also cast some light on some of the reasons why certain individuals may develop chronic hepatitis while others clear the virus. The outcome after acute HBV infection can be influenced by polymorphisms in the HLA genotypes – the class II motif DRB1:1302, for example, is associated with higher rates of clearance. Conversely, mutations in the gene for mannose binding protein (a viral opsinin) may lead to impaired viral clearance in some subjects.

An overzealous immune response is thought be the basis of fulminant hepatitis and the acute liver failure that occurs in less than 1% of HBV cases (superinfection with hepatitis D being one other cause). Such severe reactions are more likely if the patient has recently withdrawn from corticosteroids or cytotoxic drugs.

In cases of chronic active HBV hepatitis the persistent inflammatory and cytotoxic stimuli lead to the fibrosis and disordered architecture of cirrhosis. Ominously, chronic hepatitis B infection is a significant risk factor for hepatocellular carcinoma, being responsible for about 60% of cases worldwide. Suggested carcinogenic mechanisms including the cycle of chronic injury and repair, the transforming activity of the X gene products and the integration of the viral genome causing insertional mutagenesis. Recent work on transgenic mice whose livers express HBV proteins without the intact virus has shown that a chronic non-resolving HBV-specific immune response alone is sufficient to cause hepatocarcinogenesis.

Clinical features. The clinical manifestations of HBV infection vary widely. Acute, icteric infections may present with similar features to HAV, the jaundice often preceded by prodromal symptoms during the 2–6-month incubation period. HBsAg can usually be detected in the bloodstream during this prodromal phase and the onset of the overt hepatitic illness seems to coincide with the emergence of an effective host immune response. In cases of chronic infection, the clinical features are generally of little use in predicting the degree of ongoing liver inflammation, with many patients either asymptomatic or having non-specific complaints such as malaise, fatigue or arthralgia.

Some patients with chronic hepatitis B may develop extrahepatic disease associations such as polyarteritis nodosa, leucocytoclastic vasculitis or membranoproliferative glomerulonephritis. Generally, these conditions improve when the hepatitis B infection is treated.

The complications of HBV infection such as acute liver failure and, in the longer term, cirrhosis and hepatocellular carcinoma are dealt with later in this chapter.

Diagnosis. As with HAV infection, the diagnosis of HBV disease relies largely on serological tests. Liver biopsy is generally reserved for assessing the activity of chronic hepatitis or checking for the development of cirrhosis. In order to understand the serological tests for the virus, it is important to consider its natural history.

The course of an acute infection with HBV can be divided into four stages, with stages 1 and 2 making up the 'replicative' phase and stages 3 and 4 the 'integrative' phase. Initially, stage 1 is characterised by tolerance to the virus, active replication being signalled by HBeAg and HBV DNA in the bloodstream. This period lasts for about 2–4 weeks in most healthy adults, but can be more prolonged.

Stage 2 is typified by the beginning of an immune response against the virus. The involvement of T lymphocytes leads to cytolysis, cytokine production and hepatic inflammation. During this period, there is a reduction in the number of infected hepatocytes and consequently a fall in the circulating levels of HBeAg and HBV DNA. This is generally the stage of symptomatic illness, with jaundice and elevated serum transaminases, and usually lasts 3 or 4 weeks, although in those who develop chronic hepatitis it may go on for years.

Assuming that the host mounts an effective immune response, stage 3 marks the clearance of the bulk of infected hepatocytes and the beginning of what has been termed the 'integrative' phase. HBeAg disappears from the serum, replaced by an antibody against it, HBeAb, serum transaminases normalise and the levels of HBV DNA in the circulation fall dramatically (although it may still be detected in many cases by sensitive polymerase chain reaction (PCR) techniques). At this stage, HBsAg is still detectable in the patient's serum and may be produced after integration of the viral genome without viral replication occurring.

The loss of this last marker signifies the onset of stage 4, indicating an 'immune' status as testified by the development of anti-HBsAg antibodies (HBsAb) and the loss of HBsAg. HBV DNA is now undetectable in the bloodstream, although this gradual diminution may itself take several years in some cases. Progression through these stages of infection may be altered by the emergence of viral mutants (see below).

The serological tests available in most district hospital laboratories are usually HBsAg (which indicates the presence of the virus but does not distinguish chronic carriage from 'active' infection), HBcAb (with measurement of the IgM antibody used to indicate an acute infection), HBeAg (as a marker of active viral replication) and HBsAb (titres of which can be measured to give a guide to the degree of protective immunity). Many diagnostic laboratories now have the facilities to measure HBeAb and perform PCR testing for viral DNA in the peripheral blood. The typical pattern of expression of these markers is shown in **Fig. 4.51**.

In cases of chronic HBV infection, elevations in serum transaminases are relatively mild, rarely being above five times the upper limit of normal. Histological analysis (**Fig. 4.52**) may reveal 'ground glass' hepatocytes, an appearance due to the overproduction of HBV envelope proteins in the cytoplasm, and may also show 'Councilman bodies', acidophilic remnants of infected cells that have undergone apoptosis. Immunohistochemical stains can be used to demonstrate HBsAg or HBcAg in biopsy specimens.

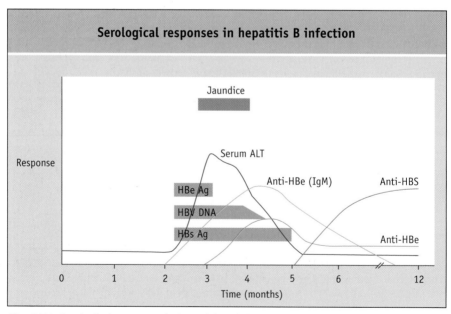

Fig. 4.51 *Serological responses in hepatitis B infection. These responses are typical of an immunocompetent adult to an acute HBV infection.*

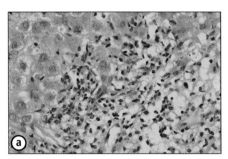 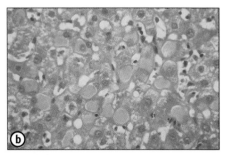

Fig. 4.52 *Histological appearance of chronic hepatitis B. Liver biopsy specimens from a patient with chronic HBV. (a) An inflammatory infiltrate and some mild steatosis. (b) 'Ground-glass' hepatocytes, so named because of the appearance of their cytoplasm, rich in HBsAg.*

Hepatitis B mutants. In recent years a number of mutant strains of HBV have been recognised. The HBeAg-negative variant, also known as the 'pre-core mutant', most commonly has a single base pair substitution that encodes a stop codon at the end of the pre-core region, preventing synthesis of HBeAg. As the virus still replicates and causes liver damage, this has underlined the value of testing peripheral blood for HBV DNA as well as HBeAg.

The pre-core mutant has been associated with fulminant hepatitis, more aggressive chronic hepatitis and accelerated graft loss after liver transplantation. It may be that loss of the circulating 'tolerogen' mentioned earlier leads to a more aggressive inflammatory reaction. The mutant may emerge late in the course of an infection with a previously HBeAg-positive strain or can be acquired *ab initio*, particularly in some Far Eastern or Mediterranean populations.

A few patients have also been found to be infected with HBV strains that bear mutations in the S gene, preventing normal synthesis of HBsAg despite replication and viraemia. These strains are capable of causing HBV infection in individuals who have been successfully vaccinated with recombinant HBsAg (the so-called 'vaccine-escape mutants') but are fortunately still rare.

Treatment. Until recently, there were few therapeutic options for chronic hepatitis B infection. Interferon therapy is well established and has recently been joined by newer antiviral drugs.

The progression from chronic hepatitis to cirrhosis and its complications can be influenced by the age of the patient, the strength of the immune system, genetic factors, coinfection with hepatitis C or D, and other hepatotoxic insults such as alcohol abuse. Environmental and geographic influences may also be relevant as the relative risk of developing cirrhosis from HBV ranges from 12 in Alaska to 79 in the Far East. Male gender and concomitant aflatoxin exposure seem particularly to increase the risks of hepatocellular cancer, which can be up to 150 times the rate seen in 'normal' populations.

The stage of HBV infection is a clear determinant in whether or not to offer immunostimulatory (interferon) or antiviral therapy. There would be little benefit in treating stage 1 disease, for example, or in offering these therapies to patients with established cirrhosis who might benefit from being considered for transplantation. Instead, the main aim is to seroconvert those patients who remain in stages 2 or 3 and diminish the ongoing liver injury.

Established and potential therapies for chronic hepatitis B

Therapy	Examples	Comments
Interferons (IFN)	IFN-α, IFN-β, IFN-γ	IFN-α most widely used Immunostimulatory and antiviral actions 'Complete' response in up to 40–50% of patients
Nucleoside analogues	Lamivudine (3TC)	Inhibits viral reverse transcriptase and DNA polymerase Can almost eliminate serum HBV DNA during treatment, but usually reappears after stopping
	Famciclovir (FCV)	Prevents priming of reverse transcription Reduces viral replication and can eliminate HBV DNA during treatment HBeAb conversion in 20% Escape mutants may occur
	Adefovir (PMEA)	Acts as DNA chain terminator, blocking reverse transcription May also have some immunostimulatory properties Viral load reduced in early studies Undergoing phase III clinical trials at present
Non-interferon cytokines	Interleukin-2 Interleukin-12	Little clinical use, but early experiments suggest may increase cytotoxic lymphocyte response Likely to be problems with delivery and possible side-effects
Potential combination therapies	Immunostimulation (using IFN or steroid-withdrawal, for example) plus nucleotide analogue	
	Combinations of more than one nucleoside analogue	Less likely to lead to viral resistance

Fig. 4.53 *Established and potential therapies for chronic hepatitis B.*

Interferon-α therapy is the best-established treatment method although response rates are generally below 50% and there are associated side-effects such as influenza-like symptoms, depression, myalgia and autoimmune phenomena. The interferons (**Fig. 4.53**) are manufactured either from cultured lymphoblasts or by using recombinant production techniques and, despite having been used clinically since 1975, little is known about their precise mechanism of action. It seems likely that the effect of interferon-α is mediated more through activation of the immune system than by its direct antiviral actions.

The best results are seen in patients who are HBeAg-positive with elevated transaminases and relatively low levels of serum HBV DNA. In these circumstances, a 3–6-month course of 5–10 megaunits, injected subcutaneously three times a week, can achieve clearance of HBeAg and HBV DNA with resolution of histological hepatitis in about 40% of patients. There is usually a long-lasting inhibition of viral replication, but reactivation may still occur later.

Recently, a number of nucleoside inhibitors have been investigated as antiviral agents in the treatment of HBV. Most trials of these drugs (principally lamivudine and famciclovir) have demonstrated a suppression of viral replication during treatment, but there is usually a return to pretreatment viraemia after stopping the course. Some patients, however, have been successfully seroconverted to HBeAb positivity. The side-effect profile of these drugs is generally very good. One earlier nucleoside analogue, fialuridine, was withdrawn after a number of trial patients developed mitochondrial toxicity with severe lactic acidosis, pancreatitis and liver failure that led to several deaths. A number of studies have failed to show any evidence of mitochondrial toxicity in patients receiving lamivudine. There have, however, been reports of severe rebound hepatitis occurring in some patients after withdrawing from lamivudine therapy.

Chronic virus-suppressing courses of nucleoside analogues may prove highly effective in reducing the long-term effects of chronic hepatitis B infection. However, escape mutants of the virus can emerge, one example being the development of mutant viral polymerase enzymes during lamivudine therapy. As seen in the treatment of HIV, combination therapies may ultimately prove more effective.

In addition to these pharmacological agents there has been renewed interest in immunostimulatory approaches and some investigators are studying therapeutic vaccines based on injections of HBV DNA sequences.

Prevention. Hepatitis B infection can be prevented by active or passive immunisation, the latter being of use in certain clinical situations described below. Despite an effective vaccine against HBV having been available since the early 1980s, little real progress has been made in eradicating this worldwide infection. Those low-endemicity countries that have introduced vaccination in targeted 'high-risk' groups have seen only a stabilisation in incidence but no reduction in the numbers of new cases. Hence, universal vaccination seems the most effective way of controlling the spread of HBV and this has been adopted in a number of western nations including the USA, France and Italy. The efficacy of universal vaccination in areas of endemic HBV infection has perhaps been best demonstrated in Taiwan, where all neonates have been immunised since the early 1980s. Recent data analysis has shown the rate of HBV carriage has dropped from 9% to 1% and there has been a marked fall in the incidence of hepatocellular carcinoma in later childhood.

The current HBV vaccines are based on recombinant HBsAg protein. Efficacy can be measured by assaying anti-HBs antibody titres, although the need for pursuing this for population-wide vaccination schedules has been disputed. Local side-effects occur after the vaccine injection in about 20% of people, but these are usually mild and transient. Controversy still rages as to whether there is an association between HBV vaccination and subsequent demyelinating disease or autoimmunity, which may rarely occur after people in older age groups are vaccinated. There have been no documented cases of demyelinating disease occurring after neonatal vaccination.

Immediate but relatively short-lived 'passive' immunity to HBV can be conferred by infusing specific immunoglobulin (HBIg). This is useful (in conjunction with contralateral active immunisation) in protecting neonates born to HBV-positive mothers, who have an 85% chance of becoming infected if she is HBeAg-positive. Such a combined vaccination approach has an efficacy of >90% in protecting the offspring.

Passive immunisation can also protect non-immune individuals who have a known episode of HBV exposure and is additionally used in liver transplant units to try and prevent previously HBV-positive patients from infecting their new graft. These transplant recipients need to continue the HBIg long-term, as subsequent active immunisation does not protect them from HBV recurrence in the new liver.

Hepatitis C

Epidemiology. Following the discovery of the hepatitis A and B viruses in the late 1960s and early 1970s, it soon became apparent that there must be at least one other transmissible agent responsible for the significant numbers of patients with what was variously termed 'post-transfusional' or 'non-A, non-B' (NANB) hepatitis. Indeed, the introduction of donor-testing for HBV only reduced the risk of developing post-transfusion hepatitis by about 25%.

The discovery of the hepatitis C virus (HCV) in 1989 was a triumph for medical science and resulted from some ingenious experimental methods. Serum from known NANB hepatitis patients was transferred to chimpanzees, who then developed a hepatitic illness. Extracts of RNA from the chimpanzees' bloodstream were used to create cDNA libraries whose gene products were tested for reactivity with the sera of NANB patients. The isolation of the relevant genetic sequence then led to the identification of the virus.

HCV is a major cause of morbidity and mortality throughout the world, with an estimated 200 million people infected. In Europe and North America it is the commonest cause of chronic viral hepatitis and HCV cirrhosis accounts for 30–40% of referrals to liver transplant centres. As the virus is most easily transmitted via blood and blood products, the highest-risk groups are intravenous drug abusers and, to a reducing extent, those exposed to infected blood products such as pooled clotting factor concentrates (**Fig. 4.54**). In the UK, virtually every haemophiliac (at least 3200) who received pooled factor VIII in the early 1970s became HCV-positive. The risk of acquiring HCV from transfusions has since been greatly diminished, if not eliminated, by the introduction of viral-inactivated products, the availability of recombinant factor VIII and the testing of blood donors for HCV (**Fig. 4.55**).

Seroprevalence rates vary widely throughout the world and within certain sections of each society's population. Most prevalence studies are based on blood donors, who by virtue of their pre-selection may not reflect the rates seen within populations indulging in intravenous drug abuse, for instance. In northern Europe and the USA, the reported prevalence rates are between 0.1 and 1%, although in the USA it is estimated that the true figure in the wider population may be as high as 1.8% – indicating a reservoir of almost 3.9 million infected Americans. Prevalence rates are generally higher in southern Europe (1–1.5%) and equatorial Africa (5–6%) and as high as 20% in Egypt. Most studies from eastern Asia have shown an HCV prevalence rate of just 1–3%, generally much lower than that of HBV.

The reasons for these wide variations in incidence are largely unknown. Unlike HBV, vertical transmission of HCV from mother to infant is uncommon and accounts for less than 3% of cases in the western nations. Despite the numbers quoted in **Fig. 4.54**, the risks

Exposure-prone behaviour reported in new cases of hepatitis C infection over a 5-year period in the USA

Risk factor	Proportion reporting (%)
Intravenous drug abuse	43
Sexual or household contact	17
Occupational	4
Transfusion	3*
None identified	33**

*Only reported in the early years of the study, with no recent cases.
**A high proportion of those patients who denied the established risk factors did have surrogate indicators such as a history of imprisonment, sexually transmitted diseases or non-injected illicit drug abuse.

Fig. 4.54 *Exposure-prone behaviour reported in new cases of hepatitis C infection over a 5-year period in the USA.*

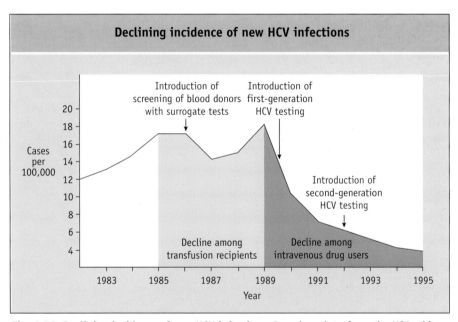

Fig. 4.55 *Declining incidence of new HCV infections. Based on data from the USA, this graph shows the fall in de novo HCV infections since the discovery of the virus, the introduction of screening of blood products and changes in the behaviour of intravenous drug abusers. Despite this fall in the acquisition of hepatitis C, the long natural history of the virus means that it will continue to cause significant morbidity and mortality for many years to come.*

of sexual transmission are actually quite low. Excluding shared habits such as intravenous drug abuse, the long-term sexual partners of HCV-positive individuals acquire the virus in less than 5% of cases (see p. 217).

Iatrogenic transmission of HCV has certainly been a factor in many countries. Prior to the introduction of effective screening of blood donations, the risk of NANB hepatitis was as high as 10% in the Far East, for example. Similarly, many patients with renal disease were exposed to the virus during haemodialysis procedures. Some of the older patients with 'unknown' risk factors may have acquired the virus through unsafe childhood vaccination schedules or by 'alternative' medical tonics previously injected into multiple recipients in many countries.

More worrying for health authorities than the prevalence of hepatitis C, however, is its increased tendency to cause chronic liver disease when compared to HBV. Estimates vary, but some 50–65% of those with HCV develop chronic liver disease and, in the USA, the virus is currently causing 8–10 000 deaths and accounting for over 1000 liver transplants per annum.

Virology. HCV is a single-stranded RNA virus related to the flaviviridae family. Its 9400-base genome encodes three structural proteins used for the viral envelope and nucleocapsid (encoded by the E1, E2 and C regions of the genome), together with a number of non-structural proteins such as the c100 membrane-associated protein, helicase, protease and RNA polymerase (**Fig. 4.56**). Importantly, the E1 and E2 (the latter also known as NS1) regions are hypervariable which can give rise to quasispecies (see below) and escape mutants that contribute to evasion of the immune system. The detection of host antibodies to the c22 and c100 proteins can be used for diagnostic serological tests (see **Fig. 4.63**).

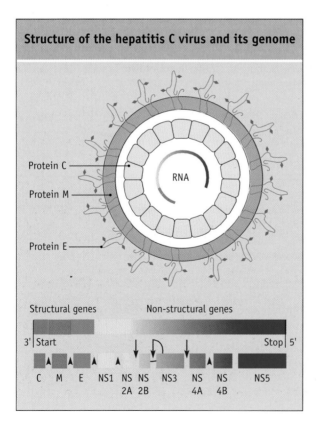

Structure of the hepatitis C virus and its genome

Protein C

Protein M

RNA

Protein E

Structural genes   Non-structural genes

3' Start   Stop 5'

C   M   E   NS1   NS NS   NS3   NS   NS   NS5
                            2A 2B   4A   4B

Fig. 4.56 *The structure of the hepatitis C virus and its genome.*

HCV, like many other RNA viruses, has an inherently variable genome due to the error-prone incorporation of nucleotides during viral replication and relatively inefficient mutation repair system. The HCV RNA polymerase enzymes lack the 'proofreading' function of their DNA virus cousins (such as HBV) and so new mutations in the viral genome arise approximately once every 1000–10 000 nucleotides in each replication cycle – about a hundred times more commonly than for DNA viruses.

Almost as soon as the HCV genome was first sequenced it became apparent that there were major differences between viruses affecting different geographical populations. These different strains, with a less than 72% sequence homology, are known as genotypes. Furthermore, it was soon observed that an individual patient may harbour multiple strains of HCV, known as quasispecies, that are more closely related to each other, usually with a homology of > 86%. HCV mutants that have homologies of between 72 and 86% make up the various subtypes of the six major genotypes described (Fig. 4.57).

Pathogenesis. Acute HCV hepatitis is usually mild and subclinical in most cases, but it is the long-term effects of the virus that are of most clinical consequence.

The pathogenesis of liver damage in HCV is complicated and still the subject of intensive research. It reflects the influence of a number of factors relating to the host (such as immune competence and the relative cellular and humoral responses, alcohol use, iron overload, coinfection with HIV or HBV) and viral influences (such as its direct cytopathic effects, replication efficiency, quasispecies, viral load and duration of infection).

There is a growing body of evidence to show that, as with HBV infection, the immune system plays a major role in causing the hepatocellular injury in chronic hepatitis C. Infected patients have circulating HCV-specific antibodies with a marked expansion of B lymphocytes in the peripheral blood signifying a strong humoral response. Specific cytotoxic T cells and CD4 proliferative cellular responses can be detected against HCV antigens and there is evidence that enhanced local production of cytokines (such as interleukin-2 and interferon-γ) may be an important mediator of liver injury.

At a histological level (Fig. 4.58), HCV leads to some changes that are common to chronic hepatitis of viral or non-viral aetiologies such as a mononuclear cell infiltration of the portal tracts, interface hepatitis and bridging necrosis (where the necroinflammatory response extends between portal tracts or links the portal tracts and the centrilobular veins). Unlike autoimmune hepatitis, however, HCV infection is often characterised by bile duct destruction (ductopenia), which together with steatosis and portal lymphocyte

Hepatitis C genotypes	
Classification	**Most common distribution**
1a	Western Europe, North America
1b	Southern and Eastern Europe, North America, Japan and Far East
1c	Europe, North America
2a, 2b	Europe, North America, West Africa, Japan
3a, 3b	Europe, North America, Nepal
4a	North and East Africa, Middle East
5a	Southern Africa
6a	Southeast Asia

Fig. 4.57 *Hepatitis C genotypes.*

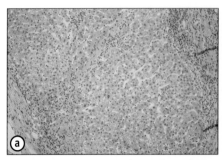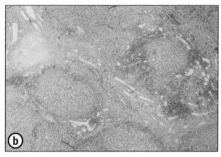

Fig. 4.58 *Chronic hepatitis and cirrhosis due to HCV infection. (a) Liver biopsy specimens showing fibrosis, portal lymphocyte aggregates and necroinflammation. (b) The longer-term development of nodularity and scarring seen in hepatitis C cirrhosis.*

aggregates is highly suggestive of hepatitis C. In order to standardise the assessment of HCV liver injury and guide the use of antiviral therapies, pathologists may use a histological activity index (HAI) such as the Knodell or Ishak scoring systems, which grades the degree of necroinflammatory and fibrotic response. In the longer term, the histological appearances of cirrhosis and hepatocellular carcinoma may be seen.

Clinical features. An 'acute' hepatitic illness due to HCV is usually subclinical. After an incubation period of 6–12 weeks (or sooner if the viral load is very large, such as after an infected blood transfusion) an icteric illness develops in only 5–15% of patients.

What is more significant is the tendency of HCV to establish chronicity. Although a small number of patients (perhaps 10–15%) will effectively clear the virus, the majority develop a persistent infection. Of these, a high proportion will develop chronic liver damage (**Fig. 4.59**), although the natural history can be difficult to predict for a given individual.

HCV is not a recognised cause of fulminant hepatitis and acute liver failure. Some isolated reports of this occurring have come from areas of high HCV endemicity and may have reflected an acute coinfection with other viruses or a supervening non-viral insult. Because the chronic liver disease induced by HCV may take many years to become apparent, most patients are asymptomatic although some have non-specific complaints such as fatigue, arthralgia or some of the extrahepatic manifestations mentioned below. The patient's first clinical features may eventually be those of liver failure and portal hypertension such as ascites, bleeding, jaundice or encephalopathy. From the time of infection, it may be 10–20 years before cirrhosis develops and 15–25 years before the peak incidence of hepatocellular cancer. Estimates of the exact risk of liver cancer in HCV cirrhosis vary, but many hepatologists screen their patients for its development with a 6–12-monthly ultrasound scan and α-fetoprotein estimation.

Extrahepatic disease. There are a number of extrahepatic disorders associated with HCV (**Fig. 4.60**), many with an autoimmune basis, although the evidence of association is stronger for some than for others. Some of the rarer associations may reflect higher background rates of HCV infection in the relevant populations being studied. There is good evidence to support an association with small vessel vasculitis in particular (**Fig. 4.61**), and HCV is the most common cause of the associated mixed essential cryoglobulinaemia. Evidence of HCV infection should be actively sought in patients with membranoproliferative glomerulonephritis, nephrotic syndrome, peripheral neuropathy, porphyria cutanea tarda and the antiphospholipid syndrome. As the side-effects of interferon-α therapy (see below) include certain autoimmune phenomena, it should be

Comparison of natural histories of HCV and HBV infections in adults (UK)		
	Hepatitis C	**Hepatitis B**
Estimated prevalence*	0.3% 171000 ↓	0.2% 114000 ↓
Progression to chronic liver disease	50% 85000 ↓	10% 11400 ↓
Progression from chronic liver disease to cirrhosis	20–50% 17–43000 ↓	15% 1710 ↓
Development of hepatocellular carcinoma	10% 1700–4300	10% 171

* Prevalence of HCV may be up to 1% of UK population.
Prevalence of HBV may be lower than 0.2% suggested

Fig. 4.59 *Comparison of natural histories of HCV and HBV infections in adults. Population figures refer to the UK, but estimates of disease progression rates are also applicable to other European and North American populations. It is apparent that HCV is a much more significant cause of cirrhosis and liver cancer in the developed nations than HBV.*

borne in mind that while many of these extrahepatic manifestations improve with treatment of the underlying HCV infection, some may actually deteriorate (**Fig. 4.62**).

One other important association of HCV is the development of non-organ-specific autoantibodies. A consequence of this may be possible diagnostic confusion with autoimmune hepatitis (see below) and in particular the type 2 form. This variety of autoimmune hepatitis is characterised by anti-liver, kidney microsomal antibodies (anti-LKM) and there have been reports linking this syndrome to chronic hepatitis C. However, in most cases of HCV infection where the antibodies are present, they are generally of low titre and there seems to be little difference in the natural history of these patients' liver disease compared with similar HCV patients who do not have the autoantibodies. This is a controversial area, but there are undoubtedly a few patients with HCV who have high titres of anti-LKM antibodies and some clinical features of autoimmunity. They can be difficult to manage as the therapeutic options for the two diseases appear to be mutually exclusive.

Diagnosis. Symptoms and/or physical signs are not sufficiently sensitive or specific to make a diagnosis of HCV infection. Likewise, the degree of elevation of serum transaminases is a poor guide to the activity of hepatic inflammation in chronic HCV.

The most widely used diagnostic tests in hepatitis C are anti-HCV antibodies and tests based on the detection of HCV RNA (**Fig. 4.63**). Anti-HCV antibodies are not protective and their presence is not an indication of immunity to the virus. Instead they merely reflect previous exposure to the virus – and while a small proportion of patients will have cleared the virus, most people with positive anti-HCV antibodies will have an ongoing infection.

The latest generation of serological tests is generally very reliable, with sensitivities of more than 95%. Initial testing is usually an enzyme immunosorbent assay against four HCV

Extrahepatic diseases associated with hepatitis C

Endocrine	Hypothyroidism Hyperthyroidism Thyroid autoantibodies Hashimoto's disease Diabetes mellitus

Autoimmune and vasculitic	Mixed essential cryoglobulinaemia
	Small vessel vasculitis
	Polyarteritis nodosa
	Pulmonary fibrosis +/– pulmonary vasculitis
	CREST syndrome (**c**alcinosis, **R**aynaud's
	    phenomenon, **o**esophageal disease, **s**clerodactyly
	    and **t**elangiectasia)

Haematological	Aplastic anaemia Idiopathic thrombocytopenia Antiphospholipid syndrome Non-Hodgkin's B-cell lymphoma
Renal and rheumatological	Glomerulonephritis Rheumatoid arthritis Myopathy Arthralgias
Dermatological	Leucocytoclastic vasculitis Porphyria cutanea tarda Lichen planus Erythema nodosum Erythema multiforme Pruritus Urticaria
Miscellaneous	Hypertrophic cardiomyopathy Dilated cardiomyopathy Sialadenitis Uveitis Corneal ulceration Peripheral neuropathy Autoantibodies

Fig. 4.60 *Extrahepatic diseases associated with hepatitis C.*

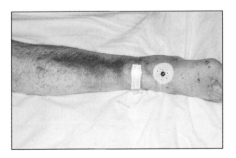

Fig. 4.61 *Vasculitic rash in a patient with chronic hepatitis C and mixed essential cryoglobulinaemia.*

Responses of various extrahepatic manifestations of hepatitis C to treatment with interferon-α

Disorder	Response
Vasculitis and cryoglobulinaemia	Improvement/no change
Thyroid dysfunction +/− autoantibodies	Deterioration/no change
Glomerulonephritis	Improvement/no change
Porphyria cutanea tarda	Improvement/no change
Lichen planus	Improvement/no change/deterioration
Thrombocytopenia	Improvement/deterioration
Non-Hodgkin's lymphoma	Improvement
Corneal ulceration	Improvement
Latent myopathy	Deterioration

Fig. 4.62 *Responses of various extrahepatic manifestations of hepatitis C to treatment with interferon-α.*

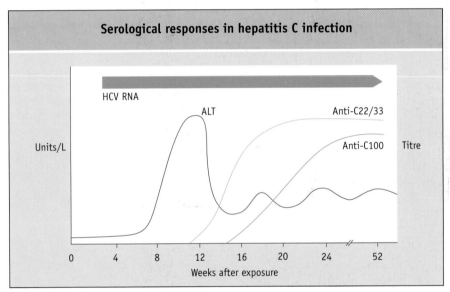

Fig. 4.63 *Serological responses in hepatitis C infection. Note the usual 3- to 4-month delay before anti-HCV antibodies are detectable. During this time there may be a variable elevation in serum transaminases and viral RNA may be detectable using PCR techniques.*

target proteins (including the c33, c22 and c100 components in **Fig. 4.63**) which, if positive, can be confirmed using a radioimmunoblot assay (RIBA) to give greater specificity.

However, if one considers that a patient with anti-HCV antibodies may possibly have cleared the virus, particularly if the serum transaminases are normal, then tests that detect viraemia are clearly useful. In most instances, this involves a *qualitative* PCR to detect HCV RNA in the patient's blood. The quality of PCR testing can vary between laboratories and false results can occur. Importantly, patients with HCV may be only intermittently viraemic and a negative PCR test alone does not exclude the disease. PCR testing is of further use in monitoring the efficacy of antiviral treatments and the clearance of viraemia is an important endpoint in clinical management.

Although used largely as research tools, it is also possible to offer *quantitative* PCR methods, which can be used to measure viral load, as well as sequence-based techniques to assess genotypes or quasispecies. However, these investigations are not essential to the routine management of most patients and are relatively expensive.

Given that the serum transaminases are normal in about 50% of HCV cases and are seldom raised above 3–4 times the upper limit of normal in most patients, a liver biopsy is the best guide to the degree of HCV liver damage. The risks of the procedure should be weighed against the potential benefits of treatment, but as a rule of thumb, a liver biopsy should be performed if there are two or more of a positive anti-HCV antibody, a positive HCV PCR or raised serum transaminases. Histological activity indices can be used to quantify the degree of inflammation and fibrosis.

Serial biopsy studies have demonstrated that patients who have a histologically mild hepatitis with no fibrotic changes have an approximately 50% risk of progression to more severe disease over a 10-year period, with perhaps a 10% risk of cirrhosis. On the other hand, patients whose liver biopsies show severe inflammation and septal fibrosis have a 60–70% risk of developing cirrhosis over the same timescale.

The diagnostic approach to suspected hepatitis C is summarised in **Fig. 4.64**.

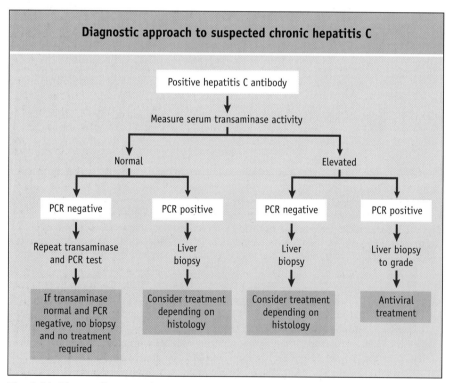

Fig. 4.64 *Diagnostic approach to the patient with a positive anti-hepatitis C antibody test.*

Treatment: patient education. Counselling and patient education feature prominently in the treatment of patients with chronic viral hepatitis. A careful explanation of the natural history of HCV should be given and if antiviral treatment is considered, a realistic assessment of the response rates and side-effects. Many patients will benefit from the leaflets offered by patient support groups such as the British Liver Trust or the American Liver Foundation.

Sexual transmission of the virus, is relatively low, with a seroprevalence rate of about 5% in long-term partners of HCV patients. A change to barrier methods of contraception is perhaps not necessary as long as higher-risk activities, such as intercourse during menstruation, are avoided. Barrier methods should, however, be used with new partners. Maternal–fetal transmission rates are low, unless the mother is also infected with HIV or has a particularly high viraemia, and there have so far been no reports of the virus being transmitted by breast-feeding.

Drug treatment. The two drugs currently licensed for treatment of HCV are interferon and ribavirin, which are most successful when used in combination – and recent guidelines have advocated using combination therapy as first-line treatment. The most extensive clinical data, however, have been accumulated on interferon *monotherapy*, particularly IFN-α_{2a} and IFN-α_{2b}. Interferon-α is a recombinant or lymphoblastoid cytokine. A commonly used regimen has been 3 mega-units of IFN injected subcutaneously three times a week for 6 months. Early studies of this treatment showed that 50% of patients would normalise their serum transaminases by the completion of the course, but of these about half would relapse within 6 months of stopping treatment, giving an overall response rate of about 25%. In the longer term, there were further cases of relapse and, based on studies which used the more accurate PCR test as a marker of viraemia, it appears that the true incidence of a sustained response (**Fig. 4.65**) to the 'standard' IFN regimen was only 10–20%.

Many variations of this protocol have been assessed over the years, with success rates generally not differing widely from the original studies. It has been shown that the majority of those patients who do go on to clear the virus and achieve a sustained response do so within the first 4–6 weeks of IFN treatment. Hence, if patients still have a positive PCR test after 3 months, there is little likelihood of them clearing the virus after 6 or 12 months of therapy. In view of this, some practitioners have consolidated the initial dose of IFN so that patients may receive 6 megaunits three times weekly for the first 3 months and then revert to a lower dose for the remainder of the course if the virus is initially cleared.

A number of factors have been identified that can help to predict the likely response to interferon therapy. Patient factors include young age (particularly <45 years), disease duration (ideally <5 years), absence of cirrhosis or the presence of only mild fibrosis on biopsy, normal or low hepatic iron content and no alcoholism. Viral factors include genotype (preferably not type 1), quantitatively low level of viraemia, low genetic diversity (few quasispecies) and lack of coinfection with HBV or HIV. Many of these factors may be interdependent, such as disease duration. Many hepatologists exclude patients with cirrhosis from interferon treatment, as response rates are generally lower and consideration should be given to liver transplantation. However, there is some evidence that patients with well-compensated cirrhosis who have evidence of active inflammation histologically may derive significant benefit from interferon therapy. Furthermore, it has recently emerged that interferon therapy can remove fibrosis and perhaps reverse the cirrhotic process in certain cases. IFN should be avoided, however, in patients with decompensated cirrhosis. In another controversial area, there have been conflicting reports as to whether or not a course of IFN in patients with cirrhosis decreases their subsequent risk of hepatocellular carcinoma.

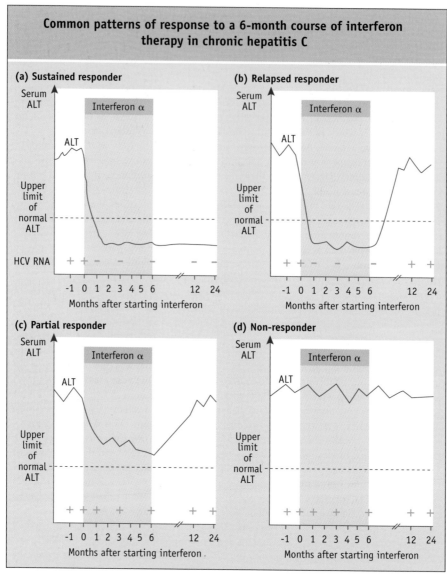

Common patterns of response to a 6-month course of interferon therapy in chronic hepatitis C

(a) Sustained responder

(b) Relapsed responder

(c) Partial responder

(d) Non-responder

Fig. 4.65 *Common patterns of response to a 6-month course of interferon therapy in chronic hepatitis C. (a) There is a successful, sustained response with normalisation of the transaminase, ALT, and elimination of circulating viral RNA. (b) The patient has an initially similar course, but relapses after stopping treatment. (c and d) Neither patient is able to clear their viraemia, but (c) is at least able to reduce the ALT level temporarily.*

Interferon therapy is associated with a number of side-effects of variable significance (**Fig. 4.66**). The most troublesome is a syndrome of 'flu-like symptoms that usually resolve with continued treatment, but can be intolerable for some patients. Depression and blood dyscrasias are also relatively common and so patients need to be closely monitored with

Adverse effects of interferon therapy

Systemic and constitutional	'Flu-like' illnesses, fever, myalgia, fatigue, backache, arthralgia, nausea, diarrhoea, headaches, anorexia
Neuropsychological	Depression, sleep disturbance, seizures, tinnitus, vertigo, reduced concentration, irritability, paranoid ideation, decreased libido
Haematological	Thrombocytopenia, leucopenia, anaemia
Immunological	Development of autoantibodies, hypothyroidism, hyperthyroidism, possible increased susceptibility to bacterial infections
Dermatological	Lichen planus, hair loss, lupus-like syndromes
Miscellaneous and rarities	Pneumonitis, proteinuria, cardiac arrhythmias, retinal haemorrhages

Fig. 4.66 *Adverse effects of interferon therapy.*

frequent outpatient clinic appointments and regular blood tests, particularly in the early stages of treatment. Given the occasional overlap between HCV and autoimmune liver disease, a worsening of liver function tests after starting interferon should lead to immediate withdrawal of the drug.

The broad-spectrum, orally active antiviral purine nucleoside analogue ribavirin has entered clinical practice recently. If given alone for HCV, it reduces the serum transaminases and has some effect in reducing histological inflammatory activity, but has no effect on viral clearance. When used in combination with IFN, however, there is a dramatic improvement in the short- and long-term therapeutic responses. The proportion of sustained responders is approximately doubled to around 40–50% of those treated.

Consensus guidelines issued by the European Association for the Study of the Liver (EASL) in 1999 have suggested that dual therapy with IFN and ribavirin should now be the first-line treatment for HCV. A typical regimen would be to use 3 mega-units of interferon three times a week with ribavirin given in a total daily dose of 1–1.2 g, for a 6-month period. Some authorities advocate a 12-month course for those infected with genotype 1 as this duration of treatment is associated with higher long-term response rates.

As well as its success in 'naive' patients, there is also a body of evidence that combination treatment may be beneficial for those who have relapsed following an apparently successful course of IFN monotherapy and also for a proportion of IFN non-responders.

Ribavirin is generally well tolerated, its main side-effect being a reversible haemolysis which is usually clinically insignificant, although about 10% of patients will have a fall in haemoglobin concentration of more than 4 g/dL, which could be particularly hazardous in those with ischaemic heart disease.

Liver transplantation. This remains an option for those who develop HCV cirrhosis and chronic hepatitis C is fast becoming one of the most common (if not *the* most common) underlying causes of transplantation in many western countries. However, viral recurrence is almost universal:

- HCV infection of the new liver occurs in >95% of cases
- Histological appearance of recurrent HCV may be similar to that of chronic rejection
- The natural history of post-transplantation HCV may differ from that in the 'native' liver

- 20–30% develop chronic hepatitis by year 5
- 15–20% develop cirrhosis by year 5
- However, the need for retransplantation is at a similar rate to other hepatic diseases

Prevention. Public health measures aimed at limiting transmission of the virus are the mainstay of HCV prevention. There is currently no available vaccine, a result of the high mutagenicity of the virus as well as difficulties in developing suitable in vitro and in vivo experimental models. Recombinant HCV envelope proteins have been the subject of some immunogenicity studies, and DNA vaccination (the injection of fragments of viral DNA rather than the proteins which they encode), such as with the E2 envelope protein sequence, may offer some future promise.

Hepatitis C, haemophilia and HIV. Worthy of special mention is the cohort of haemophiliacs infected with HCV by pooled clotting factor concentrates in the 1970s. Coinfection with HIV has also been a significant problem, with about 1200 haemophiliacs having both viruses. The consequence is a worsened natural history for both infections:

- An increased HCV replication rate
- Accelerated HIV progression
- 21 × increase in the incidence of liver failure
- 30 × increase in the rates of liver cancer development
- A diminished response to antiviral treatments

Hepatic disease is the eventual cause of death in around 10% of HIV and HCV coinfected individuals. As the liver is the source of clotting factor production, transplantation offers the potential of treating both the haemophilia and the HCV liver damage. In a large published series, haemophiliacs had no more perioperative bleeding complications than other liver transplant recipients and had normalised their clotting factor levels by a mean of 18 hours postoperatively; survival rates were 90% at 1 year (reduced to 83% if also HIV-positive) and 67% at 3 years (reduced to 23% if HIV-positive).

Hepatitis D

Epidemiology, clinical significance and virology. Previously known as the Delta agent, hepatitis D (HDV) is an unusual virus in that it cannot replicate without HBV also being present. The HDV particle is coated by HBsAg (**Fig. 4.67**) and it can only be acquired by coinfection with HBV or by superinfection of a patient already infected with HBV.

HDV is particularly common in Mediterranean countries, the Middle East, South America and Asia. Overall, it is estimated that around 5% of the world's HBV carriers are also infected with HDV. The significance of this is that HDV coinfection worsens the hepatitic illness; it is a well-recognised cause of fulminant hepatic failure and HDV superinfection should always be suspected if there is a sudden deterioration in cases of chronic HBV hepatitis. Individuals infected with both viruses are more likely to develop cirrhosis.

Transmission, like HBV, is through parenteral routes such as intravenous drug use and sexual intercourse.

HDV has a single-stranded circular RNA genome of 1758 bases in length. It is surrounded by the hepatitis D antigen (HDAg) and HBsAg.

Diagnosis. As with the other hepatitis viruses, it is possible to identify antigens, antibodies and viral genome sequences for diagnostic purposes. HDAg can be detected by radioimmunoassay and specific IgM antibodies can now be used as a marker of acute infection.

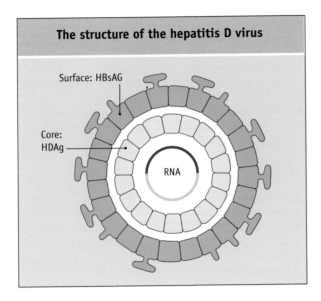

The structure of the hepatitis D virus

Surface: HBsAG

Core: HDAg

RNA

Fig. 4.67 *The structure of the hepatitis D virus.*

Treatment and prevention. There is no specific antiviral therapy for HDV. While it could be expected that therapies directed against HBV might also be effective against HDV there is no certainty that this is the case. HDV depends on the presence of HBSAg and this antigen can still be present at very high levels despite effective anti-HBV therapies being used. Interferon therapy may lead to some transient reduction in HDV activity, but it is neither curative nor long-lasting. Researchers have identified a number of HDV metabolic processes (such as HDAg dimerisation, isoprenylation and HDAg-RNA binding) that might be suitable for future therapeutic targeting.

There is currently no active or passive immunisation available for HDV. Such a vaccine would clearly be advantageous for chronic HBV carriers. Active immunisation against HBsAg also prevents HDV infection in those not already HBV-positive.

Hepatitis E

Virology and epidemiology. Discovered in 1983, hepatitis E virus (HEV) is now known to be the cause of what was formerly known as enterically transmitted non-A, non-B hepatitis. Its genome is approximately 7500 bases long and consists of single-stranded RNA.

HEV is endemic in Africa, the Middle East, Asia and Central America and is associated with poor sanitation and socioeconomic deprivation. In these countries between 10–40% of adults demonstrate seropositivity for HEV although the rate is only about 5% in childhood. Consequently, outbreaks can affect thousands of individuals, with the most significant group being pregnant women (see below).

The virus is transmitted by the faeco-oral route, with contaminated water supplies the greatest danger. HEV can also be acquired as a zoonosis, with sheep and pig faeces being possible sources of infection.

Clinical features. The incubation period is about 2–8 weeks. Symptoms and signs are similar to other causes of acute viral hepatitis and in most patients the hyperbilirubinaemia and raised transaminases resolve over a 3-week period. As with HAV, chronic hepatitis does not occur.

Those at greatest risk of serious hepatitic illness due to HEV are pregnant women, particularly in the third trimester. The disease pursues a more aggressive course in them, with a 25% mortality rate.

Diagnosis. This is largely based on detecting specific IgM anti-HEV antibodies, although false negative tests do occur. In such cases it is possible to detect HEV RNA in serum, liver or faecal samples by PCR.

Prevention. Public health measures are the most important preventative approaches and should be aimed at ensuring a clean drinking water supply and safe disposal of sewage. Trials of recombinant vaccines against HEV are being carried out in primates.

Hepatitis G

Despite the discovery of hepatitis viruses A–E, there are still some unexplained cases of presumed viral hepatitis for which the infective agents have yet to be discovered. The term 'hepatitis F', for example, has been used to represent the presumed viral cases of acute liver failure for which no known virus is found. Recently, an RNA virus has been identified and given the name hepatitis G (HGV), it is a possible cause of some parenterally transmitted non-A–E hepatitis.

The virus is a member of the flavivirus family with an approximately 30% homology to HCV. Viraemia with HGV has been detected in patients with a variety of disorders, including chronic hepatitis and acute liver failure, and in organ transplant recipients, individuals who have received blood transfusions and also the normal population. The virus can be detected in 0.8–1.5% of apparently healthy blood donors in the USA, although prevalence rates may be higher in certain risk groups (up to 20% of intravenous drug abusers) or geographical areas (an estimated 5% prevalence in Vietnam, for example).

It remains to be established whether HGV is actually a cause of significant disease. While the virus can certainly be transmitted by blood transfusion and may persist for many years, it is doubtful that it accounts for many cases of post-transfusional hepatitis (being found in just 3 out of 79 cases in one US study). An initial association with fulminant hepatitis appears to have been related more to the virus being transferred by blood products subsequently received during the hospital admission rather than having caused the illness in the first place. There is no evidence that HGV coinfection worsens the course of hepatitis C.

Work on possible disease associations is continuing, but at the present time the pathogenicity of HGV remains dubious.

ALCOHOL-RELATED LIVER DISEASE

Chronic ingestion of alcohol can cause fatty liver, alcoholic hepatitis and cirrhosis. An intake of more than 160 g of ethanol per day for men and 80 g of ethanol per day for women over a 10-year period is likely to lead to cirrhosis. However, not all individuals who have a history of chronic alcohol abuse develop significant liver injury. The type of alcoholic drink consumed does not appear to affect hepatotoxicity. Of course there are individual variations, but UK government guidelines suggest that safe levels of alcohol consumption are 21 units of ethanol per week for men and 14 units per week for women. One unit of alcohol is equivalent to:

- 10 g of ethanol
- 125 ml glass of wine
- Half a pint of beer
- Schooner of sherry
- Standard pub measure (1/6 gill) of spirits

Recently, it has been recommended that the limits should be revised upwards to 28 and 21 units per week respectively. It is estimated that around 28% of men and 14% of women drink more than these guidelines recommend. Furthermore, some 5–10% of men and 3–5% of women become dependent on alcohol.

There may be a genetic predisposition to alcoholism. The A1 allele of the dopamine D_2 receptor occurs in 77% of alcoholics, compared to 28% of non-alcoholics. Furthermore, male offspring of alcoholics are more likely to develop alcoholism than the general populus.

While popularly associated with liver cirrhosis (**Fig. 4.68**), ethanol excess can be poisonous to every cell in the body. There is no organ system that cannot be affected in some way by acute or chronic alcohol ingestion (**Fig. 4.69**).

Alcohol consumption is not completely without benefit, however. A number of large studies have confirmed the existence of a 'J-shaped curve' relating mortality to alcohol consumption. In other words, excessive drinking (beyond the recommended levels above) is undoubtedly harmful, but mild to moderate drinking is associated with a lower mortality than complete abstinence. Much of this is related to a protective effect of alcohol against ischaemic heart disease, although the incidence of this also rises with excessive consumption.

Ethanol-induced liver injury

Ethanol is metabolised by alcohol dehydrogenase to acetaldehyde, which forms protein adducts by binding at lysine residues, causing membrane damage and disruption of cellular homeostasis. Redox changes may also occur, ethanol increasing hepatic oxygen requirements. Oxygen tension may decrease in the centrilobular region as a result.

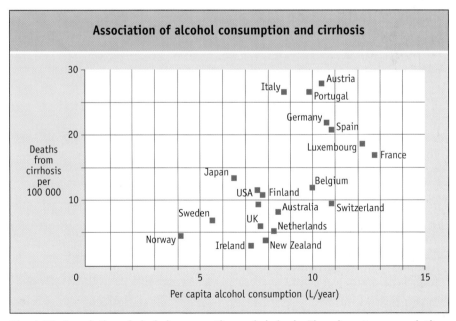

Fig. 4.68 Association of alcohol consumption and cirrhosis. There is a strong correlation between the average per capita alcohol consumption and the incidence of death due to liver cirrhosis in many countries.

Acute and chronic toxic effects of alcohol consumption	
Neurological	Acute intoxication CNS depression Alcohol withdrawal syndromes Seizures Dementia Cerebellar degeneration Peripheral neuropathy Autonomic neuropathy Nutritional deficiencies (e.g. Wernicke-Korsakoff syndrome) Increased risk of head injuries Hepatic encephalopathy
Musculoskeletal	Proximal myopathy Osteopenia Avascular necrosis of femoral head Fractures and malunion Gout
Cardiovascular	Hypertension Secondary vascular disease (e.g. stroke) Cardiomyopathy Arrhythmias
Respiratory	Increased incidence of infections (e.g. tuberculosis) Chronic bronchitis Bronchial carcinoma more common
Haematological	Macrocytosis Thrombocytopenia Neutropenia, lymphopenia Haemolysis Folate deficiency Anaemia due to blood loss

Fig. 4.69 *Acute and chronic toxic effects of alcohol consumption.*

The toxic acetaldehyde is metabolised to acetate by the enzyme aldehyde dehydrogenase 2 (ALDH2). Inhibition of this enzyme therefore causes acetaldehyde to accumulate, which can cause flushing, nausea and palpitations after drinking alcohol. This property is exploited therapeutically using the ALDH2-inhibiting drug disulfiram to maintain abstinence as part of a withdrawal and rehabilitation programme.

A defective gene encoding ALDH2 is quite common in some parts of the Far East, so that these aversive symptoms occur soon after drinking alcohol. This has the net effect of keeping alcoholic cirrhosis rates relatively low.

Hepatic steatosis (the fatty liver)

The finding of a raised serum γGT level or of a high mean corpuscular volume (MCV) on the blood film is the usual first screening procedure in patients with a history of alcohol excess, but these abnormalities may not necessarily indicate any underlying liver damage. Hepatic steatosis (**Fig. 4.70**) is the commonest histological abnormality, affecting about 50% of patients who abuse alcohol. There is perivenular accumulation of intracellular fat which displaces the hepatocyte nucleus.

Acute and chronic toxic effects of alcohol consumption (Cont)

Reproductive and genitourinary	Fetal alcohol syndrome Spontaneous abortion Impotence Hypogonadism and subfertility Renal tract infections IgA nephropathy Renal tubular acidosis
Dermatological	Increased skin infections Psoriasis Nutritional deficiency (e.g. pellagra) Porphyria cutanea tarda Skin signs of chronic liver disease
Gastrointestinal*	Gingivitis and dental caries Mallory–Weiss tear Increased risk of oesophageal cancer Alcoholic gastritis Motility disorders Enteropathy and malabsorption Increased risk of colonic cancer
Hepatopancreaticobiliary	Fatty liver Alcoholic hepatitis Cirrhosis Hepatocellular carcinoma Overt expression of latent porphyrias Acute pancreatitis Chronic pancreatitis

*Discussed in more detail in chapter 7.

Fig. 4.69 *(Cont).*

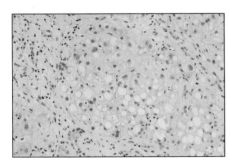

Fig. 4.70 *Hepatic steatosis. High-power view of H & E-stained liver biopsy specimen, from a patient with a history of alcohol excess, showing vesicles of fat within hepatocytes.*

Most patients are asymptomatic, but there may be right upper quadrant pain in patients who have fatty liver. This is usually because of capsular distension. Mild nausea and sometimes vomiting can be accompanying features. The liver can be tender to palpation. The hepatic transaminases may be normal, but often the ratio of AST to ALT is greater than 2. At ultrasound, there is increased echogenicity (brightness) of the liver.

Treatment is aimed at trying to ensure abstinence, but patients who have accompanying hyperlipidaemia may need treating for this in addition. Given a period of 4–6 weeks without alcohol, the steatosis will usually resolve. Patients who are physically dependent on alcohol need to be admitted to hospital and given a reducing course of a benzodiazepine, such as chlordiazepoxide, to guard against withdrawal seizures, together with high doses of thiamin to prevent Wernicke's encephalopathy.

Alcoholic hepatitis

This condition often accompanies an acute step-up in alcohol intake or a return to drinking after a prolonged period of abstinence. Patients with alcoholic hepatitis may be asymptomatic or have fatigue, weight loss, a low-grade spiking fever and right upper quadrant pain. The liver may be tender to palpation and some patients may have a hepatic bruit. Often patients are deeply jaundiced with a markedly raised serum bilirubin, alkaline phosphatase and γGT.

Hepatic decompensation with a prolonged prothrombin time, encephalopathy and ascites is not unusual. At clinical presentation, 50% of patients with alcoholic hepatitis have cirrhosis and 50% of the remainder subsequently develop cirrhosis during recovery and abstinence from alcohol. The AST/ALT ratio usually remains greater than 2 well into the recovery period.

The histological features of alcoholic hepatitis are shown in **Fig. 4.71**. The salient features are perivenular hepatocellular necrosis and polymorphonuclear leucocyte infiltration of the sinusoids. There may be intracellular accumulation of Mallory's hyalin and this is usually manifest in patients with more severe disease and a worse prognosis. Reasons suggested for the development of alcoholic hepatitis include malnutrition, alcohol-induced centrilobular hypoxia, direct toxic effects of alcohol and autoimmune mechanisms.

The clinical course of alcoholic hepatitis is variable and does not necessarily correlate with histological findings. Poor clinical prognostic factors include a serum bilirubin over 170 μmol/L, uraemia, prolonged prothrombin time unresponsive to correction with vitamin K, the presence of ascites, encephalopathy and spontaneous gastrointestinal bleeding. Mortality approaches 50% under these circumstances, but even with a normal prothrombin time and no physical signs of hepatic decompensation, it may be of the order of 1–2%.

'Discriminant function' may be used to identify patients at a high risk of mortality in alcoholic hepatitis:

- Discriminant function = 4.6 × (Prothrombin time in seconds – control) + bilirubin (in mg/dl)
- Discriminant function >32 indicates a 1 month mortality rate of 50% or over
- Calculation may be unnecessary if encephalopathy present – suggests high mortality rate itself.
- Calculation can be used to select patients for corticosteroid therapy (also need to exclude patients with active gastrointestinal bleeding, renal failure or sepsis)

Therapy involves supportive care aimed at the prevention of withdrawal seizures and the replacement of vitamin deficiencies. Specific treatment with corticosteroids (60 mg of prednisolone per day in the first instance) remains controversial, with some studies showing little benefit. However, recent meta-analyses of trial data have suggested that corticosteroids improve short-term survival for certain well-defined groups of patients. Where there is profound hepatic decompensation, liver transplantation should be considered.

Alcoholic cirrhosis

Patients may be entirely asymptomatic or present either during an episode of alcoholic hepatitis or because of the complications of portal hypertension such as ascites or variceal bleeding. Physical signs include parotid enlargement, proximal-muscle wasting,

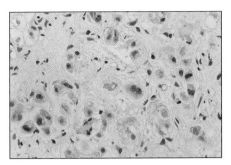

Fig. 4.71 *Mallory's hyalin in alcoholic hepatitis. Liver biopsy from a patient with alcoholic hepatitis. The eosinophilic cytoplasmic clumps within the hepatocytes (centre) are Mallory's hyalin, made up of condensed intermediate filaments. Also known as Mallory bodies, these lesions are found in about 75% of liver biopsies for suspected alcoholic disease. They may also be found in some cases of primary biliary cirrhosis and Wilson's disease.*

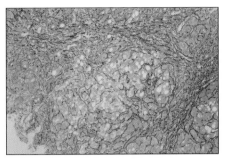

Fig. 4.72 *Alcoholic cirrhosis. Low-power view of a liver biopsy specimen from a patient with alcoholic cirrhosis. A reticulin stain has been used to enhance the appearance of fibrosis and there is obvious distortion of the liver architecture, with the scarring and regenerative hepatocyte nodules that are characteristic of cirrhosis.*

Dupuytren's contracture, spider naevi (see **Fig. 4.17**), gynaecomastia (see **Fig. 4.18**), testicular atrophy and loss of body hair. As with all patients with cirrhosis, there is an increased risk of development of hepatocellular carcinoma. Histological features of alcohol-related cirrhosis are shown in **Fig. 4.72**. Abstinence is important. The treatment of alcoholic cirrhosis centres around therapy for the complications of liver disease, but most liver transplant units will consider patients with a history of alcohol abuse for liver transplantation provided that there has been a period of proven abstinence and the psychological profile is favourable (see p. 274).

NON-ALCOHOLIC STEATOSIS OR STEATOHEPATITIS (NASH SYNDROME)

Alcohol is not the only cause of a fatty liver. Other causes include:

Most common

- Obesity
- Diabetes mellitus (particularly type II)
- Starvation
- Jejunoileal bypass surgery
- Rapid weight loss
- Drugs – e.g. amiodarone, sulphasalazine, nifedipine, methotrexate

Less common

- Chronic malabsorption
- Total parenteral nutrition
- Chronic viral hepatitis
- Wilson's disease
- Gastric bypass surgery
- Abetalipoproteinaemia

Intrahepatocyte lipid accumulation, with or without inflammatory changes, is a non-specific hepatic response to a whole range of disorders. Most individuals with this condition are asymptomatic, but some may develop upper abdominal pain due to mild hepatomegaly. The condition is usually discovered incidentally after abnormal liver function tests. Typically, the γGT level is raised and there may be a mild (< 2–3 times normal) rise in serum transaminase activity. Diffuse fatty change can be detected on ultrasonography as a hyperechogenic appearance, although areas of focal fatty-sparing can sometimes be confused with neoplasms.

The lipid that accumulates within the hepatocyte is usually triglyceride, the result of imbalances in the uptake and synthesis of fatty acids, increased production of triglyceride and decreased release of triglyceride into the bloodstream. On liver biopsy, the usual appearance is one of macrovesicular steatosis – where there is a single large cytoplasmic fat vacuole in the hepatocyte – or there may also be a variable degree of microvesicular steatosis with many small fat droplets visible in each cell. The histological appearance often resembles that of alcohol-induced fatty change and inflammatory activity can easily lead to diagnostic confusion with alcoholic hepatitis. Treatment is that of the underlying cause, such as improved diabetic control, withdrawal of precipitating drugs and gradual weight loss in the obese. However a too-rapid fall in weight can lead to a worsened steatohepatitis. There is evidence that some individuals have progressive fibrosis and that NASH may be a cause of cirrhosis.

MICROVESICULAR STEATOSIS

Some degree of microvesicular steatosis may occur in the conditions that cause NASH, but this is also the main histological finding in a group of more serious liver disorders. Examples include the acute fatty liver of pregnancy (see p. 250), Reye's syndrome, certain drug reactions (notably sodium valproate), viral hepatitis and some rare inherited metabolic defects (including Alpers syndrome, urea cycle defects and cholesterol ester storage disease). The aetiological final common pathway in many of these conditions is believed to be mitochondrial dysfunction.

GENETIC HAEMOCHROMATOSIS

Haemochromatosis, the excessive deposition of iron throughout the body, can occur as a secondary event following a number of pathological processes. Examples include iron overload after multiple blood transfusions for haemoglobinopathies (see **Fig. 4.43**) and occasionally after excessive oral or parenteral iron therapy. An increase in hepatic iron content is often seen in alcoholic liver disease, porphyria cutanea tarda and in some cases following portocaval anastomosis. Primary haemochromatosis, however, is the result of an autosomal genetic defect.

Aetiology and pathogenesis

The normal adult body contains 3–4 g of iron. Most of this (60–70%) is present as haemoglobin, and only about 1 g is present in the tissues. Normal daily losses of iron are about 1 mg in males (mostly in the stool, but also some smaller amounts from the skin and urine) and an average of 2–2.5 mg per day in menstruating women. As the typical daily diet contains around 15 mg/day and the ability to excrete iron is limited, the body is really only able to regulate its iron content by limiting intestinal absorption.

In the early stages of primary haemochromatosis, there is excessive absorption of dietary iron, although as iron overload occurs later in the disease, the rate of absorption may slow to normal levels (and yet still inappropriately high in the setting of iron excess). Uptake of luminal iron into the enterocytes proceeds as normal, but an excessive amount is allowed to pass into the circulation rather than being retained within the cell for subsequent shedding into the gut.

The genetic basis of this phenomenon has been localised to the 'HFE' gene on the short arm of chromosome 6 close to the HLA-A locus. The most common mutation that leads to haemochromatosis is a single base substitution leading to replacement of a cysteine residue with tyrosine at position 282 (the 'C282Y' mutation).

Although the haemochromatosis gene has been identified, it is still not clear exactly what mechanism is responsible for the excessive tissue iron that occurs in homozygotes. Phenotypically, the condition is influenced by other factors which affect iron balance such as menstruation or dietary iron content. It is estimated that approximately 50% of male homozygotes and 25% of female homozygotes will develop potentially life-threatening clinical complications of haemochromatosis. About a quarter of heterozygotes demonstrate mild biochemical abnormalities (such as high serum ferritin or transferrin saturation levels) but they do not develop hepatic iron overload unless other liver pathology is present.

Hepatic injury due to excess iron deposition may be summarised as follows:
- Iron-dependent lipid peroxidation damages hepatocyte cellular membranes
- Subsequent impairment of membrane functions such as mitochondrial oxidative metabolism, microsomal enzymes (e.g. cytochrome p450) and lysosomes
- Hepatocellular injury leading to activation of Kupffer cells
- Kupffer cell-derived cytokines trigger stellate cells to produce fibrosis.

If left unchecked, the hepatic fibrosis develops into established cirrhosis with all its possible complications. Patients with cirrhosis due to haemochromatosis are particularly at risk of developing hepatocellular carcinoma, which can be multifocal in origin. Consequently, surveillance with ultrasound scanning and serum α-fetoprotein estimation is required.

Epidemiology

The measured prevalence of primary haemochromatosis rather depends on how it is defined. Early studies that relied on the classical physical signs described below led to the disease being considered rare. With the advent of genetic testing it is known that homozygous C282Y mutations are found in about 1 in 300 of the population, with the heterozygous carrier frequency being as high as 1 in 10. In populations of northwestern European origin, it is the most common recessively inherited genetic disorder.

Clinical features

In the early stages, most patients are asymptomatic, although some may have non-specific complaints such as fatigue or malaise. Thereafter, the clinical features depend on the particular organ systems damaged by excessive iron deposition (**Fig. 4.73**).

Overall, the total body iron content may be increased 20–40-fold, but this average figure hides the disproportionate amount deposited in some tissues. Excess iron is deposited in the liver, pancreas, endocrine organs (particularly the pituitary but also the thyroid and adrenal glands), heart and joint synovia. Very little iron is found in the bone marrow, spleen or small bowel mucosa.

The classical presentation with 'bronze diabetes' does occur, but lethargy, arthralgia and loss of libido are the most common symptoms. On examination, the most frequent signs are hepatomegaly, skin pigmentation and loss of body hair. The clinical manifestations of advanced disease tend to occur in men typically at age 40–50 years, with the protective effect of menstruation (and usually a lower iron intake) leading to female patients generally presenting at an older age.

Diagnosis

It is likely that the recently developed genetic tests for haemochromatosis will play an increasing diagnostic role. Currently, a combination of biochemical blood tests and liver biopsy characteristics is used (**Fig. 4.74**). Raised serum ferritin and transferrin saturations are strongly suggestive of haemochromatosis. However, ferritin levels in particular can be raised in other illnesses (as an acute-phase response in many inflammatory conditions including alcoholic liver disease) and these should be considered if the transferrin saturation is normal. The serum iron level is also subject to wide fluctuations, including diurnal variations, and so is unreliable. Routine liver function tests are normal in most cases of haemochromatosis, particularly precirrhosis.

Clinical features and complications of haemochromatosis

Liver involvement	Iron deposition leads to fibrosis and cirrhosis Hepatomegaly common Jaundice and ascites infrequent Increased incidence of hepatocellular carcinoma (may be as high as 30% lifetime risk in cirrhosis)
Pigmentation	Due to excess production of melanin Worst in sun-exposed areas and skin creases May also be found on oral mucosa Reduces with iron-removal therapy
Diabetes mellitus	Present in ~60% of cases with established cirrhosis May be type I or II Subclinical, impaired glucose tolerance common Pancreatic fibrosis accompanies iron deposition Diabetic control may improve after iron removal
Cardiomyopathy	Myocardial iron deposition leads to muscle degeneration and fibrosis Arrhythmias common Cardiomyopathy may improve with iron removal
Hypogonadism	Iron deposition in anterior pituitary gland Hypogonadotrophic hypogonadism Impotence, testicular atrophy, loss of body hair Amenorrhoea Usually fails to improve after iron removal
Arthropathy	Most commonly affects second and third metacarpophalangeal joints, knees, hips, shoulders Chondrocalcinosis and pseudogout common Usually fails to improve after iron removal

Fig. 4.73 *Clinical features and complications of haemochromatosis.*

If the serum ferritin and transferrin saturations are found to be raised, a liver biopsy should be performed – not just to ascertain the presence of iron overload, but also to determine whether or not cirrhosis has developed. As well as the usual histological features (including Perl's stain, see **Fig. 4.43**), a biochemical analysis can be requested to measure hepatic iron content.

In the absence of known causes of secondary iron overload, the current criteria for diagnosing haemochromatosis are at least two of the following:
• Perl's stain of grade 3 or above
• Hepatic iron content > 80 µmol/g dry weight
• Hepatic iron index > 2
• More than 4 g iron already removed by venesection
The histopathological grade of Perl's staining is proportionate to the amount of iron present. Most cases have a grade of 2–4, with predominantly periportal hepatocytes bearing the brunt of the iron overload. In more severe cases (grade 4) there may be fibrosis and deposition of iron within Kupffer cells.

Investigations used in hereditary haemochromatosis

Investigation	Characteristics	False positives	False negatives
Transferrin saturation	Serum iron ÷ total iron-binding capacity > 55% in 90% of cases	Oral iron therapy	If total iron-binding capacity raised
Serum ferritin	Raised in > 95% of cases	Almost any inflammatory disorder Alcoholic liver disease	Uncommon (< 5%)
Serum transaminases, alkaline phosphatase, bilirubin, γGT	May be helpful in detecting liver damage, but of little diagnostic use	Very common	Very common
HLA-A3	Associated with haemochromatosis Useful in testing sibling of known cases, but not for *de novo* diagnosis	HLA-A3 found in about 25% of normal population	Only occurs in about 75% of haemochromatosis cases
Hepatic iron index	Dry-weight liver iron content ÷ age > 2 in 90% of cases	Very rare	Uncommon
Genetic testing	> 90% of UK cases homozygous for C282Y mutation	No	Less than 10% in UK, perhaps more in southern Europe

Fig. 4.74 *Investigations used in hereditary haemochromatosis.*

Given that age-related iron accumulation can be a feature of many diseases, the specificity of intrahepatic iron as a marker of haemochromatosis can be increased by expressing it as the hepatic iron index: the hepatic iron content divided by the patient's age. Consequently, a mild degree of iron deposition is of greater significance in a 25-year-old than in a 60-year-old.

MRI scanning of the liver can be used to demonstrate hepatic iron overload (**Fig. 4.75**) and has been suggested by some authors as an alternative to liver biopsy. Although there is some correlation between MRI appearances and intrahepatic iron levels, it tends to be more accurate in heavily overloaded livers, with reliability dipping considerably for more mild cases. While MRI can provide some structural and therefore prognostic information it is not as definitive as a liver biopsy in diagnosing cirrhosis.

Treatment

The most important aspects of managing this condition are to diagnose and treat it before the development of complications such as cirrhosis. Excess iron is most effectively removed

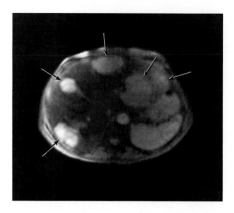

Fig. 4.75 *Iron overload on hepatic MRI. A gradient-echo MRI scan of a patient with haemochromatosis who also has liver metastases from a colorectal cancer. The difference between the iron-overloaded hepatic parenchyma (the dark areas) and the non-iron-containing metastases (arrowed) is quite obvious.*

by phlebotomy, each venesection of a 500 ml unit of blood removing about 250 mg of iron. Given that some patients with haemochromatosis have iron stores of up to 60 g, it may take a considerable number of venesections to return to normality. Healthy young patients should tolerate an initial venesection rate of twice weekly, although older or more frail patients may only be able to withstand weekly or even fortnightly phlebotomy. There is a good deal of evidence that the quicker the iron can be removed, the better the prognosis. Sequential liver biopsy studies have shown that reversal of early fibrotic changes is possible after iron removal.

Patients undergoing venesection should have their haemoglobin and full blood count measured at each phlebotomy, with serum iron, ferritin and transferrin saturation measured approximately every 3 months. Phlebotomy should continue until the serum ferritin is within normal limits, the transferrin saturation is below 50% and the haemoglobin level reduced to a state of mild anaemia. These indices can be kept at the lower end of the normal range by maintenance venesections of a frequency dictated by the blood tests, but usually between two and six occasions per year.

Some patients, particularly those with heart failure, may not be able to withstand the haemodynamic instability of regular venesection. An alternative therapy is the iron-chelating agent desferrioxamine. Given by intravenous infusion, it is more time-consuming and costly than phlebotomy, but the subsequent improvement in cardiac function may allow venesection to be introduced later.

The removal of excess iron stores prior to the development of cirrhosis leads to the restoration of a normal life expectancy. This cannot be said for patients with established cirrhosis, but weekly venesection is still important in improving symptoms such as fatigue and abdominal pain as well as diabetic control. Unfortunately, male impotence and arthralgia are likely to persist.

Patients with haemochromatosis are at high risk of developing hepatocellular carcinoma and should undergo regular surveillance.

In common with other causes of chronic liver disease and cirrhosis, liver transplantation remains an important therapeutic option for haemochromatosis.

Given the genetic basis of the condition it is vital that counselling and screening of the patient's first-degree relatives be carried out. All should have their ferritin and transferrin saturation measured and siblings should also have HLA haplotyping performed. HLA-identical siblings will almost certainly be homozygous for the haemochromatosis gene in view of its linkage to the HLA locus. A liver biopsy is advisable for first-degree relatives with elevated iron studies. HLA-identical siblings with normal iron indices should have these repeated at regular intervals (every 2–3 years) as they will remain at high risk of developing future phenotypic expression. Ferritin and transferrin saturation can also be used to screen members of the extended family. In the future, the commercial availability of genetic testing for the C282Y mutation is likely to make this method of screening much more common.

WILSON'S DISEASE

Wilson's disease, sometimes referred to as hepatolenticular degeneration, is an autosomal recessive disorder of copper metabolism leading to its accumulation in the body. This results in a number of possible hepatic, haematological, neurological and psychiatric sequelae.

Epidemiology

Because of its autosomal genetic transmission, Wilson's disease affects men and women at equal rates. Only homozygotes develop the disease. In western Caucasian populations, the gene is carried by approximately 1%, with the prevalence of the disease being about 1 in 30 000. Most patients present in the second decade of life with liver disease, although the remainder that present in the third or fourth decade tend to have neuropsychiatric involvement. There is often overlap between these two patterns of presentation.

Aetiology and pathogenesis

Normally, the body contains between 100 and 150 mg of copper, most of it stored in the liver. Copper's main metabolic role is as a catalyst in a number of biochemical reactions, such as collagen synthesis, normal erythropoiesis and cytochrome oxidation. Most of the 2–5 mg of copper taken in the daily diet is not absorbed, some 70% passing straight out again in the faeces. Of the copper taken up by the small intestine, around 16% is retained within the enterocyte and subsequently shed into the bowel lumen. The majority of the copper carried in the bloodstream is ultimately excreted into the bile, with a small amount (around 4%) passed in the urine. The liver is able to either incorporate copper into the blood-borne transport protein caeruloplasmin or secrete it into the bile in a protein-bound form that is not reabsorbed.

The Wilson's gene has now been localised to chromosome 13q14.3 and encodes a membrane-bound ATPase copper-transport protein that is normally required for both the effective biliary excretion of copper and its incorporation into caeruloplasmin. Consequently, in homozygotes for the Wilson's gene mutation, the body's copper content steadily rises, with deposition initially in the liver followed by accumulation in the central nervous system, cornea and kidneys. Excess copper damages cells in a number of ways, including disruption of lysosomal and plasma membranes, depletion of glutathione and interference with cytoskeletal proteins.

Clinical features

By and large, Wilson's disease becomes symptomatic in childhood and early adulthood. It is rare for symptoms to start before the age of 5 and only about 10% of cases become symptomatic after 25 years of age. Although rare, it is not unknown for a few patients to present as late as aged 50.

The symptoms and signs depend on the predominant pattern of organ involvement. Liver damage due to Wilson's disease may mimic any of the other causes of acute or chronic hepatitis and is the first sign of Wilson's disease in about 60% of patients. An acute or remitting-relapsing hepatitic illness often occurs and Wilson's may even present as fulminant hepatic failure. In this latter scenario, the prognosis is uniformly poor and death is almost inevitable without liver transplantation.

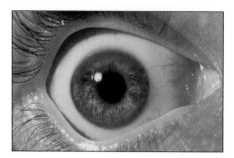

Fig. 4.76 *Kayser–Fleischer rings in Wilson's disease. The rings typically appear as gold-brown discolouration around the corneal margin. (Courtesy of AVS Department, Imperial College School of Medicine at St Mary's Hospital).*

A mild Coomb's test-negative haemolytic anaemia is a frequent companion to the hepatitis although it can be severe in some cases, particularly when associated with acute liver failure.

Haemolytic episodes are thought to be triggered by episodic release of large amounts of copper into the blood, presumably from the liver, although what causes this release is unknown.

Chronic hepatitis may lead to the eventual development of cirrhosis and clinical features such as ascites, bleeding episodes or encephalopathy. Curiously, hepatocellular carcinoma is very uncommon in cirrhosis due to Wilson's disease, leading to speculation as to whether copper has some 'protective' effect against oncogenesis.

Neurological or psychiatric disease is the presenting feature in about 40% of cases of Wilson's disease. Features are often vague initially and may include subtle personality change, impaired academic performance and clumsiness leading to more obvious changes such as tremor, rigidity, altered gait, excessive salivation and slurred speech. The condition may present as a psychiatric illness with neurosis, psychosis, manic depression or dementia.

The neurological involvement is characterised pathologically by damage to the corpus callosum, putamen, cerebral and cerebellar white matter and in some cases degenerative changes in the frontal cerebral cortex.

Many of these patients have visible Kayser–Fleischer rings (**Fig. 4.76**), a physical sign pathognomonic of Wilson's disease. Copper deposition in the superior and inferior margins of the cornea leads to the green-brown or gold-brown discolouration. Slit-lamp examination can be used to detect more subtle deposition, although this slightly lowers the specificity of the rings for Wilson's disease, with similar slit-lamp findings in some cases of primary biliary cirrhosis or autoimmune hepatitis.

Copper deposition may also lead to renal damage, although this is usually relatively mild. Renal tubular damage may result in proteinuria, hypercalciuria, glycosuria or amino aciduria.

Diagnosis

Wilson's disease is not difficult to diagnose, given the ideal set of circumstances; for instance, a combination of hepatitis, neurological disease and a Coomb's-negative haemolysis, perhaps with a family history of an affected sibling or Kayser–Fleischer rings. However, these classical patterns are not present in many patients and many of the investigations (**Fig. 4.77**) are subject to frequent false positives and negatives. A simple genetic test has been difficult to develop because there are a number of different possible mutations in the gene.

Although the serum copper and caeruloplasmin may be low, the specificity of these measurements is relatively poor. An estimation of 24-hour urinary copper excretion, ideally followed by comparison with a penicillamine challenge, is somewhat more accurate although neither approach is perfect.

Tests used in the diagnosis of Wilson's disease

Investigation	Findings	False positives	False negatives
Caeruloplasmin	Usually low or even absent	May be low in some heterozygotes	May be raised in advanced Wilson's
Serum copper	Low in most cases	May be low in some heterozygotes	May be elevated in fulminant Wilson's
24-hour urinary copper excretion	Rarely less than 100 µg/24 hours Sensitivity increased by penicillamine challenge – increases copper excretion (> 1000 µg/24 hours)	Copper excretion may be raised in other liver diseases, particularly chronic cholestasis Special container needed to avoid copper contamination	Rare
Slit-lamp examination for Kayser–Fleischer (KF) rings	Pathognomonic for Wilson's disease if visible clinically	Slit-lamp abnormalities may be detected in primary biliary cirrhosis and autoimmune hepatitis	KF rings tend to be found in those cases of Wilson's disease with neurological involvement
Liver biopsy	Histopathology may show chronic hepatitis or early cirrhotic changes Not very specific Special stains (e.g. rubeanic acid) to show copper Measurement of dry-weight copper content can be performed (usually > 250 µg/g)	Intrahepatic copper often increased in primary biliary cirrhosis and autoimmune chronic active hepatitis	Occasionally

Fig. 4.77 *Tests used in the diagnosis of Wilson's disease.*

Histopathological study and biochemical analysis of liver biopsy specimens can be diagnostic, although copper deposition can occur non-specifically in certain other diseases such as chronic cholestasis or autoimmune hepatitis.

However, a combination of blood tests, urinary copper studies and liver biopsy allows an accurate diagnosis in the majority of cases.

Treatment

If left untreated, Wilson's disease is a fatal condition. The availability of copper-chelating agents such as penicillamine has resulted in the disorder being easily treatable, with neurological complications potentially avoidable as long as Wilson's disease is diagnosed and treated early enough. Advanced neuropsychiatric disease, however, is seldom successfully treated.

Penicillamine is the drug of choice for Wilson's disease. Most patients require 1–1.5 g daily in divided doses and therapy is continued indefinitely. Penicillamine is excreted, together with its bound copper, in the urine and a prompt cupriesis develops with urinary levels usually above 2000 µg/24 hours.

Adverse reactions occur in up to 50% of patients at some stage, although most of these cases can be managed by either a brief dose reduction or temporary withdrawal of the drug. Between 5–10% of patients, however, are unable to tolerate penicillamine.

In some cases there may be an initial worsening of established neurological disease or it may be provoked for the first time by penicillamine therapy. In most cases this is transient. Acute sensitivity reactions are relatively common, including fever, blood dyscrasia, nephrotic syndrome and skin rashes. The drug seems safe in pregnancy and outweighs the risk of exacerbating the Wilson's disease by withdrawing it.

For those unable to take penicillamine, alternative copper-chelating drugs, such as trientine, are now available.

α_1-ANTITRYPSIN DEFICIENCY

The protein α_1-antitrypsin (AAT) is normally produced by the liver. Its main physiological role is to inhibit neutrophil elastase and thereby limit the degree of tissue damage that occurs in an acute inflammatory response. Around 1 in 2000 of the population are homozygotic for mutations in the AAT gene and, depending on the type of mutation, may develop liver disease due to excessive hepatocyte storage of the abnormal protein and/or emphysema due to pulmonary damage from unopposed neutrophil elastase.

Aetiology and pathogenesis

More than 60 different AAT gene mutations have been described. In the normal individual, serum AAT levels are under the control of two codominant alleles, one inherited from each parent.

Four variant forms account for almost all of the expression patterns seen in humans. They are known as Pi (or protein inhibitor) alleles and are further delineated according to the electrophoretic mobility of their protein product. Hence, they can be listed as:
1. PiM (for medium) – the most common form, found in 86–99% of normal populations
2. PiS (slow)
3. PiZ (ultra-slow)
The latter two variations are the two commonest aberrant forms. It is only rarely that the AAT allele is deleted completely and this fourth variant is termed 'Pi null'. Consequently, an individual may inherit any combination of two of these alleles, which will then lead to the relevant level of serum AAT activity (**Fig. 4.78**).

Panlobular emphysema is one consequence of lowered serum concentrations of AAT. In contrast, the liver disease that develops is the result of the accumulation of AAT in hepatocyte endoplasmic reticulum. Not all the AAT variants behave in the same way, however. Those who have one or two alleles of the Z type have an amino acid substitution in the AAT molecule that makes it more likely to be retained in the endoplasmic reticulum and cause hepatocyte damage. The protein produced by the S allele, whilst also leading to a lack of AAT secretion, is degraded within the hepatocyte and so does not accumulate. Furthermore, the null allele leads to no protein being produced at all and hence no hepatocyte damage. Hence, although all may lead to a reduced serum level (and increased tendency to emphysema), only the Z variants such as ZZ, SZ or MZ develop liver disease.

α_1-Antitrypsin phenotypes and their corresponding enzyme levels

Phenotype	Serum α_1-antitrypsin level (% of normal)
MM (i.e. 'normal' pattern)	100
MS	80
MZ	60
SS	60
M null	50
SZ	40
ZZ	15
Null null	0

Fig. 4.78 α_1-Antitrypsin phenotypes and their corresponding enzyme levels.

Clinical features

A wide spectrum of liver disease may be produced depending on the particular pattern of AAT deficiency, ranging from barely significant hepatic involvement to end-stage liver disease with cirrhosis and hepatocellular carcinoma.

Liver disease due to PiZZ homozygosity was first described in children and only later recognised as a cause of chronic liver disease in adults. A neonatal hepatitis may be seen in about 15% of cases and some may go on to follow a progressive course with cirrhosis developing in late childhood. The majority of PiZZ individuals survive childhood and are then more likely to present much later in life. Overt liver disease tends to become apparent in the 50–60 years age group although a small proportion may have developed pulmonary complications around 10 years earlier. Approximately a third of PiZZ cases will not develop any clinical evidence of liver disease at all.

Those individuals who are heterozygotic for the Z allele may occasionally develop liver disease at an even later age. There is also some evidence that Z heterozygotes are at increased risk of developing cirrhosis when exposed to other causes of chronic liver injury.

Diagnosis

The serum AAT should be measured in all suspected cases of chronic liver disease. While a low level (typically below 0.5 g/l) is almost always found in ZZ homozygotes, it can be affected by inflammatory processes and so is not completely reliable. The AAT phenotype can be determined by protein electrophoresis.

Treatment

There is currently no specific treatment for AAT deficiency, although researchers are exploring different techniques of possible gene therapy. Management consists of the same supportive care given to individuals with chronic liver disease of other aetiologies. Liver transplantation is an important therapeutic option for those patients with cirrhosis.

ACUTE HEPATIC PORPHYRIAS

The porphyrias are characterised by abnormalities of haem biosynthesis and can be broadly grouped into hepatic and erythropoietic varieties. In the hepatic types (acute intermittent porphyria, porphyria variegata, hereditary coproporphyria and aminolevulinic acid dehydrase deficiency), disordered porphyrin metabolism occurs in the liver.

Clinical features

There are a number of different possible presentations. Patients may develop an acute colicky abdominal pain that resembles an acute abdomen. There may also be vomiting, back pain, diarrhoea, tachycardia and hypertension. Neurological presentations include convulsions, confusion, paraesthesiae, peripheral paralyses and psychotic disorders. If these are left untreated, a generalised paralysis and tetraparesis may occur.

Diagnosis

A correct diagnosis is vital as the condition can be worsened by various drugs as well as surgery and anaesthetics. It is based on detecting increased production of the porphyrin precursors porphobilinogen and δ-aminolevulinic acid in the urine. A 20 ml sample is usually sufficient. Classically, the excess porphobilinogen in the urine causes a pink colour to develop when Ehrlich's reagent is added and this cannot be removed by organic solvents (the Watson–Schwartz test). Establishing the exact type of porphyria requires further biochemical analysis of porphyrin metabolites in faeces, urine and blood.

Treatment

Any drugs that may have precipitated the acute attack should be withdrawn. Typical examples include phenytoin, barbiturates, oestrogens, alcohol and sulphonamides, but there are many others.

Specific treatment involves suppressing the activity of the aminolevulinic acid synthetase enzyme, by negative feedback, with an intravenous infusion of haematin (or haem arginate).

PORPHYRIA CUTANEA TARDA

Porphyria cutanea tarda (PCT) is the commonest of all the porphyrias. Characterised by a deficiency of uroporphyrinogen decarboxylase, it exists in a familial and a sporadic form, the latter being more frequent. While the familial form is expressed in all the tissues, the biochemical abnormality is confined to the liver in the sporadic type. Unlike in the acute porphyrias, neurological involvement does not occur.

There is a strong association with hepatitis C, iron overload and alcohol excess. The main symptoms relate to the skin, with erythema and vesicular eruptions occurring in sun-exposed areas. Alopecia and excessive or reduced skin pigmentation may also develop.

As well as the hepatic disease associations already mentioned, the main differential diagnoses are photosensitive drug reactions, variegate porphyria and coproporphyria. Urinary and faecal porphyrin studies usually clinch the diagnosis.

PCT can be treated by regular venesection, with the removal of 500 ml of blood every 1–2 weeks until there is a marked fall in the urinary uroporphyrin levels or the blood haemoglobin concentration drops below 11 g/dl.

AUTOIMMUNE HEPATITIS

Autoimmune hepatitis is a group of conditions of unknown cause, characterised by the presence of certain autoantibodies, that can result in acute and/or chronic liver disease. A number of different subtypes have been recognised and more is being learned about the relevant targets of these autoantibodies. Effective immunosuppressive treatment is essential to avoid the development of cirrhosis.

Epidemiology

Autoimmune hepatitis (AIH) typically causes a chronic inflammatory disease of the liver, but acute presentations do occur. The condition is commonest among young women, with the usual age of onset somewhere between 20 and 40 years, although it may affect both sexes at any age.

The prevalence of AIH varies around the world. It is responsible for about a third of all cases of chronic hepatitis in Germany, over 60% of cases in Australia and just 1% in the Far East. In the UK, the annual incidence is just less than 1 case per 100 000 population.

Aetiology and pathogenesis

The aetiology of autoimmune hepatitis is still unknown. It is hypothesised that some form of environmental or infectious agent triggers the inflammatory response in a genetically predisposed individual, but the precise mechanism remains elusive. It seems likely that AIH is a heterologous group of disorders whose respective aetiologies may differ from each other.

Based on clinical and serological data, four main subtypes of AIH can be identified (Fig. 4.79). In some cases, the target antigens of the associated autoantibodies are known, but their role in the pathogenesis of liver injury is unclear. It is possible that the autoantibodies may be a consequence, rather than a cause, of the tissue damage.

One can speculate, however, that exposure of these target antigens on the surface of hepatocytes leads to an immune injury mediated by humoral factors (such as complement fixation) or T lymphocytes. For example, the cytochrome component that is the immunodominant epitope in type 2 AIH (cytochrome p450 IID6) has some amino acid sequence homology with the intermediate – early protein of herpes simplex virus type 1. It has been suggested that infection with the virus may subsequently trigger this form of autoimmune liver disease. However, this explanation may be a little oversimplistic given that many patients with anti-LKM antibodies are seronegative for herpes simplex.

Clinical features

The classical AIH, type 1 or 'lupoid' hepatitis (unconnected with systemic lupus erythematosus), usually presents with initially vague symptoms such as malaise, fatigue, anorexia and nausea. In common with the other types of AIH, there is often a preceding

Classification of autoimmune hepatitis

Type	Autoantibodies	Target antigen	Clinical features
Type 1	Antinuclear Anti-smooth muscle	Unknown F-actin	Classical 'lupoid hepatitis' Responds to corticosteroids
Type 2	Anti-LKM (liver, kidney microsomal)	Cytochrome p450	Common in mainland Europe Strong association with hepatitis C Responds to corticosteroids
Type 3	Anti-soluble liver antigen	Subunits of glutathione-S-transferase	Similar to type 1 Responds to corticosteroids
Type 4	None described	Unknown	Similar features to type 1 Responds to corticosteroids

Fig. 4.79 *Classification of autoimmune hepatitis.*

239

history of autoimmune or chronic inflammatory diseases in either the patient or his/her family members. These include keratoconjunctivitis sicca (35% of AIH patients), renal tubular acidosis (25%), peripheral neuropathy (10%), Hashimoto's thyroiditis (7%), ulcerative colitis (4%) and rheumatoid disease (2%).

Some patients may develop a pseudo-Cushingoid appearance with striae, truncal obesity, moon-like facies and a 'buffalo' hump. Most patients, however, have spider naevi and palmar erythema (see **Fig. 4.20**), although jaundice is uncommon in the early stages. About 40% of patients have a more rapid presentation that can be similar to an acute viral hepatitis with jaundice, tender hepatomegaly and multiple spider naevi. As well as a more marked elevation of serum transaminases, some impairment of synthetic liver function is often found in these acute cases. Many of these cases are thought to represent an acute exacerbation of an underlying subclinical chronic hepatitis.

In the majority of patients, AIH runs a remitting and relapsing course and, if untreated, may progress to the development of cirrhosis. Occasionally, patients may not present until this stage has been reached and complications such as portal hypertension, ascites and encephalopathy have developed.

Type 2 AIH has a slightly different natural history. It is particularly common in mainland Europe (making up 20% of adult AIH in Germany and France compared to less than 5% in the UK and USA). Type 2 AIH usually has its onset in childhood and is more likely to have an acute presentation and a more rapid progression to cirrhosis. Up to 30% of patients with hepatitis C infection have detectable anti-LKM antibodies, although in most cases they are of different epitope reactivity to the antibodies found in type 2 AIH.

The clinical appearances of AIH types 3 and 4 are similar to that of type 1.

Diagnosis

Autoimmune hepatitis is characterised by the presence of periportal hepatitis (interface hepatitis or piecemeal necrosis) on liver biopsy, hypergammaglobulinaemia and liver-associated autoantibodies in the serum. Alternative diagnoses which may present with similar features need to be excluded, such as chronic viral hepatitis, Wilson's disease, AAT deficiency and drug-induced hepatitis. In addition, certain 'overlap' variants of AIH exist, where the serological and histological features may share some characteristics with primary biliary cirrhosis, primary sclerosing cholangitis or viral hepatitis.

Patients with AIH usually have a polyclonal increase in gamma globulin, predominantly of IgG and, in order to fit the diagnosis of AIH, the level must be at least one and a half times the upper limit of normal. The autoantibodies (such as anti-smooth muscle, antinuclear or anti-LKM) should be present in titres of at least 1:20 in children and 1:80 in adults.

In the classical type 1 form of AIH, around 60% of patients have anti-smooth muscle antibodies and 40–70% have antinuclear antibodies. Many patients have both detectable in their sera.

On liver histology, the hallmark of AIH is periportal hepatitis, although it is not completely specific for this condition. There is disruption of the portal tract limiting plate by an infiltration of mononuclear cells together with loss of hepatocytes by apoptosis (and hence the change from the previous descriptive term 'piecemeal necrosis'). The presence of bridging necrosis or multilobular necrosis implies a poorer prognosis, with a greater risk of developing cirrhosis.

Treatment

Effective immunosuppression with corticosteroids and/or azathioprine is the mainstay of treating AIH. Initial doses are usually high in order to control the ongoing inflammation.

Most adults should be started on prednisolone 60 mg/day and this can usually be reduced to 40 mg/day after 2 weeks or so. Thereafter, changes in dosage are governed by disease activity, but most patients remain on a typical maintenance dose of between 10 and 20 mg/day for several months before the dose can be brought down any further. Steroids are of proven benefit in cases of severe AIH (10-fold elevation in serum transaminases and bridging necrosis on liver biopsy), cutting mortality from 30% to around 5%. The benefits of treating mild degrees of AIH are less well established, but most hepatologists would treat cases with elevated serum transaminases or histological evidence of interface hepatitis.

Azathioprine can be used as a steroid-sparing agent and is usually prescribed at a dose of 1–1.5 mg/kg/day. Although of little benefit in suppressing active disease it is very effective in maintaining remission. Cyclosporin can be used in patients who are intolerant or unresponsive to azathioprine and steroids.

Patients should be kept on immunosuppressive therapy for at least 1–2 years and consideration should then be given to performing a further liver biopsy to assess disease activity. If there is no evidence of ongoing inflammation, steroids can be withdrawn and around 35–50% of patients are able to tolerate this without relapse. In the remainder, however, relapse usually occurs early, particularly in the first 3 years. Those patients who still have significant inflammatory activity after 1–2 years of immunosuppression are at relatively high risk of developing cirrhosis and their therapy should be increased.

For those with end-stage liver disease, transplantation is the most effective therapeutic option. Post-transplant survival rates for these patients are currently over 80% at 5 years and, although recurrence of AIH has been described, it is rarely a clinical problem.

PRIMARY BILIARY CIRRHOSIS

Primary biliary cirrhosis (PBC) is a chronic disorder of unknown aetiology in which there is an insidious and progressive cholestasis with damage to the intrahepatic biliary tree, leading to fibrosis and, eventually, cirrhosis.

Epidemiology

PBC is most commonly found in middle-aged women, with the female to male ratio of affected patients being 9:1 and the median age at onset somewhere between 50 and 55 years. There are marked geographical variations in prevalence, with some 240 cases per million population in the UK and 50–150 cases/million in most of Europe and North America; the condition is relatively rare in Africa and Asia.

Clustering of cases has been well described, leading to suggestions of possible environmental triggers. While some studies have shown no obvious HLA associations, there does appear to be a weak association with HLA-DR8. An autoimmune aetiology has been proposed, particularly in view of some of the extrahepatic diseases associated with PBC:

Common (50–60%)
- Sjögren's syndrome

Less common (5–20%)
- Fibrosing alveolitis
- Raynaud's phenomenon
- Scleroderma
- Thyroid disease (Hashimoto's thyroiditis, hyperthyroidism and hypothyroidism)
- Small joint arthropathy
- Urinary tract infections

Uncommon (less than 5%)
- Addison's disease
- Myasthenia gravis
- CREST syndrome
- Coeliac disease
- Vitiligo
- Renal tubular acidosis
- Autoimmune haemolytic anaemia

241

As with many presumed autoimmune diseases, the reason for the disproportionate number of women affected has yet to be explained. One hypothesis is that some of these autoimmune conditions may represent a low-grade 'graft versus host' type of response due to microchimerism with persistent fetal lymphocytes after pregnancy. There are certainly a number of biochemical and histological similarities between PBC and the hepatic graft versus host disease seen after bone marrow transplantation. Further studies are under way.

Aetiology and pathogenesis

The aetiology of PBC is unknown. An autoimmune basis could be supported by the presence of serum autoantibodies (antimitochondrial antibodies in particular), circulating immune complexes and histological evidence of granulomas and lymphocytic infiltrations.

Levels of serum immunoglobulins are usually raised, particularly IgM and, to a lesser degree, IgG. Antimitochondrial antibodies, the hallmark of PBC, are reactive against the inner multi-enzyme complex of mitochondria and specific antigens described include pyruvate dehydrogenase (recognised by the M2 subtype of antimitochondrial antibody, specific to PBC) and 2-oxo-glutarate dehydrogenase. Autoantibodies directed against the gp210 nuclear pore protein are found in about 15% of PBC patients. Numerous other autoantibodies have also been reported to varying degrees, including antinuclear, antithyroid and anti-centromere antibodies.

The precise pathogenesis of the liver injury is not clear. Histological appearances vary depending on the progression of the disease and some histopathologists have classified the condition into four stages:
- Stage 1 – Initially, bile duct damage and inflammation occur in the small and medium-sized intrahepatic ducts. There is usually an expansion of the portal tracts with infiltration of lymphocytes and often the development of granulomas. At this stage, the limiting plate is intact and inflammation is confined to the portal tracts
- Stage 2 – Inflammation spreads beyond the portal tracts, gradual loss of bile ducts begins to occur and cholestasis becomes more prominent. Granulomas (**Fig. 4.80.**) and Mallory bodies may be seen
- Stage 3 – Increasing fibrosis, which may link adjacent portal tracts, and cholestasis
- Stage 4 – Cirrhosis with paucity of bile ducts

Clinical features

Fatigue and pruritus are the archetypal symptoms of PBC. Both can vary in significance and may be quite debilitating. Severe fatigue or pruritus unresponsive to medical therapy can in itself be an indication for liver transplantation in PBC.

The underlying mechanism for the pruritus is unknown but is thought to be related to changes in the endogenous opioid neurotransmitter system, with an increased central opioidergic tone and upregulation of opioid receptors in patients with PBC.

Overall, pruritus is the first symptom to develop in about half of all patients with PBC, with the next commonest symptoms being fatigue, arthralgia and non-specific abdominal discomfort. Up to 20% of patients may develop symptomatic liver disease as the first manifestation, with jaundice, variceal bleeding or ascites. On examination, scratch marks are common and there may be signs of chronic liver disease such as spider naevi or palmar erythemas (see **Figs 4.19** and **4.20**). Associated diseases such as small joint arthropathy (see **Fig. 6.12**) or scleroderma may be visible. Some patients have cutaneous deposits of lipid, in the form of periorbital xanthelasmas or peripheral xanthomata, but these are found in less than 25% of cases. Abdominal examination may reveal a palpable liver and/or splenomegaly perhaps with ascites if there is portal hypertension.

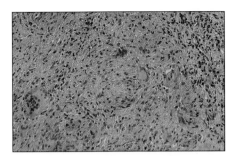

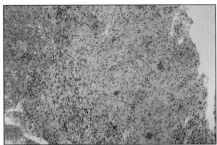

Fig. 4.80 *Histopathology of primary biliary cirrhosis. Liver biopsy specimen showing a typical epithelioid granuloma (with multinucleate giant cell formation) in a case of advanced PBC. There is extensive fibrosis, with disruption of the liver microarchitecture. Although commonly found in PBC, hepatic granulomas are not specific for this disease and may also be found in a wide range of conditions including tuberculosis, syphilis, brucellosis, histoplasmosis, schistosomiasis, sarcoidosis, inflammatory bowel disease and certain drug reactions.*

Fig. 4.81 *Hepatic sarcoidosis. Sarcoidosis may lead to similar histological changes to primary biliary cirrhosis on liver biopsy specimens. This low-power view from a patient with hepatic sarcoidosis demonstrates granuloma formation, fibrosis, cholestasis and a lymphocytic infiltrate.*

Bone disease due to osteoporosis and osteomalacia may result in fractures and there may be clinical evidence of previous vertebral collapse.

Diagnosis

The liver function tests will usually show a 'cholestatic' pattern – principally an elevation of the alkaline phosphatase (at least double the normal limit in 95% of cases) and γGT. There may be a mild rise in the serum transaminases and as the condition progresses there is usually a steady rise in serum bilirubin. Deteriorating synthetic liver function in the later stages of the illness may manifest as coagulopathy and hypoalbuminaemia.

As mentioned above, immunological blood tests will typically show antimitochondrial antibodies (in 95% of cases) and usually a raised serum IgM (in 80%).

Liver histology may show the typically focal damage of interlobular and septal bile ducts together with various combinations of fibrosis, granulomata and lymphocytic infiltration. Biopsy findings should be interpreted together with the clinical and serological data, as some of these features may be found in other conditions (**Fig. 4.81**). The differential diagnosis of PBC includes hepatic sarcoidosis, ductopenic or cholestatic drug reactions, autoimmune hepatitis, cryptogenic cirrhosis and primary sclerosing cholangitis.

Treatment

The management of patients with PBC requires a combination of supportive care and specific treatment. Symptomatic relief from pruritus may be gained by using cholestyramine, at a typical dosage of 4 g orally three times a day. Ursodeoxycholic acid (UDCA, see below) or rifampicin may also be effective and, in severe cases, plasma exchange may be beneficial.

Supplementation of fat-soluble vitamins should be given and osteopenia prevented by the use of bisphosphonates, calcium supplements or hormone replacement therapy.

Results of ursodeoxycholic acid therapy for primary biliary cirrhosis	
Symptoms	Pruritus ↓↓ Fatigue ↓ Gastrointestinal ↓
Laboratory values	γGT, AP ↓↓ Bilirubin ↓ AST, ALT ↓ AMA → IgM ↓ Cholesterol (↓)
Histology	Improved in some studies
Mortality rate/ Liver transplantation	Reduced

Fig. 4.82 *Results of ursodeoxycholic acid therapy for primary biliary cirrhosis. AMA = antimitochondrial antibodies, AP = alkaline phosphatase, AST, ALT = serum transaminases.*

There are no specific treatments for lethargy, but contributing factors such as hypothyroidism, anaemia and sedative drugs (such as antihistamines) need to be eliminated.

Many drugs have been investigated for their possible benefits in altering the natural history of PBC. Immunosuppression has been extensively studied and the use of corticosteroids, cyclosporin, azathioprine or methotrexate has shown little success.

Instead, the mainstay of drug therapy for PBC is UDCA. It has a more polar structure than other bile acids, which may be important in displacing some of the more toxic non-polar bile salts that can worsen cholestasis. Its precise mode of action is unknown but there is experimental evidence to support the following effects:

- Choleretic effects – stimulation of bile salt exocytosis
- Alteration of bile salt pool, probably by competition for ileal bile salt uptake receptors
- 'Cytoprotective' action – incorporation of UDCA into cell membranes, increasing fluidity and reducing biliary injury
- Immunomodulatory role – reduces intrahepatic aberrant expression of HLA class 1 molecules and decreases pro-inflammatory cytokine production

Clinically, there is evidence that UDCA may have a beneficial effect on symptoms, laboratory blood tests, liver histology and prognosis (**Fig. 4.82**), although the true degree of benefit is controversial.

The prescribed dose is typically between 10 and 15 mg/kg/day and this is usually well tolerated, the main side-effect being diarrhoea. This occurs in 2–5% of patients and is usually transient, resolving either spontaneously or following a reduction in dosage.

UDCA therapy reduces the severity of pruritus in about 50% of patients and usually leads to some improvement in LFTs, which can even become normalised in 5–10%. A number of multicentre studies have shown that UDCA can prolong patient survival and lengthen the time before liver transplantation becomes necessary.

The optimum timing of liver transplantation in PBC is of great importance. Previously, it was said to be indicated if the serum bilirubin level had risen above 100 μmol/l, but it is now possible to use more refined mathematical scoring systems. One example is the Mayo Clinic prognostic index, which uses a formula based on the patient's age, serum bilirubin, serum albumin, prothrombin time and the severity of peripheral oedema. In general, the same rules apply as to selecting other cases for transplantation (see p. 274) and patients with decompensated liver disease, uncontrolled portal hypertension, encephalopathy, intractable pruritus or severe fatigue should clearly be considered.

The results of liver transplantation for PBC are perhaps better than for most other forms of chronic liver disease, reflecting the relative lack of other visceral organ damage in most cases. Post-transplant survival rates are around 80% at 5 years and quality of life is usually much improved. PBC may reoccur in the engrafted liver and up to 15% of patients will have some evidence of disease recurrence 10 years after transplantation, although this is rarely of any great significance.

PRIMARY SCLEROSING CHOLANGITIS (PSC)
PSC is a chronic cholestatic disorder in which there is inflammation, fibrosis and gradual obliteration of the intrahepatic and extrahepatic biliary tree. Eventually it may lead to secondary biliary cirrhosis, portal hypertension, liver failure, cholangiocarcinoma and death.

Epidemiology
The prevalence in North American and European populations is around 6–10 cases per 100 000 population. In contrast to PBC, PSC is commonest in young men; the male to female ratio is 2:1 and PBC tends to present between the ages of 25 and 40 years, although it can occur at any age.

There is a striking association with inflammatory bowel disease and with ulcerative colitis in particular. Around 60–70% of PSC patients have ulcerative colitis and, conversely, the incidence of PSC in individuals with UC is about 6%. However, only 1% of patients with Crohn's disease develop PSC, which may possibly reflect the lower incidence of colonic involvement in this condition.

Pathogenesis
The aetiology of PSC remains unknown. On the basis of currently available evidence, it appears that the condition is an immunologically mediated disease that occurs in a genetically susceptible individual, perhaps triggered by an infectious or toxic agent. The close association with ulcerative colitis has given rise to the view that these agents may gain access to the portal circulation via the inflamed bowel.

Possible aetiopathological factors in the development of PSC include:

- Portal bacteraemia
- Absorbed colonic toxins
- Bile acid toxicity
- Viral infections
- Genetic susceptibility
- Immunological injury
- Microvascular ischaemia

The development of PSC has been linked with inheritance of the HLA haplotype Al B8 DRW 52A, which is also found more commonly in certain other organ-specific autoimmune diseases. Furthermore, around 60–80% of PSC patients have a positive perinuclear antineutrophil cytoplasmic antibody (pANCA) on serological testing, a finding also seen in around a third of UC patients. Other immunological abnormalities found in PSC include the impaired clearance of circulating immune complexes, increased activation of the complement system and a significant increase in the ratio of CD4 to CD8 lymphocytes.

Importantly, a similar pattern of injury to that seen in PSC can also occur following various other insults to the biliary system:
- Choledocholithiasis and subsequent cholangitis
- Previous bile duct surgery +/– strictures or cholangitis
- Injection of formalin into hydatid liver cysts
- Intrahepatic arterial infusion of cytotoxic drugs (e.g. floxuridine)

- Occasionally following percutaneous alcohol injection of hepatic tumours
- AIDS cholangiopathy (most likely related to *Cryptosporidia* or cytomegalovirus)

At a histological level, PSC is characterised by inflammation and fibrosis of the bile ducts, ranging from microscopic intralobular ducts to the major extrahepatic conduits. It is often a diffuse process, but PSC can also be very focal with just one or two obvious strictures particularly in the early stages of the disease. This patchy involvement means that a normal liver biopsy does not exclude the condition. The typical features on biopsy, however, are an 'onion skin' fibrosis of interlobular and septal bile ducts, often with early evidence of obliteration.

In the longer term, chronic cholestasis develops, often exacerbated by multiple episodes of acute or chronic cholangitis, dominant strictures of major bile ducts and sludging of the biliary tree. Progressive fibrosis and hepatocyte injury secondary to the cholestasis eventually result in cirrhosis and its complications.

Clinical features and natural history

Many patients with PSC are asymptomatic at the time of diagnosis, having been found to have abnormal LFTs (such as a persistently raised alkaline phosphatase level) during the course of their UC.

For the remainder, the clinical presentation of PSC varies widely. Many have vague non-specific symptoms such as fatigue, pruritus, right upper quadrant abdominal discomfort or mild weight loss. It is unusual for PSC to present as an acute cholangitis, although this is recognised.

Signs of chronic liver disease are found in about half of PSC patients at diagnosis and most commonly include jaundice and hepatomegaly/splenomegaly.

The natural history of PSC is one of progressive damage to the biliary tree, usually over a 10–15-year period. A number of studies have shown that the median period of survival from the time of diagnosis to death or liver transplantation is around 10 years. Asymptomatic patients may have a more favourable outcome, about 75% of this group surviving over 15 years.

Unfortunately, patients with PSC have a strong predisposition to developing cholangiocarcinoma. This malignancy carries an extremely poor prognosis, with 5-year survival rates well below 10%, and its development is a contraindication to liver transplantation, owing to its virtually universal recurrence.

Diagnosis

If the causes of secondary sclerosing cholangitis have been excluded (particularly previous biliary surgery or choledocholithiasis) then PSC can be diagnosed on the basis of the following radiological or histological appearances.

The typical findings on ERCP (**Fig. 4.83**) are of multiple strictures, beading and irregular dilatation of the extrahepatic and/or intrahepatic bile ducts. The stricturing can sometimes be very localised and may be particularly difficult to distinguish from a cholangiocarcinoma.

A liver biopsy may show the classical 'onion skin' bile duct fibrosis, often with oedema and expansion of the portal tracts. In the later stages there are changes typical of 'vanishing bile duct' cholestasis with fibrosis and eventually cirrhosis. However, the histological appearances are not absolutely specific for PSC and are often similar to those of other cholestatic disorders.

Blood tests also lack true specificity. There will usually be a cholestatic pattern of LFTs, with alkaline phosphatase elevated and frequently a mild rise in the serum transaminases. In the latter stages of the illness, there may be evidence of poor synthetic function with hypoalbuminaemia and coagulopathy. The pANCA autoantibody is of little diagnostic significance because of the overlap with other conditions.

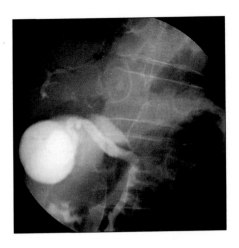

Fig. 4.83 *Radiological appearance of primary sclerosing cholangitis. ERCP showing multiple strictures, beading and irregularity of the biliary tree in a patient with PSC.*

Treatment

There is currently no medical therapy that is curative for PSC. Liver transplantation is the only effective option for suitable candidates with progressive liver disease and 5-year survival rates are now around 80–90% in many transplant centres.

As with PBC, decisions regarding the timing of liver transplantation for PSC can be made easier by using prognostic scoring systems, such as the Mayo PSC model. This is based on a mathematical formula that incorporates the histological stage, serum bilirubin, patient age and the presence of splenomegaly.

The management of PSC can be summarised as follows:

- Management of cholestasis – cholestyramine for pruritus; fat-soluble vitamin supplementation: prophylaxis against osteoporosis
- Management of cholangitis and strictures – prompt antibiotic therapy for acute cholangitic episodes: endoscopic stenting or balloon dilatation of focal obstructive biliary strictures
- Specific drug therapy – ursodeoxycholic acid may improve LFTs but has no effect on symptoms, histology, disease progression or survival: immunosuppression also ineffective
- Complications of cirrhosis – therapy for portal hypertension and ascites, similar to other causes of chronic liver disease
- Orthotopic liver transplantation – treatment of choice for patients with advanced PSC; excellent survival rates; PSC may reoccur, although significance still unknown; possibly higher incidence of post-transplant ductopenic chronic rejection

The link between PSC and cholangiocarcinoma has already been mentioned. In addition to this, patients with UC and PSC are at higher risk of developing colon cancer than those with UC alone, this risk persisting even after patients have had their PSC 'cured' by liver transplantation. Consequently, many gastroenterologists recommend annual colonoscopy with surveillance biopsies for these patients post-transplant.

The management of cholangiocarcinoma is discussed later in this chapter.

HEPATIC ABSCESSES

Pyogenic liver abscess

A liver abscess may arise from a range of sources, with localised biliary infection and portal pyaemia being the two commonest (**Fig. 4.84**). There are usually multiple small abscesses initially, and these tend to coalesce and form larger macroscopic abscesses (**Fig. 4.85**).

Causes of pyogenic liver abscesses	
Portal vein bacteraemia	Appendicitis Diverticulitis or diverticular abscess Ulcerative colitis Crohn's disease Pancreatitis Enteric infections (e.g. *Yersinia*) Gastrointestinal neoplasms Umbilical infection Pelvic inflammatory disease
Cholangitis (+/− cholestasis)	Cholecystitis Choledocholithiasis Cholangiocarcinoma Pancreatic cancer Biliary surgery Biliary strictures Parasitic infection (e.g. *Ascaris lumbricoides*) Pancreatitis
Direct extension of adjacent sepsis	Empyema of the gall bladder Perforated peptic ulceration Colonic or gastric cancer Pancreatic abscess Perihepatic abscess Perirenal abscess
Infection carried by hepatic artery	Bacteraemia of any source
Infection of pre-existing liver lesion	Neoplasia Liver cyst
Trauma	Penetrating injury (e.g. knife wound, liver biopsy, injection of tumours) Blunt trauma

Fig. 4.84 *Causes of pyogenic liver abscesses.*

Because of the heterogeneous routes by which a hepatic abscess may be acquired, there is a wide range of responsible pathogens. As most arise from biliary or intra-abdominal sepsis, Gram-negative aerobes and anaerobes tend to predominate, with *Escherichia coli* the commonest single species overall. Gram-positive infections are more likely if the abscess originates from a systemic source such as the skin or endocardium. Multiple infections are particularly common and mixed populations of bacteria are grown from most hepatic abscesses. In around 20% of cases, no organism is isolated and it is believed that most of these cases are caused by fastidious anaerobic bacteria that are difficult to culture.

The classical presentation of a liver abscess is with abdominal pain, fever and nausea. The liver may be palpable and is frequently tender. Blood tests will usually show a neutrophil leucocytosis, raised liver enzymes (particularly alkaline phosphatase) and an acute-phase response with low albumin and high inflammatory markers. A chest radiograph may show a raised right hemidiaphragm, but ultrasonography is usually diagnostic, confirming the presence and location of the abscess. The organism may be isolated from cultures of blood and from guided aspiration of abscess contents.

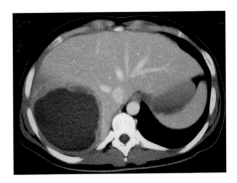

Fig. 4.85 *Pyogenic liver abscess. Abdominal CT scan demonstrating a large pyogenic abscess occupying most of the right lobe of the liver in a young woman. Cultures of the abscess contents grew a* Klebsiella *species that responded to antibiotic therapy and drainage, but the original source of the bacteria could not be identified.*

The effective treatment of a pyogenic liver abscess requires percutaneous complete drainage of the cavity (by needle or indwelling catheter) together with broad-spectrum antibiotic therapy to cover likely organisms while sensitivities are awaited. One suitable intravenous regime is the combination of a third-generation cephalosporin with metronidazole, but the advice of the local microbiologist should be sought regarding the best empirical treatment. Surgery for complicated abscesses is rarely necessary. The underlying cause of the abscess should, of course, be sought and treated.

Amoebic liver abscess

Liver abscesses due to amoeba mainly occur in endemic tropical countries – but not exclusively so. Although they are often a consequence of amoebic colitis, there is no history of intestinal disease in about half the cases of amoebic liver abscess.

The clinical presentation can be indistinguishable from pyogenic abscesses. Usually, there is a single abscess confined to the right lobe of the liver, but multiple lesions can also occur and chronic abscesses can persist for months or even years. Spread of the amoeba elsewhere often results in abscesses in the lungs or pleura.

Specific anti-*Entamoeba histolytica* antibodies can be found in the sera of over 90% of patients with an amoebic liver abscess and the organism can be detected in stool samples or on rectal biopsy in cases of amoebic colitis.

Treatment of the hepatic abscess is usually with a 10-day course of metronidazole followed by a similar course of diloxanide furoate. Aspiration can be performed, although this tends to be reserved for large abscesses in the left lobe, particularly if there is concern about impending rupture into the pericardium, pleura or peritoneum.

Hydatid disease

Hydatid cysts of the liver are caused by infection with *Echinococcus granulosus*, a dog tapeworm for which humans, sheep and cattle may be intermediate hosts. After *Echinococcus* ova are ingested, embryonic oncospheres are released which penetrate the intestinal wall and disseminate. About 60% will lodge in the liver, with around 20–30% impacting in the lung and the small remaining proportion reaching distant sites such as the kidney, bones or brain. The larvae then develop into cystic lesions, which are usually unilocular, although the less common *E. multilocularis* variant may produce multilocular cysts.

The parasite is most commonly acquired in childhood and may take years or even decades to become clinically apparent. Consequently, cysts can be quite large by the time of presentation and often cause symptoms by virtue of their mass effect. Liver cysts tend to cause abdominal pain, hepatomegaly and a palpable swelling. Rupture of the cysts into the pleura, peritoneum or biliary tree may present acutely with fever or an anaphylactic reaction that can be life-threatening.

A plain radiograph may demonstrate the typical calcification around the hydatid cyst as well as elevation of the diaphragm. Ultrasonography may also show the presence of 'daughter' cysts and the presence of hydatid 'sand' as sludge within the lesions. Diagnostic aspiration carries the risk of anaphylaxis if cyst contents are allowed to leak and so specific serology is the mainstay of diagnosis.

Traditionally, surgical excision of cysts has been the treatment of choice. Recently however, a number of randomised trials have shown that percutaneous therapeutic aspiration, combined with the antiparasitic drug albendazole, is effective and safe for uncomplicated echinococcal cysts.

LIVER DISEASES RELATED TO PREGNANCY

Pregnant women may present with liver disease either as a result of pre-existing hepatic diseases, or with coincidental illness or with certain conditions that are specifically related to the pregnancy itself (Fig. 4.86). Pregnant women are also more likely to develop gallstones, their prothrombotic tendency means that Budd–Chiari syndrome is more likely and hepatitis E infection is more likely to pursue a fatal course (see p. 221). Many of the other gastrointestinal effects of pregnancy are discussed in chapter 7.

Intrahepatic cholestasis of pregnancy (obstetric cholestasis)

This condition of unknown aetiology is characterised by a cholestatic disorder that tends to occur in the third trimester (sometimes in the second) and spontaneously resolves soon after delivery. It is the second commonest cause, after acute viral hepatitis, of jaundice in pregnancy.

Affected patients often have a family history, suggestive of a genetic basis, and cholestasis may be precipitated by the oestrogen-induced mild impairment of biliary transport that occurs in pregnancy. Patients who have had this condition are more likely to develop a cholestatic reaction to the oral contraceptive pill.

Cholestasis occurs in around 1% of all expectant mothers and there is a 70% risk of recurrence in future pregnancies.

Clinically, the condition usually presents with pruritus, often accompanied by mild jaundice (present in about a third of cases). The derangement in LFTs is rarely severe, but the alkaline phosphatase is typically raised with a secondary elevation in serum transaminases that is rarely above five times the upper limit of normal. In some cases, there may be a cholestatic vitamin K deficiency, which requires treating before delivery or Caesarean section is contemplated.

The prognosis for the mother is benign, although there is an increased risk of stillbirth and prematurity. The risk of stillbirth can be minimised by elective delivery at 37–8 weeks.

Acute fatty liver of pregnancy

The acute fatty liver of pregnancy (AFLP) is a severe and potentially life-threatening illness that is fortunately uncommon, affecting 1 in 15 000 pregnancies. It is most likely to occur in the first pregnancy and where there are multiple gestations.

The precise aetiology is unknown, but a significant proportion of affected women have been found to be heterozygous for deficiency of long-chain 3-hydroxyacyl coenzyme A. This enzyme normally catalyses the oxidation of fatty acids and it has been hypothesised that such a deficiency renders the mother and fetus more vulnerable to metabolic stresses (such as pre-eclampsia and the HELLP syndrome) during pregnancy. AFLP is more likely to develop if the father is also heterozygous for this enzyme deficiency and the fetus is a

Liver diseases associated with pregnancy

Intrahepatic cholestasis of pregnancy	Affects 1% of pregnancies Onset most commonly in third trimester Slightly increased risk of prematurity and stillbirth Usually recurs in subsequent pregnancies Responds to ursodeoxycholic acid
Hyperemesis gravidarum	Liver dysfunction may occur if severe Resolves as vomiting settles Fluid resuscitation often enough to improve LFTs
HELLP syndrome (microangiopathic **h**aemolysis, **e**levated **l**iver enzymes and **l**ow **p**latelets)	Associated with pre-eclampsia Overlap with haemolytic uraemic syndrome and thrombotic thrombocytopenic purpura Third trimester, typically around 32/40 May even occur up to 48 hours post-partum Usually nausea, vomiting, hypertension, oedema and abdominal pain Intravascular haemolysis, hepatitic LFTs Treatment is with resuscitation and early delivery, usually by emergency Caesarean section 3% maternal mortality 35% infant perinatal mortality
Acute fatty liver of pregnancy	Onset confined to third trimester May be triggered by pre-eclampsia Complications include encephalopathy, acute liver failure, disseminated intravascular coagulation and pancreatitis Potentially high mortality for mother and baby – treatment consists of supportive care and prompt delivery

Fig. 4.86 *Liver diseases associated with pregnancy.*

homozygote. Histologically, the condition is characterised by a widespread microvesicular hepatic steatosis (**Fig. 4.87**).

The initial clinical features are often non-specific and include malaise, nausea, fatigue and abdominal pain. There is usually a rapid progression over hours or a few days to encephalopathy, jaundice, bruising, bleeding and hypoglycaemia. Fulminant hepatic failure may occur. Almost half of the patients with AFLP have proteinuria, hypertension and oedema, suggestive of an associated pre-eclampsia.

Blood tests usually show a marked (7–10-fold) elevation in transaminases with a lesser rise in alkaline phosphatase and bilirubin. There is often a neutrophil leucocytosis, and disseminated intravascular coagulation (DIC) develops in about 75% of cases.

A liver biopsy may be difficult to perform in view of the coagulopathy that is frequently present, but if carried out it typically shows a marked microvesicular fatty change that is worst around the central veins of the lobule. The microvesicles can sometimes be difficult to spot on routine H&E slides and so special stains for fat (as in **Fig. 4.87**) must be used.

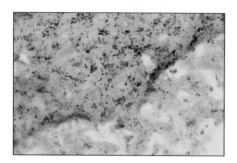

Fig. 4.87 *Acute fatty liver of pregnancy. Liver biopsy specimen, treated with a special Oro stain to detect fat, taken from a patient with acute fatty liver of pregnancy. Widespread microvesicular steatosis is clearly visible as reddish-brown deposits within the hepatocytes.*

After resuscitation and correction of DIC and hypoglycaemia, the optimum treatment is rapid delivery of the baby, usually by emergency Caesarean section. The supportive care is otherwise similar to that of other causes of acute liver failure. After delivery, the mother's liver returns to normal and recurrence of AFLP in future pregnancies is very rare.

DRUG-INDUCED LIVER DISEASE

The liver can be affected by an adverse reaction to almost any drug, either by direct toxicity or immunological injury. The liver damage caused by most drug reactions tends to be idiosyncratic but can present in very similar ways to other liver diseases, principally as hepatitic or cholestatic processes.

Examples of predictable, dose-related liver injuries are those seen with overdosage of paracetamol (acetaminophen), phenytoin or vancomycin. Idiosyncratic, usually immunologically mediated, reactions can occur to a wide range of therapeutic agents (**Fig. 4.88**).

Drug reactions should always be considered in the differential diagnosis of liver disease. A full drug history should always be taken – including recent or ongoing use of prescribed medication, over-the-counter drugs, herbal remedies and recreational substances. Chronic liver disease increases the risk of adverse reactions to many drugs, including aminoglycosides, non-steroidal anti-inflammatory drugs (NSAIDs) and β-lactam antibiotics.

A hepatic adverse drug reaction may obviously be suggested by a clear history relating exposure to a hepatotoxic agent and the illness itself. Unpredictable, idiosyncratic reactions can be more difficult to diagnose, as they are not related to dosage and may occur at varying intervals after initial exposure. Hypersensitivity responses may be suggested by the presence of rashes, arthralgia, fevers or a peripheral blood eosinophilia. In doubtful cases, a liver biopsy usually confirms an eosinophilic infiltration or may show other changes such as granulomas or ductopenia.

The causative drug must be withdrawn in cases of severe liver injury. In some milder instances it is possible to reintroduce essential therapy – for example, in the case of mild elevations of serum transaminases on an enzyme-inducing drug such as rifampicin. Suspected adverse reactions to drugs should be notified to the appropriate regulatory authorities (in the UK, the Committee on the Safety of Medicines).

THE COMPLICATIONS OF CHRONIC LIVER DISEASE

The response of the liver to injury is relatively predictable in *histological* terms. A wide variety of causal agents, including alcohol, drugs, hepatotropic viruses, genetic and autoimmune disorders, may provoke the same series of events that ultimately lead to cirrhosis (see **Fig. 4.73**). Irrespective of the original causal agent, the liver responds to injury in broadly the same way, with alteration to both its structural and functional

Examples of the more common drug-related liver diseases

Adverse reaction	Implicated drugs
Acute liver failure (fulminant hepatic necrosis)	Paracetamol overdosage, halothane, ecstasy (3,4-methylenedioxyamphetamine), monoamine oxidase inhibitors, gold, nitrofurantoin, NSAIDs, sulphonamides, phenytoin, antituberculous drugs, herbal remedies (e.g. germander, pyrrolizidine alkaloids)
Acute hepatitis	Paracetamol overdosage, aspirin, halothane, penicillins, cyclophosphamide, hydralazine, isoniazid, vincristine, co-amoxiclav, phenytoin, tricyclic antidepressants
Chronic hepatitis	Methyldopa, hydralazine, co-amoxiclav, isoniazid, nitrofurantoin
Granulomatous hepatitis	Sulphonamides, phenytoin, nitrofurantoin, sulphonylureas, allopurinol, phenylbutazone, carbamazepine
Hepatic steatosis	Amiodarone, methotrexate, glucocorticoids, tetracyclines, zidovudine, sodium valproate
Acute cholestasis	Carbamazepine, co-amoxiclav, chlorpromazine, cotrimoxazole, captopril, azathioprine, phenytoin, sulpiride
Vanishing bile duct syndrome	Carbamazepine, chlorpromazine, co-amoxiclav, flucloxacillin, methyltestosterone, arsenicals
Cirrhosis	Methyldopa, methotrexate, amiodarone
Neoplastic change	Oral contraceptive pill, anabolic steroids
Increased risk of gallstones	Oral contraceptive pill, octreotide, clofibrate

Fig. 4.88 *Examples of the more common drug-related liver diseases.*

organisation. Cirrhosis of the liver is characterised by fibrosis and the regeneration of the hepatic parenchyma in a nodular formation, the latter feature being classified by some pathologists as micronodular (nodules predominantly < 3 mm in size) or macronodular (> 3 mm) cirrhosis. The histological features of cirrhosis are:

- Combination of fibrosis and nodular regeneration
- Distortion of lobular architecture
- Variation in size of hepatocytes
- Increase in thickness of liver cell plates
- Excess of hepatic venous tributaries

However, the *clinical* spectrum of liver injury is broad, extending from the asymptomatic individual with well-compensated cirrhosis to those patients with inexorable functional decompensation, manifested by jaundice, ascites, portal hypertension and their resultant complications.

The accurate delineation of hepatic function in patients with cirrhosis is important for management purposes, including the timing of liver transplantation. The degree of injury is conventionally assessed using tests that reflect its structure (tissue biopsy), cellular permeability (serum transaminase concentrations) and synthetic activity (prothrombin time, plasma albumin and serum bilirubin levels).

The Child–Pugh scoring system

The most widely used index of the functional severity of chronic liver disease is the Child classification (or one of its modifications). This system (**Fig. 4.89**) grades liver function in patients with cirrhosis.

Decompensated disease

Ten years after the initial diagnosis of cirrhosis, the probability of developing decompensated disease is approximately 60% with a survival rate of 50%. Once clinical decompensation has occurred, the prognosis is poor, with a 16% probability of survival at 5 years. The major complications of decompensated cirrhosis with portal hypertension are variceal bleeding, ascites and spontaneous bacterial peritonitis (SBP), the hepatorenal syndrome and hepatic encephalopathy.

Portal hypertension

The exact definition of portal hypertension has varied, but generally a portal venous pressure of greater than 10 mmHg can be said to be diagnostic. If the gradient between portal and hepatic veins can be measured (by hepatic venous catheterisation and wedge pressure analysis), then it can be defined as a gradient of more than 5 mmHg, with variceal bleeding tending to occur when this figure reaches 10–12 mmHg.

The fluid pressure in any vascular system is equal to the flow rate multiplied by the resistance (Ohm's law). Hence, portal hypertension may occur when there is an abnormal increase in portal venous blood flow and/or vascular resistance (**Fig. 4.90**). Worldwide, the obliteration of presinusoidal hepatic blood vessels by schistosomiasis is the commonest cause of portal hypertension. In Europe and North America, hepatic cirrhosis is by far the commonest cause although non-cirrhotic portal hypertension may occur in the setting of Budd–Chiari syndrome (obstruction of the large hepatic veins, with or without vena caval involvement, which may present either acutely or insidiously with chronic portal hypertension – **Fig. 4.91**) or compression of the portal vein by tumours and nodules.

The Child–Pugh scoring system for functional severity of cirrhosis			
Criterion	**1**	**2**	**3**
Bilirubin	Less than 28 µmol/L	28–51 µmol/L	More than 51 µmol/L
Prothrombin time	1–3 s prolonged	4–6 s prolonged	More than 6 s prolonged
Albumin	Greater than 35 g/L	28–35 g/L	Less than 28 g/L
Ascites	None	Slight	Moderate
Encephalopathy	None	I–II	III–IV

The patient is rated from 1–3 for each of the five categories. The Pugh's score varies from 5 (best function) to 15 (worst function). Child's grade A = 5–6 (compensated disease); Child's grade C = 10+ (decompensated disease); Child's grade B = 7–9 (intermediate grading).

Fig. 4.89 *The Child–Pugh scoring system for functional severity of cirrhosis.*

Classification and causes of portal hypertension

Type of portal hypertension	Location of obstruction	Hepatic venous pressure	Portal venous pressure	Common causes
Extrahepatic	Portal vein	Normal	Increased	Portal vein thrombsis
	Splenic vein	Normal	Normal	Splenic vein thrombosis*
Intrahepatic	Presinusoidal	Normal	Increased	Schistosomiasis
	Postsinusoidal	Unable to measure	Increased	Budd–Chiari syndrome
		Normal	Increased	Veno-occlusive disease
	Mixed	Increased	Increased	Liver cirrhosis

*Splenic venous thrombosis may cause a localised venous hypertension that can cause gastric varices in particular – although it is not strictly a cause of portal hypertension, given that the portal pressure is usually normal.

Fig. 4.90 *Classification and causes of portal hypertension.*

Cardiovascular physiology in patients with cirrhosis is further complicated by a hyperdynamic state (**Fig. 4.92**) that is influenced by circulating vasoactive factors (such as glucagon, prostaglandins, substance P and endothelins) and diminished responses to vasoconstrictors.

In an effort to bypass the hypertensive portal circulation, venous collaterals develop at sites where the portal and systemic venous systems communicate. As a consequence, engorged varices may occur, particularly in the oesophagus and proximal stomach, and the shunting of blood around the liver may enable substances normally removed by the liver to gain access to the wider circulation. This latter feature is important in the pathogenesis of hepatic encephalopathy (see below).

Risks of varices and variceal bleeding

The most ominous complication of portal hypertension is oesophageal variceal bleeding. Patients who bleed have a poor long-term prognosis, irrespective of treatment, and few survive more than 5 years. However, only 40% of patients with oesophageal varices will bleed, but for every bleeding episode, the mortality can be up to 50%. The risk of recurrent bleeding ranges from 50–70% within 2 years of the index haemorrhage and is at its highest during the first week.

Risk factors for variceal bleeding seen at endoscopy include large varices, red wale markings and cherry red spots (see **Fig. 1.44**). Additional factors are Child's grade C cirrhosis and a portal pressure greater than 12 mmHg.

Varices may also occur in other sites (duodenum 17%, jejunum and ileum 18%, colon 15%, rectum 9%, ileostomy or colostomy 27%, other sites 14%).

Examples of the endoscopic appearances of portal hypertensive lesions are shown in **Figs 4.93–4.97**.

Management of variceal bleeding. Acute variceal haemorrhage is a medical emergency and appropriate management demands a combination of prompt resuscitation, medical therapy and endoscopic intervention. Radiological or even surgical procedures may be required in difficult cases and the supportive care of the patient with decompensated cirrhosis is vitally important.

Budd–Chiari syndrome

Aetiology	Around 50% of cases have underlying prothrombotic disorder Pregnancy Oral contraceptive use Connective tissue disease (systemic lupus, Behçet's disease, antiphospholipid antibody syndrome) Haematological disorders (myeloproliferative disease, paroxysmal nocturnal haemoglobinuria, deficiencies of protein S or protein C) Paraneoplastic (renal carcinoma) Direct compression by hepatic cysts or infiltration by malignancy Abdominal trauma Congenital webs of vena cava or hepatic veins
Pathogenesis	If acute, leads to marked centrilobular congestion and venous infarction of hepatocytes May cause fulminant hepatic failure Mild or more chronic obstruction may lead to sinusoidal dilatation, fibrosis and cirrhosis as well as portal hypertension Caudate lobe drains directly to vena cava and may be spared
Clinical features	Classical acute presentation as abdominal pain, ascites and hepatomegaly Fulminant hepatic failure occurs in 10% Often vague onset with malaise, discomfort and gradual ascites Variceal bleeding Marked lower limb oedema if vena caval involvement Main differential diagnosis is right heart failure
Diagnosis	Doppler ultrasound of hepatic vessels CT or MRI may be useful Hepatic venography is gold standard – defines vascular anatomy and offers interventional therapy Liver biopsy useful in chronic cases – establishes reversibility of damage
Treatment	Vascular decompression – Radiological intervention (e.g. balloon dilatation), TIPSS, surgical shunts Medical therapy – management of liver failure, treatment of variceal bleeding, some success with thrombolysis, lifelong anticoagulation in most patients Liver transplantation – In some cases of acute liver failure or chronic Budd–Chiari complicated by cirrhosis

Fig. 4.91 *Budd–Chiari syndrome.*

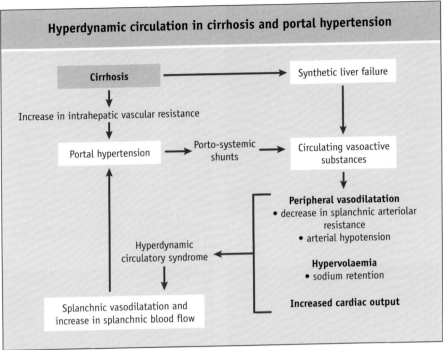

Hyperdynamic circulation in cirrhosis and portal hypertension

Cirrhosis ──────────────→ Synthetic liver failure

Increase in intrahepatic vascular resistance

Portal hypertension ──→ Porto-systemic shunts ──→ Circulating vasoactive substances

Peripheral vasodilatation
• decrease in splanchnic arteriolar resistance
• arterial hypotension

Hyperdynamic circulatory syndrome

Hypervolaemia
• sodium retention

Splanchnic vasodilatation and increase in splanchnic blood flow

Increased cardiac output

Fig. 4.92 *Hyperdynamic circulation in cirrhosis and portal hypertension.*

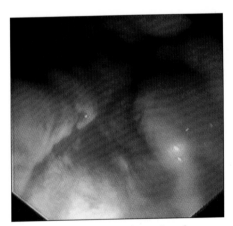

Fig. 4.93 *Bleeding oesphageal varices.*

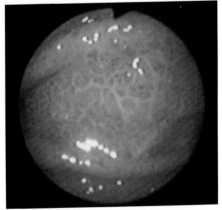

Fig. 4.94 *Portal hypertensive gastropathy. Endoscopic view of the gastric body, demonstrating the classical 'snakeskin' appearance of portal hypertensive gastropathy. Histologically it is characterised by vascular ectasia in response to raised portal pressures and may itself be a source of bleeding.*

257

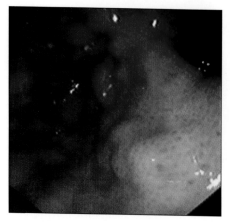

Fig. 4.95 *Gastric fundal varices. Retroflexed view, demonstrating fundal varices and surrounding portal hypertensive gastropathy in a patient with hepatitis C cirrhosis. Most gastric varices occur in patients with oesophageal varices, although they can be found in isolation if there is a regional cause of portal hypertension such as a splenic vein thrombosis. Bleeding gastric varices are generally more difficult to manage than their oesophageal counterparts, responding less well to the usual sclerotherapy or banding approaches. Tissue adhesives or bovine thrombin have been successfully used as sclerosants although reduction of portal pressure is the treatment of choice in the longer term.*

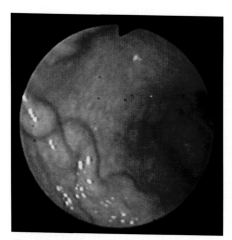

Fig. 4.96 *Gastric antral varices. Large antral varices in a patient with non-cirrhotic portal hypertension, due to a portal vein thrombosis. Gastric varices generally occur more commonly in the fundus and cardia than the antrum.*

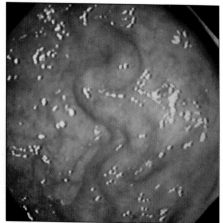

Fig. 4.97 *Colorectal varices. Sigmoidoscopic view of a proximal rectal varix in a patient with alcoholic cirrhosis.*

Resuscitation and general care of the patient with variceal bleeding involves:
- Adequate assessment of blood loss
- Pulse, BP, postural drop, peripheral perfusion
- Prompt, large-bone intravenous access and infusion of blood, clotting factors and platelets as appropriate
- Use of colloids or crystalloids while awaiting arrival of blood transfusion
- Central venous access and pressure monitoring (N.B. Supine pressure may be falsely high if tense ascites present)
- Close monitoring of cardiovascular and renal function
- Medical therapy to lower portal pressure – somatostatin or vasopressin analogues

- Care of decompensated liver disease (lactulose for encephalopathy, vitamin therapies, early identification and treatment of sepsis. etc)

Emergency endoscopy should be performed after the initial resuscitation. It can be a hazardous procedure in the emergency situation, however, and there should be a low threshold for protecting the airway with an endotracheal tube in patients with significant ongoing haematemesis. As well as offering a diagnostic role (a non-variceal source is identified as the cause of bleeding in about a third of cirrhotic patients), variceal sclerotherapy or band ligation can be undertaken.

Injection sclerotherapy (**Fig. 4.98**) controls the acute bleeding in up to 95% of cases. There is probably a reduction in the early rebleeding rate, but there is no proven effect on survival. There are some important complications associated with variceal sclerotherapy (generally more common with paravariceal than intravariceal injection of sclerosant) including ulceration, stricture formation, perforation (in 0.5% of cases and usually delayed by 5–7 days), mediastinitis, sclerosant embolism and portal vein thrombosis. Mortality is 1–3%. Although most of these reactions are uncommon, virtually all patients experience some discomfort, fever or mild dysphagia immediately after the procedure. Prophylaxis against subsequent sclerotherapy ulcers can be offered by prescribing sucralfate suspension and/or a proton pump inhibitor.

If the patient rebleeds during the same admission, a further course of sclerotherapy can be performed, but there is no evidence of benefit from further injections beyond this and other interventions to lower the portal pressure (such as TIPSS) must be considered.

Management of bleeding varices may be summarised as follows:

- Resuscitation
- Pharmacotherapy – e.g. somatostatin or analogues, vasopressin or analogues
- Endoscopic therapy
- Balloon tamponade
- Interventional radiology
- Surgery (shunts, oesophageal transection, liver transplantation)
- Secondary prevention – further endoscopic approaches, medical therapy

Endoscopic band ligation (**Fig. 4.99**) controls bleeding in up to 90% of cases. There is less rebleeding (30%) and fewer complications than with sclerotherapy, but vision for the

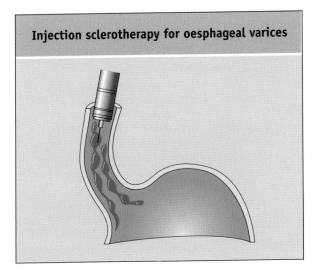

Injection sclerotherapy for oesphageal varices

Fig. 4.98 *Injection sclerotherapy for oesophageal varices. A sclerosing agent (e.g. 5% ethanolamine) is injected into each varix, although some studies have shown that much of the intended dose is delivered paravariceally because of technical difficulties during an acute bleed.*

Technique for banding ligation of oesophageal varices

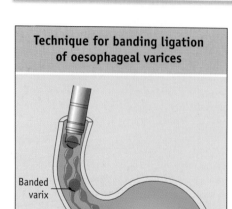

Banded
varix

(a)

Fig. 4.99 *Banding ligation of oesophageal varices. (a) Technique. (b) After the varices have been located, endoscopic suction is applied and the varix is drawn up into the ligator attached to the end of the scope. A rubber band is released from the endoscope and tightly constricts the varix, so that it subsequently necroses and sloughs off. A visible blue band (c) is applied to the varix and another blue band can be seen at the periphery of the endoscopic view, attached to the ligation apparatus.*

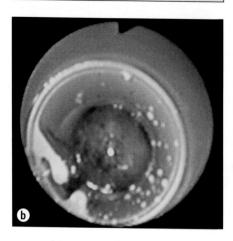

(b)

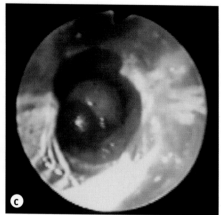

(c)

operator is more limited during an acute bleed due to the band ligation apparatus. After control of the initial bleeding episode, patients should receive further courses of banding ligation over the next few weeks until the varices are eliminated. Fewer treatment episodes are required than with injection sclerotherapy, and mortality is lower.

Due to reduced vision some gastroenterologists prefer to use injection sclerotherapy to achieve haemostasis; a subsequent course of banding is performed electively when visibility is better.

Pharmacotherapy with vasoactive drugs may improve outcome and rebleeding rates if administered during an acute presentation (**Fig. 4.100**). Octreotide is a longer-acting somatostatin analogue which decreases portal pressure and collateral blood flow, while vasopressin and its analogues (such as glypressin) cause splanchnic vasoconstriction with a similar effect on the portal pressure as octreotide.

If bleeding is uncontrolled, balloon tamponade (**Fig. 4.101**) may be used as a holding procedure until further sclerotherapy can be performed or while the patient is transferred to a specialist liver unit. However, the best outcome in these circumstances is with TIPSS as discussed below. The use of Sengstaken–Blakemore (or Minnesota) tubes for balloon tamponade is not itself without risks (**Fig. 4.102**):

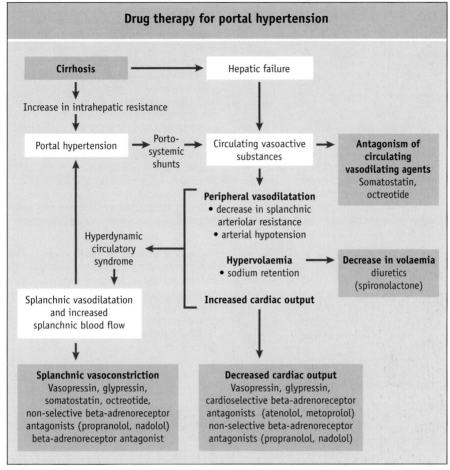

Drug therapy for portal hypertension

Fig. 4.100 *Drug therapy for portal hypertension. Analogues of somatostatin and vasopressin are the two drugs most commonly used during a bleeding episode. Beta-blockers and nitrate-based therapies such as isosorbide mononitrate can be used for prevention of further bleeding episodes.*

- Aspiration pneumonia (10%)
- Airway obstruction by misplaced or migrated balloon
- Oesophageal rupture
- Oesophageal ulceration and stricture formation
- Rebleeding (approximately 50% on removal of tube)

Transjugular intrahepatic portosystemic shunts (TIPSS). These shunts are mainly indicated for the management of uncontrolled variceal haemorrhage, but they have also been used for refractory ascites, for hepatic hydrothoraces and in the hepatorenal syndrome. They effectively reduce portal pressure and are useful for the relief of non-cirrhotic portal hypertension as well as the cirrhotic type. TIPSS allows measurement of the portal pressure and gradient and produces a marked reduction in the rebleeding rate.

The hepatic vein is cannulated, using the internal jugular and vena caval route; a small shunt can be created by connecting a branch of the hepatic vein to the portal system and

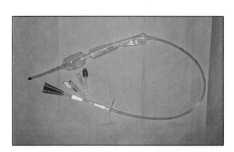

Fig. 4.101 *Balloon tamponade (Sengstaken–Blakemore) tube for the treatment of bleeding oesophageal varices. The deflated gastric and oesophageal balloons are visible at the distal end (top left); after insertion the gastric balloon is inflated and pulled back. By impacting at the gastric cardia, the inflow to the oesophageal varices is compressed and this is usually sufficient to stop the bleeding. If not, the oesophageal balloon can be inflated (to a pressure between the portal venous and arterial pressures, typically 30–40 mmHg) to compress the varices completely. The use of this balloon markedly increases the already high complication rate and it must be periodically deflated to reduce the risk of oesophageal necrosis. The tube shown here is a four-lumen device, having two channels for inflation of the respective balloons and two further channels through which the gastric and oesophageal contents can be aspirated.*

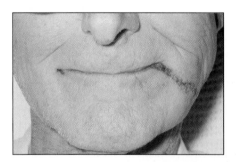

Fig. 4.102 *Skin necrosis following Sengstaken–Blakemore tube insertion. This patient developed pressure necrosis of his facial skin after an oesophageal balloon tamponade tube was left in situ for 2 days. Similar damage to the oesophagus is a relatively common complication of this procedure.*

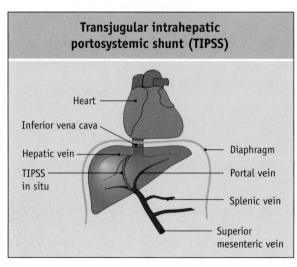

Fig. 4.103 *Transjugular intrahepatic portosystemic shunt (TIPSS).*

passing a small catheter device through the liver parenchyma (**Fig. 4.103**). An expandable metal stent (typically 8–12 mm in diameter) is left in place, creating a portosystemic shunt.

The main complications are the development of hepatic encephalopathy and shunt stenosis or occlusion (30% at 1 year, 60% at 2 years). Other complications include haemorrhage, haemolysis and infection. The technique is difficult to perform and requires radiological follow-up, but procedural mortality is low (< 1%). If hepatic encephalopathy is unresponsive to standard treatment, the TIPSS can subsequently be blocked off or reduced in size.

Surgery for variceal bleeding. The role of surgery in arresting variceal haemorrhage has gradually diminished since the advent of effective medical and endoscopic therapies and the introduction of liver transplantation.

Surgical shunts to relieve portal hypertension, devascularisation procedures and staple-gun transection of the oesophagus can all be used to arrest bleeding varices. Patients with advanced cirrhosis are not the most robust candidates for major surgery and mortality rates can be high. Encephalopathy is a further complication of shunt procedures, although its incidence can be reduced by performing selective shunts such as the distal splenorenal type.

However, the main disadvantage of these operations is that they interfere with the local surgical anatomy, and subsequent scarring or adhesions may make liver transplantation difficult or even impossible. Hence, the patient's current or future suitability for transplantation should always be considered before these operations are carried out. The TIPSS technique does not reduce the patient's chances of receiving a successful liver graft.

Secondary prevention. After the initial treatment of variceal haemorrhage, the prevention of rebleeding is best obtained with a combination of beta-blockers as maintenance treatment (isosorbide mononitrate if contraindicated or not tolerated) and serial endoscopic band ligation until variceal obliteration has been achieved. If a TIPSS has been inserted, most radiologists carry out regular surveillance of patency with a 6-monthly Doppler ultrasound scan and 6–12-monthly shunt venography.

Ascites

Patients with chronic liver disease account for more than 75% of cases of ascites (see **Fig. 4.18**). Over a 15-year period from initial diagnosis, up to 60% of patients with previously compensated cirrhosis will have developed ascites.

Theories on the mechanisms underlying the development of ascites are shown in **Fig. 4.104**.

The complications of ascites include infection (spontaneous bacterial peritonitis, SBP), tense ascites, umbilical herniation and hepatic hydrothorax.

Management of ascites. Diagnostic abdominal paracentesis with analysis of ascitic fluid is the initial step. A 10 ml aliquot should be aspirated in the flank using a green needle in all patients with new-onset ascites, in all patients being admitted to hospital and wherever there is a clinical deterioration or fever (**Fig. 4.105**). This procedure is mandatory in the management of such patients. There are no contraindications, apart from where there is clinically apparent disseminated intravascular coagulation. The coagulopathy associated with cirrhosis does not preclude paracentesis. Prophylactic transfusion of fresh frozen plasma and platelets is rarely necessary, since the risk of abdominal wall haematoma formation is less than 1%. Where there is clinical doubt about the presence of ascites, the procedure can be performed under ultrasound guidance.

Ascitic fluid should be sent for an immediate white cell count. This provides information on the possibility of SBP. A white cell count of greater than 500 neutrophils per ml of ascitic fluid is an absolute indication for treatment with intravenous antibiotics. The result should be actively pursued, because SBP is a cause of grave morbidity and mortality. Fluid should also be sent for culture (in blood culture bottles, rather than in a universal container), albumin and protein content (**Fig. 4.106**). Optional analyses include glucose, LDH, amylase, Gram stain, TB smear and culture, cytology and triglyceride levels.

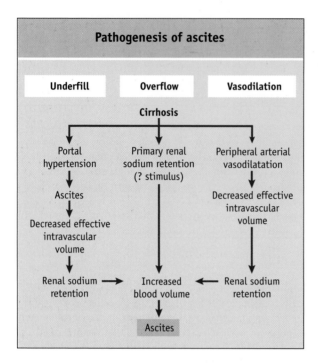

Fig. 4.104 *Pathogenesis of ascites: different theories. Three important factors in the production of ascites in cirrhosis are portal hypertension, hypoalbuminaemia and hepatic blockage of lymphatic flow with local overproduction.*

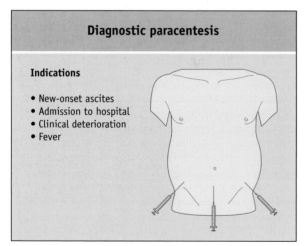

Fig. 4.105 *Diagnostic paracentesis. A 10–20 ml sample of ascitic fluid is usually sufficient for diagnostic purposes. If infection is suspected (e.g. spontaneous bacterial peritonitis) the yield of cultured organisms can be greatly increased by inoculating blood culture bottles with a sample of fluid at the bedside.*

The initial treatment of ascites involves sodium restriction, a stepwise increase in spironolactone (and frusemide if needed), and if the ascites is tense, large-volume paracentesis. There are four major approaches to the treatment of refractory ascites:
• Large-volume paracentesis
• TIPSS
• Peritoneovenous shunting
• Liver transplantation

Aetiology of ascites and the serum-ascites albumin gradient	
[Albumin] serum - [Albumin] ascites	
High (>11 g/L)	**Low (<11 g/L)**
Cirrhosis	Peritoneal carcinomatosis
Cardiac disease	Tuberculous peritonitis
Massive liver metastases	Pancreatic duct leak
Fulminant hepatic failure	Biliary leak
Hepatic outflow block	Nephrotic syndrome
Portal vein thrombosis	Serositis
Alcoholic hepatitis	

Fig. 4.106 *Aetiology of ascites and the serum–ascites albumin gradient. Like many fluid collections, ascites can be classified as an exudate or transudate based on whether its protein content is above or below 30 g/l respectively. However, many patients with ascites are hypoproteinaemic and so this distinction is less useful than the gradient between the ascitic fluid and serum albumin levels.*

Large-volume paracentesis should not be undertaken until diuretic and dietary manipulations have been tried, unless the ascites is tense. Inserting a cannula into the flank can introduce infection and, for these reasons, under no circumstances should an indwelling cannula be inserted and left there for free drainage for an extended time period (overnight, for example). The ascitic fluid tends to reaccumulate quickly and, for most patients, paracentesis only offers temporary respite.

The Barcelona regimen of attempting to drain the ascites to dryness and replenishing the intravascular volume with human albumin solution is still widely practised. The need for intravenous salt-poor albumin is debatable, but administering a sodium-rich fluid may hasten the further accumulation of ascites. With the debate over the possibility of transmissible prion proteins being present in blood products, some centres are using non-gelatine-based plasma expanders instead.

The typical intravenous albumin regimen is to give 8 g of salt-poor albumin for each litre of ascites drained, with the aim of limiting post-paracentesis circulatory disturbance. No differences have been found between albumin and the other plasma expanders when less than 5 litres of ascites is removed.

Insertion of a TIPSS may reduce portal hypertension and, for this reason, may lead to the resolution of ascites. It can certainly be useful in selected patients, but in the treatment of ascites, the benefits need to be weighed against the risks of the procedure (particularly encephalopathy).

Prior to the development of TIPSS, *peritoneovenous shunts* were a more common method of attempting to alleviate refractory ascites. LeVeen or Denver shunts are plastic tubes with a one-way valve which connect the peritoneal cavity to one of the great vessels in the neck (usually the jugular vein). The tubing is tunnelled subcutaneously and the venous end may have a titanium tip, which is designed to be less thrombogenic than a plastic one. These shunts depend on there being a large volume of ascitic fluid flowing through the tubing. They have a short useful 'life span', because blockage is an almost invariable problem, mainly at the venous insertion. Of course, the ultimate treatment for ascites is *liver transplantation.*

Expected survival after the development of ascites is approximately 50% at 2 years, with SBP the main cause of morbidity and mortality.

Spontaneous bacterial peritonitis (SBP)

The risk of developing SBP is 25% in the first year after the initial development of ascites. This is considerably increased in patients who have poor nutritional status and hepatic synthetic function. Up to 30% of patients have no symptoms, but fever, confusion and increased bilirubinaemia may be pointers towards the diagnosis. *E. coli* is the commonest causal organism, but cultures of ascitic fluid often fail to grow an identifiable organism. The diagnosis is best made by performing a white cell count on a 10 ml aspirated sample of ascitic fluid. SBP can be diagnosed if the polymorphonuclear cell (i.e. neutrophil) count is > 250/mm^3 if the patient is symptomatic (or has clinically decompensated). In the absence of symptoms, a count of > 500/mm^3 is diagnostic.

Treatment is usually with an intravenous third-generation cephalosporin. Cefotaxime 2 g three times a day for 5 days is perhaps the most widely used approach, although many hepatologists add metronidazole to the regimen. Recent studies have shown that a proportion of patients with 'uncomplicated' SBP (i.e. without renal failure, severe encephalopathy or gastrointestinal bleeding – perhaps less than a third of SBP cases overall) might be safely treated on an outpatient basis with the oral quinolone antibiotic, norfloxacin.

The development of SBP is an important prognostic sign in the course of chronic liver disease. The subsequent 1 year survival is less than 40%. Long-term antibiotic prophylaxis with norfloxacin reduces the recurrence rate from 70% to 20%.

Hepatic encephalopathy

The neuropsychiatric abnormalities affecting patients with liver disease are termed hepatic encephalopathy (HE). The condition is a reversible metabolic abnormality, typified by global depression of central nervous system function, the manifestations of which are widely variable and involve a spectrum from mild subclinical disturbance to deep coma. HE results from the development of hepatocellular failure and/or portosystemic shunting. Factors involved in the pathogenesis of hepatic encephalopathy include:

- Circulating gut-derived neurotoxins (ammonia, phenols, mercaptans, γ-aminobutyric acid (GABA), endogenous benzodiazepines, short-chain fatty acids)
- Alteration of the blood–brain barrier
- Alteration in neurotransmitter systems
  - Increased neuroinhibition (serotonin, GABA)
  - Decreased neuroexcitation (glutamate)
- Impaired energy metabolism

Research interest has been focused on the potential pathogenic role of circulating gut-derived toxins, particularly ammonia, and on changes in the functional state of cerebral neurotransmitter systems. However, it is unlikely that any one abnormality is causal, rather that a number of alterations occur which act in an additive or a synergistic fashion. Factors precipitating encephalopathy include:

- Gastrointestinal bleeding
- Drugs – e.g. sedatives, opiates, antihistamines, diuretics, NSAIDs, alcohol
- Electrolyte disturbance
- Dehydration
- Constipation
- Infection
- Deteriorating liver function
- Trauma
- Surgery
- Hypoxia

HE occurs in two distinct forms.

HE as a result of acute liver failure. Acute HE often progresses rapidly, over a period of days or even hours, and has a high associated mortality if left untreated. The predominant neuropathological picture is of cerebral oedema, due to increased permeability of the blood – brain barrier. Death frequently results from cerebral coning with herniation of the brain through the basilar foramina, as a result of increased intracranial pressure from the development of cerebral oedema.

HE as a result of surgical or spontaneous portosystemic shunting in chronic liver disease. This syndrome is termed portal-systemic encephalopathy (PSE) or chronic hepatic encephalopathy (CHE). In the majority of patients with chronic liver disease, CHE is subclinical and affects reaction times in the activities of daily living such as driving or operating machinery. The subclinical form of the syndrome is usually detected in slowing of the electroencephalogram (EEG) or as impairment of psychomotor performance. However, about 30% of patients develop clinically overt CHE and it is in these that the clinical demonstration of impaired mental state is central to the diagnosis. This usually manifests as disorientation and alteration of consciousness, personality, behaviour and intellectual function. These abnormalities may follow a chronic persistent, but usually an episodic and relapsing course. Fetor hepaticus, caused by increased circulating mercaptan levels, is a characteristic accompaniment, together with a 'liver flap' or asterixis. Neurological signs may be classed as extrapyramidal (resting tremor, dysarthria, muscle rigidity, micrographia and shuffling gait), cerebellar (intention tremor, dysarthria, nystagmus and ataxia) or pyramidal (hyperreflexia and hypertonia). Differentiation from other causes of confusional states in this patient population, particularly in alcoholic liver disease, is obviously extremely important (**Fig. 4.107**).

Diagnosis. HE is accompanied by demonstrable psychometric and electrophysiological abnormalities, but the majority of psychometric tests are too complicated for easy use at the bedside. The construction of a five-pointed star (**Fig. 4.108**) is one of the most widely used assessments, since many patients display constructional apraxia (**Fig. 4.109**).

The demonstration of EEG abnormalities may be a useful adjunct in the diagnosis and assessment of HE. In general, the EEG is typified by slowing of the normal 9 to 12 cycles per second to as few as 3 to 4 cycles per second, coupled with increments in the amplitude of the waves.

Blood ammonia concentrations are frequently increased in patients with HE and therapies aimed at reducing circulating nitrogenous compounds remain the mainstay of treatment. In healthy people, 40% of the ammonia is produced by the action of gut bacteria upon ingested food. The other 60% is derived directly from the breakdown

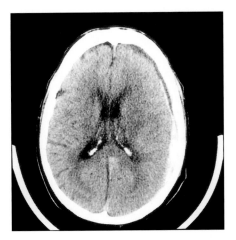

Fig. 4.107 *Subdural haematoma. Cerebral CT scan of a patient with alcoholic liver disease who presented with a confusional state. There is an obvious subdural haematoma, visible as an area of increased density between the skull and cerebral cortex.*

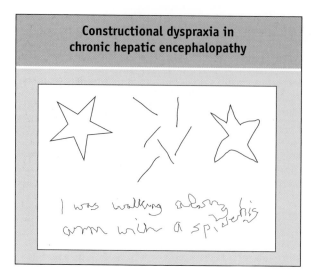

Constructional dyspraxia in chronic hepatic encephalopathy

Fig. 4.108 *Constructional dyspraxia in chronic hepatic encephalopathy. A patient has attempted to copy the drawing of a five-pointed star shown on the left, with little success. In addition, her spidery handwriting shows typical dysgraphia.*

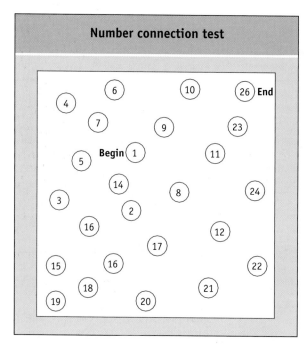

Number connection test

Fig. 4.109 *Number connection test for the diagnosis of chronic hepatic encephalopathy. The patient is asked to draw lines connecting 1 with 2, 2 with 3 and so on, as quickly as possible, and the time to completion is recorded. Serial measurements can be used to document changes in neurological status.*

products of digested dietary protein, together with the metabolism of circulating amino acids. In patients with cirrhosis, both reduction in hepatocellular function and portosystemic shunting contribute to raised ammonia concentrations in the bloodstream. However, blood ammonia levels are not always raised and do not necessarily correlate with the severity of HE (**Fig. 4.110**).

Cross-sectional imaging of the brain, in addition to excluding conditions such as subdural haematomas, may show some structural changes in chronic hepatic

Ammonia and hepatic encephalopathy

Factors supporting a role for ammonia in the pathogenesis of HE	Factors mitigating against ammonia in the pathogenesis of HE
Neurotoxicity of ammonia – ↑ brain glutamine (↓ glutamate), inhibition of chloride channels, may impair oxidative phosphorylation	Differential effects of ammonia depending on level – may cause CNS excitation rather than depression at low doses
Hyperammonaemia caused by other conditions may cause syndrome similar to HE	HE may occur with normal blood ammonia level
Reduction in blood ammonia by lactulose or antibiotics → improves HE	Poor correlation between blood ammonia levels and severity of HE
Feeding ammoniagenic substances may precipitate encephalopathy	Tolerance often seen to relatively high levels of ammonia in chronic HE

Fig. 4.110 *Ammonia and hepatic encephalopathy.*

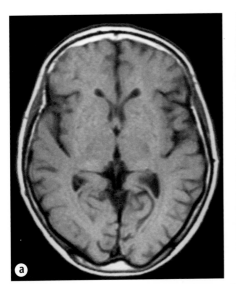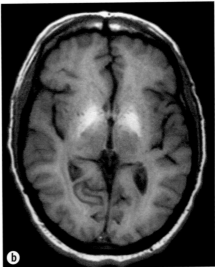

Fig. 4.111 *Intracerebral manganese accumulation in chronic hepatic encephalopathy. (a) T_1-weighted cerebral MR image from a volunteer (b) The image from a patient with chronic hepatic encephalopathy demonstrates hyperintensity of the basal ganglia. This appearance is the result of manganese accumulation. Manganese is normally excreted in bile and similar findings may sometimes be seen in chronic cholestasis. The reason for its deposition in this area of the brain is unknown.*

encephalopathy. Many patients with a lifelong history of alcohol abuse may have evidence of cerebral or cerebellar atrophy on CT scanning. Patients with chronic hepatic encephalopathy often have demonstrable evidence of manganese accumulation in the basal ganglia on MRI (**Fig. 4.111**).

Diagnostic techniques for the future.   Alterations in the blood – brain barrier, cerebral energy metabolism and neurotransmitter systems are believed to play a central role in the pathogenesis of HE. These factors may be directly assessed using techniques such as magnetic resonance spectroscopy (MRS) and positron emission tomography (PET).

Treatment of hepatic encephalopathy.   This is aimed primarily at reducing the absorption of potentially neurotoxic material from the gastrointestinal tract and is achieved by dietary alterations and by the use of agents that alter the nature and metabolism of the intestinal flora.

During a severe, acute exacerbation of HE all *dietary protein* has traditionally been stopped or curtailed. However, the scientific evidence for this treatment approach is lacking. Most patients with overt HE are actually in a catabolic state and very few benefit from protein restriction, which is best avoided. In fact, protein requirements may need to be increased in some patients. Clinical trials assessing mental state in patients with CHE have shown that in the longer term, vegetable protein is better tolerated than meat protein. However, clinical use of a vegetable protein diet is limited by poor patient compliance.

The use of the *non-absorbable disaccharide*, lactulose, has been part of the management of CHE for the past three decades, reducing intestinal absorption of potentially neurotoxic compounds by altering ammonia absorption and metabolism in the enteric flora. The synthetic disaccharide, lactitol (β galactosido-sorbitol) may produce fewer gastrointestinal side-effects.

The efficacy of oral *antibiotics* to reduce gut bacterial load in HE also remains controversial. A recent placebo-controlled study showed no clinical benefit from neomycin compared to placebo in patients with acute HE. In addition, up to 3% of an orally administered dose of neomycin is absorbed into the systemic circulation and nephrotoxicity can be produced. For this reason the long-term use of the drug in CHE is not advisable.

Several *new therapeutic agents* have been evaluated in patients with CHE, such as the administration of *Lactobacillus acidophilus* to recolonise the colon with non-ammonia forming organisms; the intravenous administration of branched-chain amino acid (BCAA) supplementation to redress the circulating amino acid imbalance; the use of the benzodiazepine antagonist, flumazenil, and of levodopa or bromocriptine to combat parkinsonian symptoms; and the administration of oral sodium benzoate or L-ornithine-L-aspartate to increase nitrogen excretion from the body. For all of these agents early promise has not yet been confirmed in controlled trials.

Control of precipitating factors which cause deterioration in mental state, such as constipation, gastrointestinal haemorrhage, electrolyte imbalance and infection, must remain the key factor in the management of HE. The fact that HE runs a fluctuating clinical course means that the benefit of any pharmacological intervention must be proven in large controlled clinical trials.

Hepatorenal syndrome and hepatopulmonary syndrome

These important systemic complications of liver disease are discussed in chapter 6.

ACUTE LIVER FAILURE

The term 'acute liver failure' (ALF), sometimes referred to as fulminant hepatic failure, is used to denote a number of clinical syndromes characterised by severe hepatic injury with a relatively short interval between the development of jaundice and encephalopathy. This jaundice to encephalopathy time has important prognostic significance and has led to the following classification of ALF which is broadly accepted within the UK:

Causes of acute liver failure	
Viral hepatitis	Hepatitis A Hepatitis B (may be acute, reactivation, or superinfection with HDV) Hepatitis D Hepatitis E Indeterminate ('non A–E') Cytomegalovirus Epstein–Barr virus Herpes simplex
Drugs and toxins	Paracetamol overdose Reye's syndrome *Amanita phalloides* Carbon tetrachloride Halothane Idiosyncratic reactions to almost any drug – e.g. nitrofurantoin, sodium valproate, isoniazid, rifampicin, ecstasy
Autoimmune hepatitis	
Cardiovascular and metabolic disturbance	Budd–Chiari syndrome Circulatory shock Heat stroke Sepsis
Wilson's disease	
Pregnancy-associated liver disease	Acute fatty liver of pregnancy HELLP syndrome
Malignant infiltration	Hepatic secondaries Lymphoma

Fig. 4.112 *Causes of acute liver failure.*

- Hyperacute liver failure – a jaundice to encephalopathy interval of less than 7 days
- Acute liver failure – jaundice for between 8 and 28 days before the onset of encephalopathy
- Subacute liver failure – jaundice for 4–12 weeks before onset of encephalopathy

ALF is a life-threatening emergency, often accompanied by multi-organ failure and sepsis, and yet because of the liver's potential for regeneration, a significant proportion of patients may make a full recovery with adequate supportive care. For the remainder, there is the possibility of liver transplantation and (perhaps soon) artificial liver support, but even so, ALF is frequently fatal.

Aetiology

Acute liver failure may be caused by a wide variety of hepatic insults (**Fig. 4.112**), but the commonest causes worldwide are the hepatitis viruses A, B, D and E. Overdosage of paracetamol is the most frequent cause in the UK and idiosyncratic drug reactions are also responsible for some cases. Toxicity due to consumption of the mushroom *Amanita phalloides* is common in central Europe and the western USA.

Pathogenesis

At a histological level, there is usually widespread hepatocellular necrosis. The clinical syndrome that develops depends on the influence of three factors: the metabolic effects of deficient liver function, the systemic toxicity of factors released into the circulation by necrotic liver and the ability of the liver to regenerate.

Acute liver failure is effectively a multisystem disease. The failure of the liver to clear circulating pathogens, coupled with an increase in gut permeability, results in sepsis and endotoxaemia. Circulatory disturbances lead to relative tissue hypoxia and multi-organ failure. Along with the defining feature (encephalopathy), coagulopathy and jaundice soon develop with progression to the complications of cerebral oedema, renal failure, electrolyte disturbance and infection. An early consequence of the endotoxaemia and sepsis is the widespread activation of macrophages, with release of many pro-inflammatory cytokines into the circulation such as tumour necrosis factor, interleukin-1 and interleukin-6.

However, not all of these features are found in every case. In paracetamol overdosage, for example, coagulopathy and encephalopathy may be severe and the condition may progress to cerebral oedema before jaundice has even developed.

Clinical features

Encephalopathy can be graded into four stages.
- Grade I: Poor concentration, mild dysphoria, reversed sleep pattern, coherent when roused
- Grade II: Increasing disorientation and confusion, though still relatively alert
- Grade III: Usually sleeping, but can be roused to commands or noxious stimuli; may become agitated or aggressive
- Grade IV: Comatose, poorly responsive to pain

The main difference from chronic hepatic encephalopathy is the greatly increased risk of developing cerebral oedema, which is particularly likely once grades III and IV are reached and can occur without signs of papilloedema.

Another distinction from chronic encephalopathy is that the flapping tremor and hepatic fetor are often absent.

The complications of acute liver failure may lead to the clinical features of respiratory failure, bleeding tendency due to coagulopathy, fever, hypertension or hypotension, cardiac arrhythmias and cerebral oedema.

Investigations

The aetiology of the hepatic failure influences the management and prognosis of the illness. Hence, the investigations should include viral serology, autoimmune markers, drug screens and an ultrasound scan with Doppler assessment of the hepatic veins. Close monitoring of haematological and biochemical parameters is vital and the prothrombin time, renal function and arterial pH have particular prognostic significance.

Management

All patients with acute liver failure should be discussed with a specialist (liver transplant) centre early in the course of their illness. Examples of the supportive care given for certain specific problems are shown in **Fig. 4.113**.

N-acetylcysteine is particularly useful in ALF, not just for treating acute or late (> 36 hours) presentations of paracetamol overdose but also for helping improve tissue perfusion and oxygen delivery in patients with circulatory disturbance. There is some evidence that it may also protect against renal impairment. The dosage for this indication is a loading bolus of 150 mg/kg intravenously over half an hour, followed by a maintenance infusion of 150 mg/kg/24 hours.

Specific complications of acute liver failure and their management

Problem	Frequency	Management
Intracranial hypertension and cerebral oedema	Occurs in 50–70% of ALF	Intensive monitoring in high-risk patients Nurse at 30° to horizontal Minimise tactile and auditory stimuli Mannitol Optimise cerebral perfusion Controlled, moderate hypothermia
Seizures (may be subclinical if comatose)	10–15%, particularly in subacute liver failure	Correct electrolyte disturbance, hypoglycaemia, hypoxia Anti-epileptic therapy
Sepsis	Bacterial in 50–85% Fungal in 30–40%	Early, aggressive use of antimicrobials
Renal failure	Occurs in 75% paracetamol-induced ALF Otherwise ~30%	Continuous haemofiltration Meticulous fluid balance N-acetylcysteine
Hypoglycaemia	Very common	Hourly blood glucose measurements Low-volume, hypertonic (10 or 20%) dextrose infusions
Hypotension	Very common	Intensive monitoring of cardiovascular function Usually pulmonary artery catheterisation with wedge pressures Combinations of inotropic or vasopressor drugs with N-acetylcysteine or prostacyclin
Respiratory failure	Common	Ventilatory support
Electrolyte disturbances	Very common	Maintain normal values of sodium, potassium, magnesium and phosphate in particular
Pancreatitis	15% of paracetamol-induced ALF	May be difficult to diagnose Severe cases may contraindicate liver transplantation
Coagulopathy	All cases	Not usually corrected unless bleeding or to cover invasive procedure

Fig. 4.113 *Specific complications of acute liver failure and their management.*

The main aim of management is to support the patient while the liver recovers and begins to regenerate. If the liver damage is so overwhelming that this cannot occur, then the patient must be kept in the optimum state for hepatic transplantation, avoiding sepsis, cerebral oedema and hyponatraemia. For paracetamol overdosage, the selection criteria for transplantation are well defined – as an arterial pH measurement of < 7.3 OR all three of a prothrombin time > 100 seconds, creatinine > 300 μmol/l and grade III–IV encephalopathy. For transplantation in ALF due to other causes, regardless of the grade of encephalopathy, the selection criteria require three of the following: age < 10 or > 40 years, a jaundice to encephalopathy interval of > 7 days, prothrombin time > 50 seconds, serum bilirubin > 300 µmol/l, or an aetiology of non-A–E (indeterminate) hepatitis, halothane hepatitis or idiosyncratic drug reaction.

Recently, a number of extracorporeal 'liver assist' devices (or artificial livers) have been developed. They usually involve some degree of haemoperfusion, but hepatocyte-based systems are also being perfected and it is likely that they will gradually be introduced as a method of supporting patients until either liver regeneration occurs or a donor organ becomes available.

LIVER TRANSPLANTATION

There are few, if any, applications of surgery which have made such an impact as organ transplantation. The ability to convert a patient with a terminal illness into an individual with a normal lifestyle and excellent 5–10 or even 20-year life expectancy has justifiably resulted in many countries investing substantially in organ transplantation and there has been a gradual improvement in the outcome of organ transplantation. The demand for donor livers in many countries falls short of the numbers required. This sometimes necessitates the consideration of non-ideal donors, where age, history and preservation time may not be optimal. Organ shortage could be solved by developing more accurate methods of assessing the viability of currently available organs or by techniques for increasing the pool of donor organs such as the use of non-heart-beating donors, split grafts or live donors.

Indications for transplantation

The major indications for liver transplantation are listed in **Fig. 4.114**. The vast majority of patients are transplanted for decompensated chronic liver disease.

Absolute contraindications to liver transplantation include AIDS, active sepsis, metastatic cancer, extrahepatic cancer (other than local skin cancer), severe pulmonary hypertension, advanced cardiac disease and advanced pulmonary disease. Relative contraindications to liver transplantation are age > 65 years, diabetes mellitus with evidence of end-organ damage, previous malignancy, active alcohol abuse, cardiac disease, advanced HIV infection, hepatitis B virus DNA positivity and previous biliary surgery.

Many transplant centres will not consider alcoholic patients for operation unless there has been 6 months' proven abstinence, owing to the possibility of recidivism. However, others will consider patients who have no record of abstinence, provided that there is an acceptable psychiatric assessment. Favourable factors include recognition of alcohol dependence by the patient with an acceptance that there is a need to do something about it; a socially stable living environment with a network of support which can be invoked to maintain continued abstinence; and a lack of intercurrent psychiatric disorders. Negative factors include:
- Pre-existing psychotic disorder
- Unstable character disorder
- Unremitting polydrug abuse
- Multiple alcohol rehabilitation attempts
- Social isolation

Transplantation of patients with chronic viral hepatitis may also be difficult because of the possibility of recurrence in the new liver, particularly in the context of immunosuppressive drugs. With hepatitis B-induced cirrhosis, good results can be obtained provided that there is no active viral replication. It is standard to give hepatitis B immunoglobulin in the perioperative period to all such patients, but specific antiviral treatment such as lamivudine can be given if individuals are hepatitis B e antigen (HBeAg)-positive and HBV DNA-positive on serology.

Indications for liver transplantation

Decompensated chronic liver disease	Intractable diuretic-resistant ascites Recurrent spontaneous peritonitis Grossly disabling lethargy Chronic persistent hepatic encephalopathy Progressive muscle wasting Worsening hepatic synthetic function with low serum albumin and progressive jaundice
Specific indications Alcohol	Proven abstinence or good psychiatric assessment with strong social support to ensure against post-transplant recidivism
Primary biliary cirrhosis	Bilirubin over 100 µmol/l Intractable itching and fatigue
Primary sclerosing cholangitis	Hilar strictures with absence of underlying cholangiocarcinoma
Malignancy Hepatocellular carcinoma	Small unifocal tumour < 4 cm diameter or up to 3 lesions with combined diameter of 3 cm, confined to one lobe of the liver
Neuroendocrine tumours	
Acute liver failure	
Budd–Chiari syndrome	
Graft versus host disease	

Fig. 4.114 *Indications for liver transplantation.*

When patients with hepatitis C are transplanted, infection of the graft by HCV is almost inevitable. Pretreatment with interferon to prevent recurrence after the operation has not met with success. Although some patients develop graft dysfunction in the early postoperative period, and this can be difficult to distinguish from allograft rejection, many patients with HCV do not develop any significant problems. Nevertheless, the same progression from mild through to severe hepatitis and ultimately cirrhosis can occur in the new liver. The unavoidable immunosuppression required to prevent allograft rejection usually results in a considerable acceleration of this process and in some individuals fibrosis can occur in the new liver within a year after the operation.

Transplantation for malignancy is relatively clear-cut. Patients with cholangiocarcinoma should not be transplanted, because these tumours always recur very quickly. The problem arises with patients with primary sclerosing cholangitis who are being transplanted for worsening of biliary strictures, because it can be difficult to exclude an underlying cholangiocarcinoma, even with good imaging techniques or with biliary brushings obtained at ERCP for cytology.

Good results with hepatocellular carcinoma can be obtained, provided patients are carefully selected; suitable candidates are those with cirrhosis and single tumours less than 3–5 cm in size. Meanwhile there have been mixed results with neuroendocrine (e.g. carcinoid) tumours. Generally these are slow-growing and such patients may be considered to be a good operative risk if there is no extrahepatic dissemination of disease.

There is little data on transplanting rare tumours such as hepatoblastomas, fibrolamellar carcinomas and epithelioid haemangio-endotheliomas, but these probably represent a better operative risk in terms of the speed and inevitability of recurrence than angiosarcomas of the liver which are highly malignant and always recur with a vengeance.

Another extremely rare indication for liver transplantation is graft versus host disease, with irreversible liver damage in patients where the prognosis is otherwise excellent from bone marrow transplantation. The liver damage is usually directed against the bile ducts and is a cause of the 'vanishing bile duct syndrome'.

Hepatic vein thrombosis (the Budd–Chiari syndrome) is an indication for transplantation if there is underlying hepatic decompensation and failure to recanalise the vein by other means such as direct installation of thrombolytic agents into the area of the clot.

Fulminant hepatic failure and subacute hepatic failure are the other main indications for transplantation. Unlike in France where the consumption of wild mushrooms may lead to inadvertent *Amanita phalloides* poisoning, in the UK paracetamol (acetaminophen) poisoning from deliberate overdosage is the commonest cause. This drug is available over the counter and it has only been in the past few years that regulations have come into force which limit the number of tablets which can be bought at any one time. Prompt administration of intravenous N-acetylcysteine is vital to prevent accumulation of hepatotoxic metabolites. All accident and emergency departments in the UK have guidelines for treatment on view for easy access, but if there is any doubt about whether to treat, it is better to err on the side of caution and do so until the serum paracetamol levels are known. Most patients present within 12 hours of overdosage, but even if there is late presentation, N-acetylcysteine administration may be beneficial. The absolute indication for transplantation is a metabolic acidosis of pH 7.3 or less, but if renal dysfunction (creatinine more than 300 μmol/l), encephalopathy and a prothrombin time of greater than 100 seconds are present, the outcome is grave without transplantation. Referring hospitals should contact specialist centres for advice if the admission pH is less than 7.35, if the patient is encephalopathic or has developed renal impairment, or if the prothrombin time has risen beyond 50 seconds. Prompt transfer may be needed.

Perioperative and postoperative graft dysfunction

The success of liver transplantation is dependent not only on the quality of the original graft, but also on its method of storage. The importance of preservation solutions is highlighted by the improved graft survival reported initially with Collins solution and more recently by the introduction of University of Wisconsin (UW) solution. Despite the use of more physiological solutions, there remain a variety of graft disorders which are attributed to preservation damage including reperfusion syndromes, primary graft non-function, delayed function and bile duct damage, all of which lead to significant patient morbidity and mortality. Primary non-function alone accounts for 6–13% of initial graft failure.

Some element of acute cellular rejection is a near-universal phenomenon in the immediate post-operative period, but this can be overcome by manipulation of the immunosuppressive regimens. The salient feature of chronic rejection in the later post-transplant period is a loss of small bile ducts (ductopenia) and on average this affects 8% of liver transplant patients, often resulting in severe cholestasis. It is usually associated with progressive graft dysfunction and may even require retransplantation. Its diagnosis rests to a large extent on histological examination of liver biopsy samples. Classically, there is loss of bile ducts in at least 50% of the portal tracts, but often considerably fewer portal tracts may be affected, which frequently makes definitive diagnosis impossible at an early stage. Furthermore, the condition affects the liver patchily and diagnosis often may only be made on comparison of serial biopsies. However, there is evidence to suggest that chronic rejection may be reversible, consequent to manipulation of anti-rejection chemotherapy.

Other post-transplant problems

Opportunistic infections may occur, particularly in the early postoperative period. Serious fungal infections may develop in the context of a complicated clinical course. Around 10–20% of patients develop cytomegalovirus infection, which can be life-threatening but is fortunately uncommon now as a result of improved prophylactic and therapeutic use of antiviral drugs.

Disease recurrence may be a problem with certain conditions, such as viral hepatitis, PBC, PSC, autoimmune liver disease and alcoholism.

HEPATIC NEOPLASIA

Hepatocellular carcinoma

Aetiology.
- Viral hepatitis
- Aflatoxins
- Cirrhosis
  - Hepatitis B
  - Hepatitis C
  - Alcohol
  - Haemochromatosis
  - Primary biliary cirrhosis
  - (Primary sclerosing cholangitis)

Hepatocellular carcinoma (HCC) (**Fig. 4.115**) is a recognised complication of chronic liver disease of any aetiology, with the development of cirrhosis being the most significant predisposing factor in countries of the developed world. Patients with autoimmune hepatitis or Wilson's disease appear to have a lower risk of developing HCC than those with most other causes of chronic liver disease.

Hepatitis B and hepatitis C infection are associated with a significantly higher risk of HCC than other causes of cirrhosis. This is reflected in the incidence of HCC, which has a marked geographical variation, being commoner in areas of the world where viral hepatitis is more prevalent (**Fig. 4.116**). In some countries, such as in southern Africa, aflatoxin, the environmental toxin obtained from food spoilage moulds and in particular from mouldy

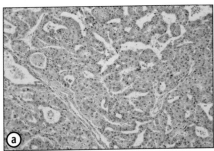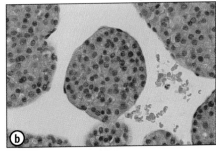

Fig. 4.115 *Hepatocellular carcinoma. Histological views demonstrating the typical appearance of the neoplastic cells with abundant cytoplasm, arranged in a trabecular pattern. (a) The low-power view also shows some adjacent cirrhosis. (b) High-power view.*

Geographical variation in the incidence of hepatocellular carcinoma in men (incidence per 100 000 people)

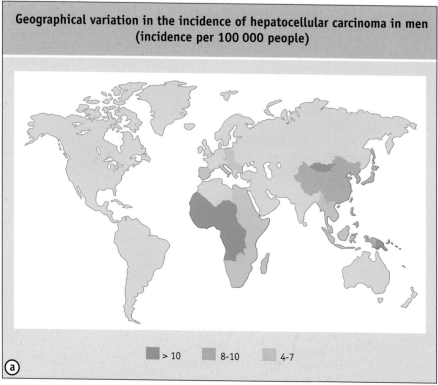

> 10   8-10   4-7

(a)

Fig. 4.116 *Geographical variation in age-adjusted incidence rates (per 100 000 people) for hepatocellular carcinoma. (a) Men. (b) Women. Overall, the tumour occurs more frequently in males, with a 3:1 M:F ratio. In the developed world, HCC is commoner in the fifth and sixth decades of life, but in some developing countries, particularly in Africa, the tumour may present much earlier without prior cirrhosis.*

groundnuts, has been strongly associated with the development of this tumour in young people, who do not necessarily progress to cirrhosis. Hepatocellular carcinomas are generally much more common in males than females.

Incidence and mortality statistics. In western Europe and the USA, most HCCs develop in patients over the age of 50, but in the Far East and Africa younger people are affected. In the Far East, the early development of HCCs has been associated with the acquisition of hepatitis B infection in childhood or by vertical transmission as a neonate. However, – the introduction of mass childhood vaccination programmes against the hepatitis B virus (HBV) for example, since 1984 in Taiwan – has led to a marked decline in the subsequent incidence of these tumours.

Hepatitis C virus (HCV) infection usually causes an asymptomatic acute hepatitis and, in about 80% of cases, the infection becomes chronic. The true prevalence of chronic infection with the HCV virus in the UK is unknown, but current estimates suggest up to 1% of the population is infected, in line with figures from the rest of western Europe and the USA. About 30% of individuals then develop cirrhosis over a variable period of up to 30 years after the initial infection. The subsequent incidence of HCC has then risen to 5%

Geographical variation in the incidence of hepatocellular carcinoma in women (incidence per 100 000 people)

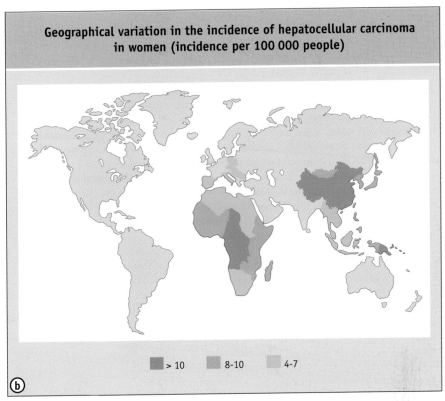

■ > 10   ■ 8-10   ■ 4-7

(b)

Fig. 4.116 *(Cont.)*

per year. Recent studies from France and Italy have suggested that the incidence of HCC is increasing in these and many other countries of the developed world, probably as a result of HCV infection. This may be associated with HCV infection from an increase in drug usage and in sharing of needles before the AIDS era when greater awareness of viral transmission and better public health measures, such as needle exchanges, were instituted.

Molecular pathology. Although less is known about the underlying genetic and biochemical abnormalities in HCC than in other gastrointestinal tumours such as colonic or pancreatic cancer, there are a number of well-described features. In particular, it seems that there are geographical variations in the molecular biology of HCCs with, for example, mutations in the p53 tumour-suppressor gene being much more common in areas where HBV is endemic. Similarly, chromosomal damage is found less often in tumours from western Europe and North America.

Based on studies of microsatellite instability, it is estimated that around a third of HCCs demonstrate defects in DNA mismatch repair enzymes.

Clinical presentation. The clinical presentation of HCC is as follows:

- Liver failure signs (ascites, jaundice, encephalopathy) 65%
- Ascites 51%
- Jaundice 32%
- Encephalopathy 17%
- Toxic syndrome 37%
- Epigastric or right upper quadrant pain 26%
- Gastrointestinal bleeding 2%

In any patient with cirrhosis who has sudden hepatic decompensation, the presence of a tumour should be considered. Nevertheless, by the time HCCs become clinically evident, the therapeutic options are often limited.

Worldwide, the 5-year survival rates for primary liver tumours remain poor and HCCs are frequently diagnosed at too late a stage for hepatic resection or liver transplantation to be a viable option. Early diagnosis can be difficult and increased vigilance in the at-risk populations, such as those patients with cirrhosis secondary to chronic viral hepatitis, is required.

Screening programmes. Screening programmes for HCC in patients with cirrhosis of all aetiologies need to be evaluated. A combination of regular 3–6-monthly hepatic ultrasound examinations and measurement of serum α-fetoprotein levels to detect HCCs at an earlier stage seems most appropriate. In some centres, the measurement of serum des-γ-carboxyprothrombin, a protein induced by the absence of vitamin K (PIVKA), has been used as an alternative to α-fetoprotein estimations. However, both of these blood tests have drawbacks, with only 70% of cases having raised levels. Furthermore, only 30% of HCCs produce very high serum α-fetoprotein levels.

Screening for tumours may become particularly important in HCV-induced cirrhosis, because the natural history of HCV infection would suggest that many of those individuals who contracted the virus from intravenous drug abuse in the late 1960s and early 1970s are developing cirrhosis and are currently at risk of HCC. Therefore the incidence of HCC in the UK is likely to increase over the next few years, in line with the published figures from elsewhere in western Europe.

Investigations. The investigation of a suspected HCC is as follows:

Screening
- α-fetoprotein
- des-γ-carboxyprothrombin
- Liver ultrasound

Investigation of a suspected lesion
- Blood tests
  α-fetoprotein
  Liver function tests
  Coagulation screen including prothrombin time
- Imaging
  Ultrasound
  CT
  MRI
  Angiogram
- Liver biopsy

Appropriate imaging is important. Ultrasound is the usual screening modality which brings the tumour to medical attention.

Spiral CT is helpful, particularly with the use of lipiodol, a contrast agent that is taken up preferentially and retained by the more vascular tumour tissue. HCCs can therefore be highlighted up to 10 days after contrast injection on follow-up CT. Selective angiography may show the tumour blush, and intra-arterial injection of lipiodol with follow-up CT has become the gold standard. The affinity of lipiodol for cancerous tissue can also be exploited for therapeutic tumour-targeting and used to deliver novel anticancer drugs in macromolecular polymers solubilised with the lipiodol.

MRI may be used to highlight tumours and newer manganese-based contrast agents may be helpful, such as manganese dipyrridole diphosphate (MnDpDp) (see **Fig. 4.35**).

However, there is usually no substitute for biopsying the lesion, since it can still be difficult to distinguish between cirrhotic nodules and HCC on imaging, even with newer developments such as ultrasound microbubble contrast agents. The theoretical drawback of obtaining a tissue diagnosis is the seeding out of tumour cells along the needle track. Nevertheless, with a careful ultrasound-guided technique and injection of an agent such as gelfoam as a plugging agent and absolute alcohol to kill any stray cells along the track, the incidence of this complication may be minimised.

Treatment. The 5-year survival of this tumour depends on the size and presence or absence of vascular invasion and micrometastases or satellite nodules within the liver. Most tumours will occur on the background of a cirrhotic liver and any underlying decompensation has also to be taken into account. The Okuda classification therefore grades tumours according to size and underlying function of the cirrhotic liver. Stage I is the smallest tumour with the best underlying liver function, while stage III describes the largest tumours with the worst underlying liver function. The median untreated survival for HCC is 12.8 ± 2.4 months for stage I, 3.2 ± 0.8 months for stage II, and 0.9 ± 0.2 months for stage III.

If tumours are small, transplantation of the liver should be a consideration. Initially, survival statistics were disappointing for patients with HCC because of subsequent tumour recurrence, but with more stringent transplantation selection criteria, such patients have a good outlook. As a general rule unifocal tumours smaller than 4 cm in diameter may be considered for transplantation or multifocal tumours provided that there are no more than three lesions confined to one lobe of the liver. Some centres have 75% 5-year survival rates under these circumstances, as good as most other indications for transplantation.

Partial hepatectomy may be considered if the tumour is larger or there are more than three lesions confined to the same lobe of the liver. The only problem is that most patients have cirrhotic livers and careful thought needs to be given as to whether there would be enough residual hepatic function in the remaining liver following the surgical procedure.

Where surgery is considered inappropriate, a number of other therapeutic options can still be used:

- Percutaneous alcohol injection
- Arterial embolisation
- Chemoembolisation (lipiodol-epirubicin)
- Thermal ablation
- Chemotherapy
- Radiotherapy

Percutaneous ethanol injection under ultrasound guidance has had some success, with published figures from Japan and Italy showing a 30% 3-year survival.

The results of chemotherapy or radiotherapy studies have been disappointing, as has the use of hormonal manipulation with tamoxifen. However, there has been some success with the use of targeted chemotherapy with epirubicin bound to lipiodol, which has a higher affinity for tumours when injected intra-arterially at selective angiography. An alternative is I^{131}-labelled lipiodol. Angiography allows tumour embolisation to be effected. Other agents which can be used to embolise the tumour include gelfoam, plastic beads or metal coils.

Alternative treatments include thermal ablation with laser fibres, cryotherapy or focused ultrasound. Recent developments with open access interventional MRI scanners allow such therapy to be monitored in an interactive fashion using heat-sensitive MR sequences (see **Fig. 4.36**).

Cholangiocarcinoma

Cholangiocarcinoma accounts for over 95% of biliary tract cancers (the remainder being even rarer tumours such as squamous cell carcinomas, leiomyosarcomas and lymphoma). It is much less common than HCC on a worldwide basis, but its main significance is that it often carries a poor prognosis, the result of being difficult to diagnose as well as treat.

Epidemiology and aetiology. Biliary tract cancer makes up approximately 10–15% of all primary hepatobiliary malignancies. In the USA, there are some 3000 new cases each year (compared to around 30 000 cases of pancreatic cancer). The tumour is slightly more

Possible risk factors for developing cholangiocarcinoma	
Chronic inflammation of the bile ducts	Sclerosing cholangitis Liver fluke infestation Caroli's disease Intrahepatic calculi (hepatolithiasis) Congenital hepatic fibrosis Choledochal cysts
Chemicals and toxins	Vinyl chloride Aromatic hydrocarbons Oxymethalone Thorotrast
Chronic liver disease	Cirrhosis Hepatitis C
Miscellaneous	Ulcerative colitis

Fig. 4.117 *Possible risk factors for developing cholangiocarcinoma.*

common in men than women and typically occurs in the sixth or seventh decade of life, although around a third of patients present below the age of 50 years.

For the most part, the aetiological agents are not understood and the tumour arises in an otherwise normal liver. This is particularly true for older patients, although those aged below 50 are more likely to have been exposed to one or more of the risk factors listed in **Fig 4.117**. The group most vulnerable to developing cholangiocarcinoma are patients with chronic cholangitis. In western Europe and the USA, primary sclerosing cholangitis, is the commonest predisposing factor. Cholangiocarcinomas are notoriously difficult to diagnose in the setting of PSC and it can be very difficult, even with sophisticated ERCP techniques, to tell whether a biliary stricture is harbouring an underlying tumour.

In Japanese and other Far Eastern populations a further predisposing cause of chronic cholangitis is hepatolithiasis, which is associated with biliary stasis and sepsis. In southeast China, the liver fluke, *Clonorchis sinensis*, is a common aetiological agent, whereas in Thailand, the predisposing chronic cholangitis is caused by another liver fluke, *Opisthorchis viverrini*. The now-obsolete radiological contrast agent, thorotrast, has also been strongly associated with the development of cholangiocarcinoma. Smoking, the oral contraceptive pill and alcohol have been causally suggested, but the evidence for this is fairly unimpressive. Cholangiocarcinoma may rarely be seen in association with cirrhosis and has been weakly linked to chronic hepatitis C infection. There is evidence that the incidence of cholangiocarcinoma is rapidly increasing in a number of western countries but the precise reasons for this remain unexplained.

Clinical features and investigation. Jaundice, weight loss, pruritus and abdominal pain are common presentations. Liver function tests are deranged and there may be an elevated serum carcinoembryonic antigen (CEA) and/or CA 19–9. Measurement of the latter was felt to hold some promise as a screening test, particularly in patients with primary sclerosing cholangitis, but its sensitivity and specificity are not high enough to be wholly reliable.

It may be difficult to visualise the tumour itself on ultrasonography, but the scan may demonstrate dilatation of the obstructed bile ducts or malignant infiltration of the hepatic parenchyma or blood vessels. Cross-sectional imaging with spiral CT or MRI is also

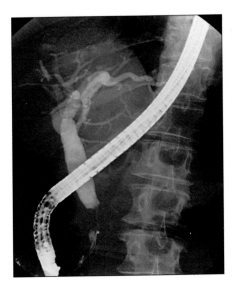

Fig. 4.118 *Obstructive jaundice due to cholangiocarcinoma. ERCP demonstrating a cholangiocarcinoma affecting the common bile duct, with marked proximal dilatation of the biliary tree (compare the width of the dilated duct to that of the endoscope). These tumours may occur anywhere in the biliary tree, but are most often found in the common bile duct or at the confluence of the hepatic ducts (the latter are often referred to as Klatskin tumours).*

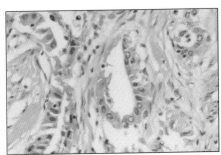

Fig. 4.119 *Histological appearance of cholangiocarcinoma. High-power H&E-stained view, with moderately differentiated cholangiocarcinoma forming variable-sized tubules.*

appropriate, but if the tumour is small, this too may be unrevealing. ERCP can demonstrate the nature and extent of an obstructing lesion (**Fig. 4.118**) as well as offering the potential to obtain samples for cytology or histology and to place a stent across the stricture. PTC may be required for more proximal lesions or if ERCP is technically unfeasible.

MRCP can highlight strictures but gives no information on tissue diagnosis. Even when tissue samples are obtained, however, the diagnosis can still be difficult. Cytology of aspirated bile has a sensitivity of only 30%, which rises to 50–60% if brushings are taken from a focal stricture. Histological biopsy (**Fig. 4.119**) may be performed, either with forceps through the endoscope or percutaneously under imaging control, but sampling errors restrict the sensitivity of even this test to 70–80%.

Treatment. Generally, the prognosis for patients with cholangiocarcinoma is grim. The overall 5 year-survival rate is around 5–10%, with only about 10% of patients being suitable candidates for potentially 'curative' surgery at presentation. However, palliative operations to decompress and bypass obstructions can also be useful and may prolong survival. Liver transplantation should be avoided as disease recurrence rates are extremely high. Endoscopic or radiological techniques allow the placement of biliary stents for palliative relief of obstructive jaundice but patients may require repeated procedures as their disease progresses. Radiotherapy and chemotherapy are of little or no benefit.

Rare primary liver tumours

These include:

- Fibrolamellar carcinoma
- Hepatoblastoma
- Malignant mesenchymal tumours
    Epithelioid haemangioendothelioma
    Angiosarcoma
    Kaposi sarcoma
    Fibrosarcoma
    Malignant fibrous histiocytoma
    Leiomyosarcoma
    Embryonal rhabdomyosarcoma
    Embryonal (undifferentiated) sarcoma

Fibrolamellar carcinomas. These are a variant of HCC, but are relatively slow-growing and therefore have a comparatively good prognosis. They are characterised by eosinophilic cells arranged in trabeculae, separated by fibrous strands (**Fig. 4.120**). These tumours generally occur in young adults on the background of a non-cirrhotic liver. The α-fetoprotein is usually normal, but there may be raised vitamin B_{12}-binding globulin and neurotensin levels in the plasma. Circulating levels of des-γ-carboxyprothrombin may also be elevated. Treatment is similar to standard HCCs, but outcome at transplantation may be better since it may take longer to develop recurrence, if at all.

Hepatoblastomas. These tumours of childhood represent about 50% of primary liver tumours in children. The aetiology is unknown. Treatment is either with resection and chemotherapy or with liver transplantation. Some liver transplant centres have reported up to 70% 5-year survival.

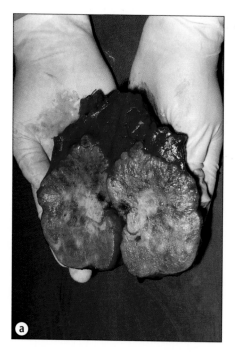

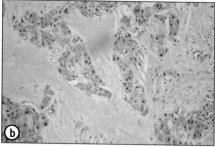

Fig. 4.120 *Fibrolamellar carcinoma. (a) Macroscopic appearances showing the tumour with dense scar tissue on the cut surface. (b) Microscopic view, demonstrating lamellar strands of thin collagen fibres with trabeculae of hepatocytes (H&E stain).*

Epithelioid haemangioendotheliomas. This very rare type of mesenchymal tumour has a variable prognosis. Some patients can live a number of years even with widespread metastatic disease and, unlike those with cholangiocarcinoma, these patients may do well following liver transplantation.

Angiosarcomas. Angiosarcomas of the liver have a very poor prognosis. The peak onset is in the sixth and seventh decades of life. There is an association with exposure to thorotrast, vinyl chloride, arsenic and anabolic steroids.

Hepatic metastases

For most tumours, the development of hepatic metastases is an extremely grave development with a poor prognosis. However, treatment strategies have been developed for metastatic colorectal cancer, which is the second commonest malignancy in the UK. Each year up to 20 000 patients die of this tumour with hepatic metastases contributing in about 50% of cases. If left untreated, most patients with hepatic metastases from colorectal carcinoma survive for a year or less. Nevertheless, surgical resection and various medical options may have a role.

Clinical presentation. Early and accurate diagnosis is clearly important. Physical examination of patients with metastatic colorectal tumours may reveal jaundice and hepatomegaly in those with weight loss. Liver function tests are usually deranged with increased serum bilirubin, alkaline phosphatase and also aspartate and alanine transaminases. Serum CEA, CA 19–9 and CA-242 may be elevated and serial measurement may be useful to detect recurrence after treatment. Imaging should be performed – initially with ultrasound and then with CT (Fig. 4.30) or MRI. Formal angiography may define the anatomy further if surgical resection is considered to be an option.

Treatment. Potentially curative surgery with complete resection of the tumour margins can be offered to patients with three lesions or less confined to one lobe of the liver. Ideally, patients should have no evidence of hilar and coeliac lymph node involvement. However, only 10–20% of cases are suitable for such treatment, which generally consists of a partial hepatectomy with or without preoperative portal vein embolisation (to cause atrophy of the area to be resected). Adjuvant chemotherapy may also be helpful.

Medical alternatives include hepatic arterial infusion therapy with direct instillation of chemotherapeutic agents such as 5-fluorouracil via an infusion pump. Other chemotherapeutic agents are the subject of current clinical trials.

Thermal ablation with cryotherapy or laser photocoagulation is technically possible, with monitoring of the thermal energy delivered using interventional MRI (as in **Fig. 4.36**). However, such methods are by no means established. Treatment in the future may be directed towards the inhibition of tumour angiogenesis or the adoption of gene therapy approaches such as genetic prodrug activation or enhancing immunotherapy.

It would seem that the best option at present is preoperative chemotherapy using 5-fluorouracil or one of its analogues, with surgical resection and intra-operative coagulation of the resection margins using a cryoprobe. Such techniques may offer 5-year survival in up to 40% of cases.

Carcinoid tumour. These serotonin-producing tumours usually arise in the gut and may cause the carcinoid syndrome if the liver becomes involved. Hepatic metastases are generally slow-growing and therefore suitable for surgical or medical treatment. If confined to the same lobe of the liver, surgical resection may be possible. Alternatives include hepatic arterial embolisation and thermal ablation. Patients should have an adequate intravenous dosage of octreotide to cover the procedure, in order to avoid the flushing that accompanies the syndrome, particularly since unpredictable hormone release can result from the necrosing tumour. The management of these tumours and the carcinoid syndrome are discussed in chapter 6.

GALLSTONES

Gallstones are the commonest cause of biliary tract disease, but are frequently an incidental finding in otherwise normal individuals. The two most important influences on the incidence of gallstones in a population are gender and age. Gallstones are 2–3 times more common in females and the overall prevalence of stones rises steadily with increasing age, affecting 30–40% of the population by the age of 80 years. Increased parity, oral contraceptive use and obesity further increase the incidence.

Composition

Around 75% of gallstones are composed mainly of sedimented cholesterol anhydride with an admixture of other lipids and bile pigment. Cholesterol is water-insoluble and its solubility in bile is dependent on the presence of other lipids, lecithin and bile acids. Bile also contains glycoproteins and calcium carbonate, the remaining 25% of gallstones thus being made up of calcium bilirubinate (pigment stones).

The serum cholesterol level correlates poorly with the risk of gallstone formation except in patients with type IV hyperlipidaemia.

Key points about gallstones include:

- The pathogenesis is multifactorial and gallstones may result from hepatic, gall bladder or intestinal defects in bile metabolism
- Gallstones are very common – but most patients (>70%) have no symptoms and do not require treatment
- The optimum treatment is surgery, but non-surgical alternatives are available for those who are unfit for operations.
- Although cholecystectomy relieves the pain due to gallstones, up to 50% of patients may continue to have digestive symptoms of some kind
- Despite the introduction of laparoscopic cholecystectomy, the overall morbidity, mortality and costs of gallstone surgery have not fallen, as more operations are carried out in patients who are older and have greater comorbidity

Pathogenesis

The old surgical maxim is that females who are fair, fat, fertile and over forty are prone to cholelithiasis. It is true that oestrogens may reduce bile acid secretion and reduce gall bladder tone, leading to gall bladder stasis. Furthermore, the propensity to stone formation increases with age. Bile that is supersaturated with cholesterol and which has a lower content of bile pigments and lecithin in order to dissolve the cholesterol is lithogenic. A nidus is usually required to spark off lithogenesis and the presence of bacteria, calcium bilirubinate and foreign bodies such as biliary stents can induce stone formation. Cholesterol crystal growth is facilitated by gall bladder mucus and is inhibited by apolipoprotein and lecithin vesicles.

Bacteria in the gut metabolise bile salts and produce secondary bile acids which have a decreased ability to dissolve cholesterol. Drugs such as cholestyramine may increase lithogenesis by reducing the bile acid pool.

Reduced enterohepatic circulation of bile acid also occurs in patients with terminal ileal disease. Crohn's disease is therefore associated with an increased incidence of gallstone formation.

Pigment stones

These stones also contain calcium phosphate, calcium carbonate and cholesterol. Those at risk of development of pigment stones are patients with haemolytic anaemias, sickle cell disease and acquired haemolysis from certain types of prosthetic heart valve.

Complications of cholelithiasis

Only the minority of patients develop complications from their gallstones (around 20%). So, the presence of gallstones on ultrasound (see **Fig. 4.26**) does not necessarily equate to cholecystitis. Evidence of gall bladder wall thickening on ultrasound examination is a more positive indication of gall bladder inflammation and is a more convincing reason for a surgeon to consider laparoscopic or standard cholecystectomy than historical grounds alone. The common complications of gallstones are.

- Acute cholecystitis
    Gall bladder perforation
    Gangrene of the gall bladder
    Gall bladder fistulae
- Choledocholithiasis
    Biliary colic
    Cholangitis
    Gallstone pancreatitis
- Gall bladder carcinoma

Acute cholecystitis. Patients present with right upper quadrant pain, fever and nausea. The pain is usually hypochondrial and constant in nature. The gall bladder may be palpable (25% of cases) and there may be a positive Murphy's sign where inspiration is arrested as the gall bladder tip is felt. There may be mild jaundice and, more often, a leucocytosis.

Patients who present with Charcot's triad (progressive jaundice, spiking fevers and colicky abdominal pain) have cholangitis secondary to obstruction of the bile ducts from an overdistended gall bladder or else from a stone in the duct itself.

Cholecystitis is usually caused by gallstones impacting in the neck of the gall bladder, obstructing bile flow through the cystic duct. However, occasionally cholecystitis may be acalculous where there has been prolonged biliary stasis, including patients on long-term total parenteral nutrition. Typhoid, tuberculosis, leptospirosis and actinomycosis can also provoke acalculous cholecystitis.

Choledocholithiasis. Around 90% of stones in the bile duct originate in the gall bladder. This can lead to biliary colic as the stone is passed out of the biliary tree (sudden onset of pain which is constant until the stone is passed through the ampulla). If the stone impacts, cholangitis or gallstone pancreatitis may result. Impacted stones can be removed at ERCP (see **Fig. 4.31**).

Cholangitis. Patients with cholangitis secondary to stones in the common bile duct must undergo urgent biliary drainage after initial stabilisation with antibiotics and rehydration. The bile duct can be cleared and the gall bladder removed surgically, but usually ERCP and sphincterotomy are effective, combined with a trawl of the bile ducts with a balloon which is inserted endoscopically up the bile ducts and inflated beyond the stone. Alternatively, the biliary tree can be decompressed at PTC.

Gallstone pancreatitis. This may occur when a gallstone becomes lodged in the ampulla. Again, urgent drainage is required using ERCP and sphincterotomy.

Treatment of gallstone-related disease.

- Analgesia – e.g. pethidine or diclofenac – for acute biliary colic
- Broad-spectrum antibiotics for acute cholecystitis, cholangitis or empyema of the gall bladder
- Cholecystectomy for symptomatic or complicated gallstone disease
- Laparoscopic cholecystectomy is associated with shorter hospital stay and more rapid return to work – but higher risk of bile duct injury and retained CBD stones (hence usually preceded by ERCP).

- If unfit for surgery, consider gallstone dissolution with ursodeoxycholic acid (need to have functioning gall bladder and radiolucent stones) but may take up to 2 years; extracorporeal shockwave lithotripsy; contact dissolution treatment (cholesterol solvent via percutaneous transhepatic catheter)
- After dissolution therapies, the recurrence rate is approximately 50% at 5 years; regular ultrasonographic follow-up and early bile acid therapy help to keep these patients free of stones in the long term

CARCINOMA OF THE GALL BLADDER

This is a rare but relatively aggressive tumour. Chronic inflammation from repeated cholecystitis appears to be a risk factor for its development and patients with a porcelain gall bladder (see **Fig. 4.25**) may be particularly vulnerable. Certain occupations with a high exposure to aromatic chemicals (rubber, textiles and wood varnishing) and raised biliary concentrations of heavy metals have also been implicated in carcinogenesis. About 85% of tumours are adenocarcinomas. Papillary tumours may progress from an adenomatous polyp to frank adenocarcinoma. Surgery offers the only hope of cure, these tumours responding poorly to chemotherapy or radiotherapy.

SPHINCTER OF ODDI DYSMOTILITY AND FUNCTIONAL BILIARY PAIN

It has only relatively recently been recognised that some patients can develop abdominal symptoms due to dysmotility of the biliary tree. Often these symptoms resemble those of gallstone disease, although no stones can be found. Sphincter of Oddi dysmotility (SOD) may be diagnosed on the basis of sphincter manometry carried out at ERCP. There is usually a high resting pressure with marked phasic contractions and often some retrograde peristalsis. Further clues to the presence of biliary dysmotility may come from a failure of contrast to drain from the biliary tree within 45 minutes and the transient development of mildly abnormal biochemical liver function tests during episodes of pain. Endoscopic sphincterotomy or balloon sphincteroplasty may give prolonged pain relief in such individuals.

chapter 5

The Pancreas

STRUCTURE AND FUNCTION

EMBRYOLOGY

The embryological origins of the liver, bile ducts and pancreas have already been dealt with in chapter 4 (see **Fig. 4.1**). Some of the important embryological defects that affect the pancreas are listed in **Fig. 5.1**.

ANATOMY

The adult pancreas normally measures 13–15 cm in length and lies in a retroperitoneal position across the upper abdomen. It is an elongated glandular organ, consisting of a head, neck and tail (**Fig. 5.2**), with the head lying in the curvature of the second part of the duodenum. The stomach lies anteriorly and the superior mesenteric vessels run just behind the pancreas, the vein uniting with the splenic vein to form the portal vein just behind the angle of the head and body of the pancreas. The organ's arterial blood supply derives from branches of the gastroduodenal, superior mesenteric and splenic arteries. Its venous drainage is to the portal circulation via the pancreaticoduodenal and splenic veins. The pancreas receives its innervation from branches of the vagus and the coeliac plexus.

Developmental abnormalities and variations of the pancreas	
Abnormality	**Significance**
Pancreas divisum	5–10% of population May be associated with chronic pancreatitis
Annular pancreas	Ventral pancreas encircles duodenum May cause neonatal duodenal obstruction Associated with duodenal atresia and Down's syndrome
Heterotopic pancreas	Up to 10% of population 'Rests' of pancreas found in stomach, small bowel, gall bladder, common bile duct, splenic hilum Most cases asymptomatic May rarely cause bleeding, pancreatitis or obstruction
Congenital cysts	Rare Usually solitary Multiple cysts may occur in polycystic renal disease

Fig. 5.1 *Developmental abnormalities and variations of the pancreas.*

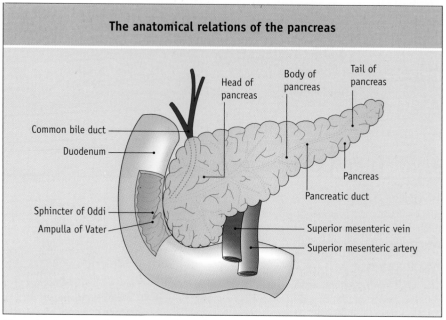

The anatomical relations of the pancreas

Head of pancreas

Body of pancreas

Tail of pancreas

Common bile duct

Duodenum

Pancreas

Pancreatic duct

Sphincter of Oddi

Ampulla of Vater

Superior mesenteric vein

Superior mesenteric artery

Fig. 5.2 *The anatomical relations of the pancreas.*

Its lymphatic vessels pass alongside the arteries and veins towards the pancreaticoduodenal and para-aortic nodes.

Histologically, the pancreas consists mostly of exocrine glands and ducts (about 80% of the organ), endocrine cells (2%) and supporting connective tissue (18%). The exocrine pancreas produces digestive enzymes and a fluid rich in bicarbonate. Secretory glands consist of pyramidal acinar cells that secrete the enzymes through their apical surface into the lumen. The acinar duct is lined with centroacinar cells responsible for the secretion of fluid and electrolytes. This fluid is carried initially in intercalated ducts that merge to form intralobular and interlobular ducts before reaching the main pancreatic duct.

The endocrine cells of the pancreas are arranged into the islets of Langerhans and include α cells, β cells, D cells and PP cells (see **Fig. 5.3**).

PHYSIOLOGY

As we have seen, the glandular pancreas has both endocrine and exocrine secretory functions (**Fig. 5.3**), the latter being of obvious importance for digestion (see chapter 2). The exocrine pancreas releases enzymes, largely in inactive forms to avoid autodigestion, together with water and electrolytes. The inorganic component of pancreatic juice is produced in response to the hormone secretin, liberating an alkaline solution rich in bicarbonate, chloride, sodium and potassium that is isotonic with plasma. Each day some 2.5 litres of fluid are produced, with a peak output of around 4 ml per minute. Like biliary electrolyte secretion, secretin causes a rise in intracellular cyclic adenosine monophosphate (cAMP) that stimulates the cystic fibrosis transmembrane regulator (CFTR) apical chloride channel. A network of apical and basolateral ion exchange transporters ensures that there is net secretion of sodium and bicarbonate.

The functions of the pancreas

Fig. 5.3 *The functions of the pancreas.*

Exocrine (acinar cells)	
Proteases	Trypsinogen Chymotrypsinogen Procarboxypeptidase A Procarboxypeptidase B Proelastase
Lipolytics	Pancreatic lipase Carboxylesterase lipase Prophospholipase A$_2$
Amylolytic	Pancreatic amylase
Nucleases	DNAse RNAse
Miscellaneous	Trypsin inhibitor Procolipase*
Endocrine (islets of Langerhans)	
Glucagon	Produced by α cells
Insulin	Produced by β cells
Somatostatin	Produced by D cells
Pancreatic polypeptide (PP)	Produced by PP cells

*Procolipase is converted to colipase in the duodenum; rather than acting as an independent enzyme, colipase forms a complex with bile salts that facilitates the action of lipase.

The pancreatic enzymes are synthesised in the rough endoplasmic reticulum of acinar cells. They are released into the acinus in response to the hormone cholecystokinin (CCK) and also to the neural release of acetylcholine, vasoactive intestinal polypeptide (VIP) and gastrin-releasing peptide (GRP). Once in the intestinal lumen, trypsinogen is hydrolysed to trypsin by the brush-border enzyme, enterokinase. This initiates a cascade whereby trypsin cleaves the other proenzymes into their active forms.

As with the secretion of gastric juices, the exocrine pancreas operates in cephalic, gastric and intestinal phases (**Fig. 5.4**). The main negative feedback influencing the levels of CCK and enzyme secretion appears to be intraluminal trypsin. Whereas during digestion, trypsin is occupied with food contents, the presence of free trypsin in the duodenum inhibits the release of CCK. Further inhibition of pancreatic secretion appears to be mediated by the islet hormone PP, acting via the reduction of vagal acetylcholine release.

The phases of exocrine pancreatic secretion and their control	
Phase	**Mechanism**
Cephalic	Mediated by vagus nerve May lead to 50% maximal secretion Neurotransmitters include acetylcholine, gastrin-releasing peptide (GRP) and vasoactive intestinal polypeptide (VIP) Further enhanced by cephalic-phase gastric acid reaching duodenum
Gastric	Vagovagal reflex Greatest response seen with gastric distension
Intestinal	Both neural and hormonal components Effects of gastric juice and food on small intestinal mucosa Secretin released when pH <4.5 and also in response to fatty acids and bile acids Cholecystokinin (CCK) released in response to fat >protein > carbohydrate Vagovagal enteropancreatic neural reflex

Fig. 5.4 *The phases of exocrine pancreatic secretion and their control.*

SYMPTOMS AND SIGNS

Symptoms and signs of diseases of the liver, biliary tract and pancreas are dealt with in chapter 4.

INVESTIGATIONS

General investigations of the liver, biliary tract and pancreas are described in chapter 4.

PANCREATIC FUNCTION TESTS

Some information about the degree of pancreatic exocrine insufficiency may be gained from the tests used in the standard diagnostic work-up of patients with suspected malabsorption (see chapter 2). If the patient is eating a diet that contains at least 70–100 g fat per day, then measurement of the faecal fat on a 72-hour collection may be well above the normal 7% level of faecal losses. It is, however, of little use in mild to moderate cases of pancreatic insufficiency and is clearly subject to the influence of other conditions that may cause fat malabsorption.

Consequently, many investigators have explored different techniques of measuring the secretory functions of the pancreas (**Fig. 5.5**). None of the tests can be said to be a true 'gold standard', but each has its merits. The direct tests of pancreatic function are clearly the most accurate when milder cases of insufficiency are included, but they are relatively invasive and so the indirect tests are more commonly used in clinical practice.

Tests of exocrine pancreatic function

Direct tests*	
Secretin	After secretin, volume and bicarbonate content of pancreatic
Cholecystokinin (CCK)	juice is measured. Following CCK, levels of amylase, trypsin
Secretin and CCK	and lipase can be assayed. Highly sensitive and specific for all grades of exocrine insufficiency, but relatively invasive and not widely available
Indirect tests**	
Pancreolauryl test	An ester, fluorescein dilaurate, is taken orally during a period of taking a set diet. Normally, pancreatic arylesterases liberate free fluorescein which is absorbed, partly conjugated in liver and excreted in urine. 24-hour urine collection performed; excreted levels correlate closely with exocrine pancreatic function. Sensitivity and specificity better for advanced pancreatic disease than for mild cases
PABA test	Similar concept to pancreolauryl test. Para-amino benzoic acid (PABA) is cleaved from an ingested precursor (NBT-PABA) by chymotrypsin and absorbed before being excreted in urine. Wide range of drugs may interfere with assay which is easily affected by hepatic disease, renal impairment and small bowel disease
Lundh meal test	Measurement of duodenal trypsin level after oral ingestion of a set test meal. Requires duodenal intubation and aspiration of contents. Lipase or amylase often measured too. More accurate at diagnosing severe pancreatic insufficiency than mild cases.

*Require intraduodenal intubation to measure pancreatic secretion after an intravenous injection of a hormonal secretagogue.
**Generally less invasive; use some form of surrogate marker.

Fig. 5.5 *Tests of exocrine pancreatic function.*

DIFFERENTIAL DIAGNOSIS

ACUTE PANCREATITIS

Acute pancreatitis is a relatively common condition whose severity can vary widely between individuals, with potentially life-threatening complications occurring in about 25% of cases. Improvements in diagnosis and treatment over the last three decades have seen the mortality rate fall from around 30% to 6–10% and there is now a greater knowledge of its pathogenesis and the optimum timing of surgical intervention. However, acute pancreatitis remains a serious condition that requires prompt diagnosis and optimum management if severe complications are to be minimised.

Aetiology

In the UK, around 40% of cases are caused by gallstones and it is likely that biliary microlithiasis may also account for a further proportion of cases. The incidence of alcohol-induced acute pancreatitis varies between countries according to the prevalence of alcohol abuse and the condition may be precipitated either by binge drinking or by a sustained regular intake. Other aetiological factors are:

- Gallstones
- Alcohol
- Trauma (penetrating or blunt)
- Post-endoscopic retrograde cholangiopancreatography (ERCP)
- Ductal obstruction (neoplasm, ampullary stenosis, duodenal diverticulum, parasites)
- Hypertriglyceridaemia (type I or IV)
- Hypercalcaemia
- Hypothermia
- Ischaemia (hypotension, vasculitis)
- Infections (mumps, mycoplasma, Coxsackie, salmonellosis)
- Drugs (azathioprine, pentamidine, didanosine, thiazide diuretics, sulphonamides, corticosteroids, tetracyclines, sodium valproate and many others)
- Miscellaneous (hereditary pancreatitis, pregnancy, cardiopulmonary bypass)

No cause is identified in about 10% of cases. Recently, two prospective studies of 'idiopathic' acute pancreatitis have shown that around two-thirds of patients had evidence of biliary microlithiasis or sludge at ERCP and that these patients responded favourably to endoscopic sphincterotomy and/or subsequent cholecystectomy.

Pathogenesis

Many authorities now consider acute pancreatitis as a two-stage disease. A first phase is characterised by a systemic inflammatory response syndrome (SIRS) which is usually initially sterile and represents the effects of numerous cytokines and vasoactive mediators (Fig. 5.6). Depending on the course of the illness, sepsis may be superimposed.

Should this phase fail to resolve (either spontaneously or with therapeutic intervention) a later, and often more prolonged, second phase ensues in which complications develop within and around the pancreas, elsewhere in the abdomen and in other distant organ systems.

The precise event that initiates acute pancreatitis depends to some extent on the aetiology of the condition. Alcohol, for example, alters the tone of the sphincter of Oddi, increases ductal permeability to pancreatic enzymes and is directly toxic to acinar cells. Gallstones may initiate inflammation by obstructing the pancreatic duct and raising pressure in the ductal system. Whatever the cause, it seems that a combination of injury caused by activated digestive enzymes (which may be exacerbated by reflux of enterokinase from the duodenum) and the release of reactive oxygen species from inflammatory cells are important pathogenic events. Local tissue damage in the pancreas attracts further inflammatory cells and the process spills over into a systemic inflammatory response driven by macrophage-derived proinflammatory cytokines such as platelet activating factor (PAF), tumour necrosis factor-α (TNF-α) and interleukin 1 (IL-1). In severe cases, this can rapidly lead to multi-organ failure with renal and circulatory dysfunction and the development of the acute respiratory distress syndrome (ARDS).

Clinical features

Almost all patients complain of abdominal pain, which is typically epigastric and may radiate through to the back or become more generalised. The pain may be confused with other acute events such as a perforated peptic ulcer or a myocardial infarction. In acute pancreatitis, the pain tends to be constant and may be relieved by leaning forwards. Importantly, the condition can sometimes occur without pain and should be considered in the differential diagnosis of any patient who presents with shock.

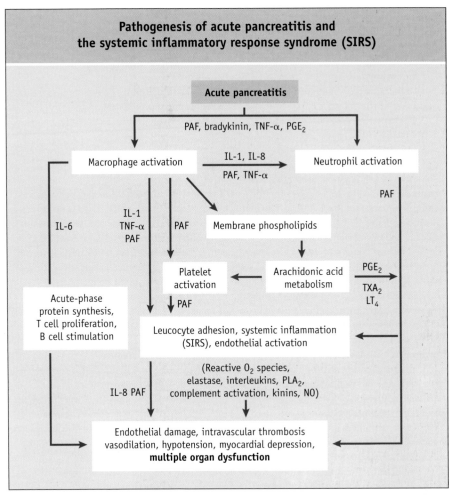

Fig. 5.6 *Pathogenesis of acute pancreatitis and the systemic inflammatory response syndrome (SIRS). PAF = platelet activating factor, TNF-α = tumour necrosis factor-α, PGE$_2$ = prostaglandin E$_2$, IL = interleukin, TXA$_2$ = thromboxane A$_2$, LT = leucotriene, NO = nitric oxide, PLA$_2$ = phospholipase A$_2$.*

Nausea and vomiting are usually prominent and 10–20% of patients are jaundiced. Other findings on examination include dehydration, confusion (which may be due to hypoxia), abdominal tenderness and hypotension. The classical features of Grey Turner's sign (discolouration of the flanks due to bleeding into fascial planes) and Cullen's sign (similar discolouration around the umbilicus) are found in less than 5% of cases, although they do tend to indicate more severe disease.

Investigation

Acute pancreatitis is usually diagnosed by a combination of clinical features, blood tests and appropriate radiology. Initial investigation of suspected acute pancreatitis consists of:

- Blood tests
  - Serum amylase
  - Urea, creatinine and electrolytes
  - Liver function tests
  - Calcium
  - Glucose
  - Coagulation screen
  - Full blood count
  - Arterial blood gases
- Plain radiology
  - Chest X-ray
  - Abdominal film
- Abdominal ultrasonography
- Electrocardiograph

Serum amylase is the test most commonly used to identify suspected cases; a value of at least three times the upper limit of normal is most useful. Significantly, there is no direct correlation between the rise in amylase and the severity of pancreatitis and levels tend to fall after the first 24 hours unless there is ongoing inflammation, pseudocyst formation or the development of a pancreatic abscess. Generally, the amylase level tends to be lower in alcohol-induced cases than those due to gallstones, but this difference is seldom clinically useful. Raised serum amylase levels may also occur with a perforated peptic ulcer, myocardial infarction, intestinal obstruction, ruptured ectopic pregnancy, mesenteric infarction, aortic aneurysm and other causes of an acute abdomen.

Measurement of the serum lipase level is claimed to have a higher specificity and is widely used in the USA and mainland Europe. Its serum level declines more slowly than amylase and so may be a better 'historical' marker for acute pancreatitis.

A urinary dipstick test for excreted trypsinogen-2 is being investigated as a further diagnostic aid and is showing some promise.

Plain radiographs of the chest and abdomen are essential. The chest film may show a pleural effusion or ARDS in severe cases and the abdominal film may demonstrate a 'sentinel' small bowel loop due to a secondary ileus or the calcified gland of chronic pancreatitis. Abdominal ultrasonography should be performed to look for gallstones and its prompt use in severe cases may help identify those requiring urgent ERCP.

Computed tomography (CT) and magnetic resonance imaging (MRI) are generally of little use in the management of mild pancreatitis, but are of great value in more severe cases, initially as a 'baseline' scan and then subsequently (repeated at least weekly) in order to identify complications such as extensive necrosis, abscess formation or pseudocysts.

Assessment of severity and prognosis

Scoring systems can be useful in identifying those patients with severe pancreatitis (and consequently those needing intensive care) as well as allowing standardisation of patient groups for inclusion in clinical trials.

The most widely used systems are the Ranson and the Glasgow scales (Fig. 5.7); there is little to choose between the two. A slight disadvantage of both is the need to collect data for 48 hours before a full assessment can be made, with the result that earlier risk estimations may lack sensitivity. In view of this, many clinicians grade patients according to the APACHE II scoring system (Acute Physiology and Chronic Health Evaluation) that is widely used in intensive care medicine; its calculation in the first 24 hours is at least as accurate as the Ranson or Glasgow scores.

Using these systems, a rule of thumb is that around one in four cases of acute pancreatitis can be classified as 'severe', and approximately one in four of these severe cases will prove fatal.

Comparison of the Ranson (USA) and Glasgow (UK) scoring systems for assessing acute pancreatitis

Ranson	Glasgow
On admission	
Age > 55 years	Age > 55 years
Blood glucose > 11 mmol/l	Blood glucose >10 mmol/l (and no
White blood cell count >16 × 10^9/l	history of diabetes mellitus)
Lactate dehydrogenase (LDH) 700 iu/l	Serum urea > 16 mmol/l (and no
Asparte aminotransferase (AST) >250 iu/l	improvement with i.v. fluids)
	White blood cell count > 15 × 10^9/l
Within 48 hours	
Arterial PaO_2 <8 kPa	Serum calcium <2.0 mmol/l
Serum calcium <2.0 mmol/l	Serum albumin <32 g/l
Haematocrit fall by >10%	LDH >600 iu/l
Rise in blood urea nitrogen >5 mg%	AST or alanine aminotransferase
Base deficit >4 mmol/l	(ALT) > 100 iu/l
Fluid sequestration >6 litres	

For both systems, disease is defined as severe when three or more factors are present.

Fig. 5.7 *Comparison of the Ranson (USA) and Glasgow (UK) scoring systems for assessing acute pancreatitis.*

Three other criteria also seem to be useful predictors of which cases will develop complications. Obese patients (and particularly those with a body mass index > 30) are at much higher risk, as are those who have left-sided or bilateral pleural effusions on admission. A serum C-reactive protein (CRP) estimation of > 120 mg/l within the first 48 hours is also highly predictive of a complicated clinical course.

Management

Supportive care. All patients with acute pancreatitis should be admitted to hospital, kept 'nil by mouth' and given full supportive care with intravenous fluid resuscitation, antiemetics and parenteral analgesia. Pethidine is generally preferred to morphine in view of concerns about spasm of the sphincter of Oddi with the latter drug, although the actual clinical significance of this has been questioned.

Close monitoring and continuous clinical assessment are vital if complications and changes in severity are to be detected. In particular, circulatory, respiratory and renal function should be monitored and regular checks made for fever or hyperglycaemia.

The degree of further intervention required differs for mild and severe forms of acute pancreatitis (**Fig. 5.8**). In particular, patients with severe gallstone pancreatitis (APACHE II score of 8 or higher, for example) should undergo ERCP and sphincterotomy as soon as possible, ideally within 48 hours, as this has been shown to improve survival.

Because of the likelihood of local complications and/or multiple organ failure, patients with severe pancreatitis benefit from multidisciplinary management in a high-dependency or intensive care unit. Radiological, endoscopic and surgical intervention may all be required. The specific care and correction of respiratory failure, renal impairment, refractory hypotension, hypocalcaemia and coagulopathy are of paramount importance.

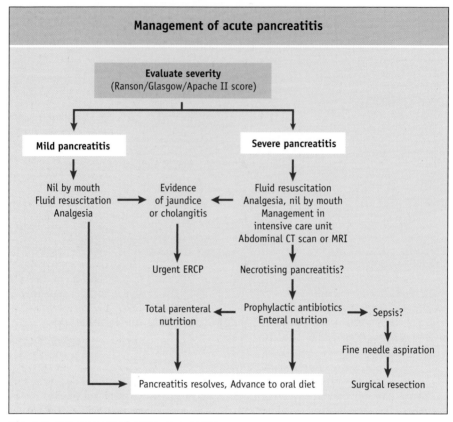

Fig. 5.8 *Management of acute pancreatitis.*

Antibiotics. Patients with mild pancreatitis and no evidence of sepsis do not require antibiotic prophylaxis, unlike those with severe disease. Sepsis is a common cause of morbidity and mortality for the latter and, although there have been few truly blind randomised trials of the use of prophylactic antibiotics, there is general agreement that patients with severe pancreatitis should receive them. The main intention is to reduce the incidence of infected pancreatic necrosis and so antibiotics with good tissue penetration of the pancreas should be used, such as imipenem, third-generation cephalosporins, fluoroquinolones and metronidazole.

Identifying an established infection of pancreatic necrosis can be difficult. Fever and leucocytosis may just be features of a sterile inflammatory response and even on CT it can be hard to distinguish the poor contrast enhancement of a necrotic area from an infected one. Even intrapancreatic gas, often a sign of anaerobic infection, is not completely specific or sensitive. Reliable diagnosis frequently requires percutaneous aspiration of necrotic pancreatic tissue and Gram staining of the aspirate, although this procedure itself carries a small risk of introducing infection.

Therapeutic antibiotics, such as the ones listed above, should be continued for at least 14 days. However, antibiotics alone are usually ineffective in treating infected pancreatic necrosis and surgical debridement is normally indicated.

'Specific' therapies. Knowledge of the early pathogenic events of acute pancreatitis has stimulated the use of specific therapies designed either to interrupt proteolytic enzyme activation or to limit the systemic inflammatory response. Somatostatin and its analogue octreotide have been used in attempts to limit pancreatic secretion and autodigestion, but trials have failed to show any benefit. Similarly, protease inhibitors such as aprotinin and gabexate have not been particularly impressive. Other unsuccessful therapies have included calcitonin, glucagon, atropine, fresh frozen plasma and therapeutic peritoneal lavage.

Recent work, focused on the early SIRS of acute pancreatitis, has shown that platelet activating factor (PAF) has a pivotal role in its pathogenesis. PAF is a bioactive lipid whose many properties include the ability to activate neutrophils and endothelial cells, promoting neutrophil 'pavementing' and migration from blood vessels. A powerful antagonist of PAF, lexipafant, has recently been shown to reduce the mortality of acute pancreatitis significantly in a large prospective randomised trial. If given within the first 48 hours of the illness, intravenous lexipafant reduced the mortality rate from 18% to 8% and also significantly lowered the incidence of pseudocyst development (see below). Earlier studies also revealed a reduced frequency of multiple organ failure. Further clinical trials are in progress.

Nutritional support. The traditional wisdom has been that the inflamed pancreas should be 'rested' and stimuli that might provoke further enzyme secretion, such as food intake, should be avoided. However, the systemic inflammatory response coupled with starvation result in a net negative energy balance and it is fortunate that most patients with mild pancreatitis are able to resume an oral diet within 5–7 days. Patients with more severe disease have generally been given total parenteral nutrition (TPN), although this is relatively expensive and comes with its own risks, such as the possibility of introducing more infection. Recent evidence has shown that TPN, as opposed to enteral nutrition, leads to increased gut permeability and a greater translocation of luminal bacteria.

There has been much recent interest in the early introduction of enteral feeding; in particular, enteral nutrition given by a nasojejunal tube (usually endoscopically placed beyond the ligament of Treitz) and started within the first 48 hours of illness has been shown to be beneficial, with substantially fewer septic episodes compared to TPN. This nurturing of the bowel wall is believed to protect its functions as a physical and immunological barrier. Prolonged or extensive ileus occasionally limits the use of enteral feeding and so TPN should be reserved for those patients who have been unable to meet their feeding goals after 48 hours.

Surgical intervention. Most patients recover with the therapeutic steps outlined above, but surgery remains an important option for some complications:

- Infected pancreatic necrosis
- Pancreatic abscess, if percutaneous drainage has failed or is not possible
- Unresolving pseudocyst, if percutaneous or endoscopic drainage procedures have failed or are not possible
- Extensive pancreatic necrosis with deteriorating clinical picture
- Significant haemorrhage

Complications

The most severe early complication, infected pancreatic necrosis, occurs in approximately 3–6% of cases, with pancreatic abscesses developing in a further 3–4%. The most common organisms responsible for these infections are enteric bacteria such as *Escherichia coli*, perhaps reinforcing the importance of bacterial translocation in much of the pathology of severe pancreatitis. Fluid collections around the inflamed pancreas can easily become the nidus of a bacterial infection.

In most cases, these small fluid collections resolve spontaneously, but if they persist beyond 4 weeks they are termed 'pseudocysts'. As their name implies, these collections do not have a true epithelial lining and are filled with a mixture of pancreatic juice, extracellular fluid and inflammatory debris. Enzymes present in the fluid can occasionally cause erosion of major blood vessels and significant haemorrhage or pseudoaneurysm formation (see **Fig. 4.28**).

More typically, the pseudocyst presents as an abdominal mass clinically or on imaging (**Fig. 5.9**) and may compress the bile duct or obstruct gastric emptying. Other clues to its presence are persistent or recurrent pain, pyrexia or hyperamylasaemia.

Pseudocysts that have persisted for 4–6 weeks are unlikely to resolve spontaneously, particularly if greater than 5 cm in diameter, and drainage is usually required:

- Radiological – percutaneous, guided catheter insertion with dependent drainage is suitable for most pseudocysts. Avoid if pancreatic necrosis present as may introduce infection. Simple aspiration alone is inferior to drainage, as reaccumulation of fluid invariably occurs
- Endoscopic – possible to create a cyst-gastrostomy or cyst-duodenostomy by the endoscopic route, ideally where a thin-walled pseudocyst bulges into the gut lumen
- Surgical – usually required if above measures fail or are impossible or if cyst communicates with pancreatic duct. Aim is usually to drain the pseudocyst into the stomach or a Roux-en-Y loop of jejunum, although partial pancreatectomy is sometimes necessary for pseudocysts in the pancreatic tail

Pancreatic abscesses may present in a similar fashion to pseudocysts, although signs of sepsis are common. Their prognosis is much more benign than infected necrosis (mortality < 5%) and diagnosis is usually made with a combination of cross-sectional imaging and microbiological assessment of aspirated fluid. Abscesses are frequently loculated, which can make percutaneous drainage difficult, and a surgical approach is often required.

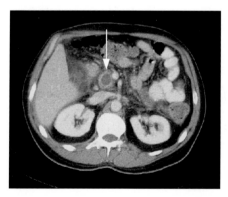

Fig. 5.9 *Pseudocyst formation in acute pancreatitis. Axial CT scan, enhanced with intravenous contrast, showing a fluid collection at the head of the pancreas (arrowed). Note also the streaky infiltration of the peripancreatic fat secondary to acute pancreatitis. An example of a much larger pseudocyst is shown in Fig. 4.29.*

Long-term management

Steps should be taken to avoid recurrence of the initial episode of acute pancreatitis. Those patients whose condition was due to alcohol excess should be given professional help to reduce their intake. Recurrent gallstone pancreatitis should be safeguarded against by referral for elective cholecystectomy and some surgeons advocate performing this before the patient is discharged from hospital.

A single episode of 'idiopathic' pancreatitis is generally unlikely to recur, although those with more than one attack should be referred for ERCP to eliminate the possibility of microlithiasis or biliary sludge as possible causes.

CHRONIC PANCREATITIS

This is a chronic inflammatory disorder, characterised by destruction and fibrosis of the pancreas with eventual deficiency in its exocrine and endocrine functions. Three subgroups of the disease have been recognised (**Fig. 5.10**), of which chronic calcific pancreatitis is by far the most common.

Epidemiology and aetiology

In the UK, chronic pancreatitis has a prevalence of around 50–70 cases per 100 000 population. A number of factors have been implicated in its development, alcohol abuse being the most common in developed nations. Some of the other known risk factors are listed below, although the condition can be idiopathic in up to 30% of cases:

- Alcohol
- Tropical pancreatitis
- Hereditary pancreatitis
- Congenital ductal strictures (e.g. pancreas divisum)
- Acquired ductal strictures or obstruction (e.g. tumour)
- Cystic fibrosis
- Hyperparathyroidism
- Hypertriglyceridaemia
- Post-radiotherapy
- Associated autoimmune disease (Sjögren's syndrome, systemic lupus erythematosus)

Types of chronic pancreatitis		
Subgroup	**Pathology**	**Comments**
Chronic calcific pancreatitis	Parenchymal fibrosis, calcification, intraductal stones and proteinaceous plugs	Most common type Alcohol is frequent cause
Chronic obstructive pancreatitis	Ductal dilatation, secondary exocrine atrophy and eventual fibrosis	Typically caused by intraductal or ampullary tumour, rarely by benign stricture <10% cases reversible
Chronic inflammatory pancreatitis	Glandular atrophy, mononuclear cell infiltrate, fibrosis	Least common Associated with Sjögren's syndrome and primary sclerosing cholangitis

Fig. 5.10 *Types of chronic pancreatitis.*

The risk of alcohol-induced chronic pancreatitis is related to the duration and the quantity of alcohol excess. Individual susceptibility varies, but a typical history would be one of more than 15 units of alcohol per day for more than 10 years, although an accelerated clinical course may occur. Most patients are males in the fourth, fifth or sixth decade of life. There is some evidence that a high intake of dietary fat may further worsen the risk of chronic pancreatitis in alcohol abusers.

Tropical pancreatitis is a distinct cause of chronic pancreatitis that chiefly occurs in areas within 30° of the equator. It tends to occur in younger age groups, equally in both sexes, and is thought to be related to multiple vitamin deficiencies and possibly a high dietary content of cassava. *Hereditary pancreatitis* is a rare autosomal dominant condition that is derived from a mutation in the cationic trypsinogen gene. Significantly, patients with this disorder have a 50-fold increased risk of developing pancreatic cancer.

For many years it was felt that acute and chronic pancreatitis were quite separate disease entities. It is now recognised that repetitive overt or subclinical acute injury to the pancreas can lead to chronic inflammation, atrophy and fibrosis.

Pathophysiology

In response to chronic injury of the pancreas, there is progressive damage to lobular acinar cells, often with atrophy of the glandular elements and fibrotic replacement. The ductal system becomes distorted and may show focal areas of dilatation or stenosis. Intraductal stones and cysts frequently develop, further exacerbating the impaired ductal transport. Stone formation and pancreatic calcification result from a combination of ductal stasis, increased viscosity of pancreatic juice, protein precipitations and diminished levels of factors that normally prevent calcium carbonate crystal formation such as citric acid and the enzyme lithostatine.

In the longer term, there may be pancreatic exocrine insufficiency with malabsorption and eventual loss of endocrine function leading to diabetes mellitus.

Clinical features

Pain is the predominant symptom of chronic pancreatitis. It can be particularly severe and unremitting, lasting for hours, days or even weeks at a time. The pain has a constant, gnawing character, usually worst in the upper abdomen, and radiates through to the back. It may be relieved by leaning forwards or in some cases by vomiting. An alcohol binge or a large meal may precipitate an episode of severe pain and patients frequently develop weight loss as a result of avoiding food. However, chronic pancreatitis may develop painlessly and insidiously, particularly in some cases of idiopathic calcific pancreatitis.

In most individuals, the clinical course is typified by recurrent episodes of acute abdominal pain, although these usually become less marked as the symptoms of pancreatic insufficiency begin to supervene. Over a decade of chronic pancreatitis, more than 80% of patients will develop exocrine insufficiency and overt diabetes mellitus occurs in approximately a third. The high functional reserve of the pancreas means that more than 90% of the glandular tissue needs to be lost before insufficiency becomes clinically apparent. Weight loss, steatorrhoea and nutritional deficiencies are often found in these patients, although there are often surprisingly few clinical signs on examination other than mild abdominal tenderness despite quite severe symptoms.

Diagnosis

In addition to compatible clinical features, chronic pancreatitis is usually diagnosed on the basis of imaging techniques that demonstrate the chronically injured pancreas. Additional tests of exocrine pancreatic function should be performed to detect insufficiency (see **Fig. 5.5**) and patients should be screened for diabetes mellitus and its complications.

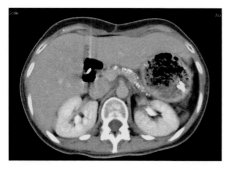

Fig. 5.11 *Chronic calcific pancreatitis. Abdominal CT scan demonstrating the typical speckled calcification affecting the pancreatic body and tail.*

Pancreatic calcification may be visible on a plain abdominal radiograph, but is generally more easily seen on CT scanning (**Fig. 5.11**). An ultrasound scan may identify changes in the size, density and shape of the pancreas, as well as revealing any biliary obstruction, but a CT scan is less operator-dependent and not vulnerable to bowel gas artefacts.

ERCP is considered by many to be the 'gold standard' of imaging in chronic pancreatitis, demonstrating tortuous or dilated duct systems and any local strictures that can be stented during the same procedure. Cytological brushings can be taken to exclude pancreatic carcinoma. Magnetic resonance cholangiopancreatography (MRCP), is being explored as an alternative imaging modality, although it lacks the interventional option.

The serum levels of biochemical markers such as amylase, trypsin and lipase are highly variable in chronic pancreatitis and are frequently normal. Occasionally, an abnormally low amylase level may be a useful pointer to pancreatic insufficiency, but these tests lack specificity and sensitivity.

Guided histological biopsies can be taken from the pancreas, but these are seldom performed and are generally best reserved for the investigation of mass lesions.

Management

It was previously thought that chronic pancreatitis, once initiated, was an inevitably progressive disease. This view has been overturned recently and although the histological and functional changes are largely irreversible, they do not necessarily progress if further pancreatic insults can be avoided. In particular, patients with alcohol-induced chronic pancreatitis should be strongly encouraged to remain abstinent.

Otherwise, the main goals of patient management are to relieve pain, replace the insufficient pancreatic enzymes, relieve ductal obstructions and try to prevent further episodes of pancreatic inflammation.

Pain relief in chronic pancreatitis. Ensuring adequate pain relief is perhaps the most challenging aspect of managing patients with chronic pancreatitis. Although difficult, it is an important goal as it will help the patient maintain an adequate nutritional intake as well as relieving a distressing symptom. Approaches are based on:

- Avoidance of alcohol
- Analgesic therapy
- Supportive therapy for acute or chronic pancreatitis
- Measures to decrease raised intrapancreatic pressure
- Reduce pancreatic secretions with H_2 antagonists, proton-pump inhibitors, pancreatic enzyme supplements, octreotide
- Relieve ductal obstruction or stenosis, using stone extraction, stenting or surgery
- Modify neural transmission
- Coeliac plexus block
- Thoracoscopic splanchnicectomy

A stepwise approach to analgesia should be adopted, initially using simple agents such as paracetamol which may later be combined with a non-steroidal anti-inflammatory drug or a weak opioid if ineffective alone. Stronger, narcotic analgesics may be necessary in some patients and carry the risk of addiction. Referral to a specialist pain clinic can be very useful.

Effective pain relief can also be achieved by blocking the afferent innervation of the pancreas. The procedures most often used are chemical blockade of the coeliac ganglion and, more recently, thoracoscopic splanchnicectomy. The coeliac plexus block can be performed at laparotomy, but is more commonly achieved by percutaneous injection of 50% alcohol (usually after a preceding diagnostic block using a local anaesthetic agent) under imaging control. Although the majority of patients achieve some relief, pain does tend to recur after approximately 3 months.

As the afferent pain fibres are carried through the thorax in the sympathetic chain, it is possible to disrupt them at thoracoscopy, using thermal ablation or simply by cutting them. There is some evidence that this technique may provide a longer duration of analgesia than coeliac plexus blockade, but it is still relatively new.

Endoscopic and surgical interventions. Some patients with chronic pancreatitis have evidence of intrapancreatic ductal hypertension. Methods of relieving these raised pressures include the clearance of obstructing stones at ERCP and endoscopic sphincterotomy. Pancreatic duct stenting can provide effective pain relief in many cases and internal drainage can also be fashioned for communicating pseudocysts.

Surgery may be necessary for some cases. The main indication is intractable pain and pancreatic resections are performed for this in some centres, although there is controversy over the most suitable surgical procedure and the respective postoperative complications. Other indications for surgery include pseudocysts and duodenal or biliary obstruction. Drainage procedures can be performed in cases with dilated ductal systems without the need for extensive resection.

Pancreatic enzyme supplementation. The development of frank malabsorption is usually a relatively late event in the clinical course, a tribute to the high degree of pancreatic functional reserve. The most obvious digestive impairment caused by pancreatic insufficiency is an inability to digest fats. In contrast, the digestion of starch may be slowed by pancreatic insufficiency, but salivary and brush-border amylases can still achieve 80% of the normal digestive capacity. In a similar fashion, protein can be effectively hydrolysed by gastric proteases and intestinal peptidases so that digestion can be at least partly maintained in the presence of a failing pancreas.

However, the intestine does not express enzymes with triglyceride-digesting abilities and extraintestinal sources (such as gastric or lingual lipases) are extremely small. There is also some evidence that the secretion of pancreatic lipase is selectively damaged at an early stage by alcohol excess and the enzyme's activity is further reduced by the impaired secretion of bicarbonate commonly found in chronic pancreatitis. As a result of these factors, steatorrhoea and deficiency of fat-soluble vitamins (A, D, E and K) occur many years before malabsorption of proteins or carbohydrates becomes apparent.

The treatment of pancreatic exocrine insufficiency therefore requires the effective delivery of enzyme replacements into the duodenum at meal times. The standard therapy is to take enteric-coated pancreatin microspheres by mouth. The enzymes, and lipase in particular, are vulnerable to inactivation by gastric acid and so the pancreatin supplements generally contain 5–10 times the amount of enzyme that would otherwise be required. Enteric coating has some effect in resisting gastric acid, but it is often necessary to co-prescribe an antisecretory drug to reduce acid output. Patients should titrate the dose of pancreatin until steatorrhoea is controlled.

The supplements are generally well tolerated, although very high doses given to some children with cystic fibrosis have been associated with the development of a fibrosing colonopathy. A similar syndrome, again associated with particularly high doses, has recently been reported in adults.

PANCREATIC CANCER

To all intents and purposes, the term 'pancreatic cancer' is synonymous with adenocarcinoma. The other malignancies affecting the organ are rare and include neuroendocrine tumours, lymphoma, metastases and pancreatoblastomas.

Adenocarcinoma of the pancreas

Few malignancies have a prognosis as grave as that of pancreatic cancer. Despite advances in molecular genetics, diagnostic imaging, surgical techniques, chemotherapy and radiotherapy, the survival figures still make grim reading, with the mortality rate almost identical to the incidence rate. The retroperitoneal location of the pancreas, coupled with a particularly malignant phenotype, encourages an insidious presentation with the disease typically too advanced for curative surgery. However, there is renewed optimism that improved knowledge of the molecular pathogenesis of pancreatic cancer may lead to more effective therapies in the near future.

Epidemiology. In Europe and North America, pancreatic cancer is the fifth most common cause of cancer death. Each year there are approximately 6000 new cases in the UK and some 30 000 in the USA.

Pancreatic cancer is more common in older age groups, with over 80% of cases developing between the ages of 60 and 80 years. Men are at higher risk than women, with an overall male to female ratio of between 1.5 and 2:1; the condition occurs more often in black populations compared to white and in urban areas rather than rural. Little is known about the aetiology of the vast majority of cases, but perhaps the most convincing association has been with cigarette smoking. Reports linking coffee consumption to pancreatic cancer now seem to have been discredited. Other reported associations (of varying strengths) have included alcohol consumption, poor dietary intake of fruit and vegetables, exposure to ionising radiation and chronic pancreatitis. There is a recognised association with diabetes mellitus, but this is more likely to be an effect of the developing cancer rather than its cause; if cases of diabetes developing less than 2 years before the cancer are excluded, the association disappears.

Familial pancreatitis is a rare but well-recognised risk factor for the development of pancreatic adenocarcinoma, as are some family cancer syndromes. However, it is difficult to identify a causal factor in the vast majority of patients who develop sporadic cancers.

Pathology. Our knowledge of the tumour biology of pancreatic cancer is perhaps second only to colonic cancer, with which it shares a 'multistep' model of carcinogenesis. Like many cancers, it appears to involve an accumulated series of acquired genetic mutations, each giving the malignant cell a higher growth rate or other selection advantage. For instance, activating mutations of oncogenes, (such as K-ras) lead to an unremitting growth stimulus being generated within the cell. Conversely, the inactivation of tumour suppressor genes (such as p53 or p16) removes the normal control mechanisms that would usually push a defective cell into apoptosis or stop it dividing. Examples of some of these mutations and their frequency are listed in **Fig. 5.12.**

In addition, pancreatic cancer cells simultaneously over-express a number of polypeptide growth factors and their receptors, so that the uncontrolled growth of adjacent cells is encouraged. Abnormalities of these growth factor systems and the altered

Acquired genetic abnormalities in pancreatic cancer		
Gene	Locus	Frequency of alteration
K-ras	12p12	90%
p16*	9p21	80%
p53	17p13	60%
DPC4**	18q21.1	50%

*Also known as CDKN2 or MTS1.
**Also known as SMAD4.

Fig. 5.12 *Acquired genetic abnormalities in pancreatic cancer.*

expression of matrix proteinases are also involved in generating a dense fibrous stroma around the malignant cells, as well as stimulating the growth of new blood vessels that both nourish the tumour and create a route for metastasis.

As a result of these changes, pancreatic cancer is able to grow rapidly, invade adjacent tissues and create distant metastases, usually before the disease is clinically apparent. Tumours that originate in the head of the pancreas may present at an earlier stage if the disease occludes the biliary tree or (in less than 5% of cases) causes an acute pancreatitis. Local invasion into the duodenum (**Fig. 5.13**), retroperitoneal tissues, mesocolon, perineural tracts or portal venous system may occur.

Macroscopically, tumours are found to originate in the pancreatic head in two-thirds of cases, the body or tail in a fifth and a combination of sites in the remainder. The vast majority (> 80%) are of ductal origin, although less common subtypes include mucinous, adenosquamous or acinar cell cancers. These share the poor prognosis of ductal lesions.

Clinical features. Abdominal pain, weight loss and jaundice are the three most common symptoms of pancreatic cancer, although it often presents in a vague and insidious manner. Pain is experienced in 60–80% of cases and is typically epigastric, often with radiation through to the back. Frequently, the pain is non-specific and difficult to localise. Weight loss is a common feature at presentation and can be quite severe even with a small tumour burden. As described above, invasion or compression of the lower common bile duct leads to obstructive jaundice, which is the presenting symptom in around a third of cases of pancreatic cancer. In accordance with Courvoisier's law, a palpable gall bladder in the presence of obstructive jaundice implies that gallstones are not the cause and instead suggests a neoplasm of the head of the pancreas.

Other presentations include lethargy, anorexia, nausea, new-onset diabetes mellitus and thrombotic episodes.

On examination, around 25% of patients have a palpable abdominal mass, 50% have hepatomegaly and about a third are jaundiced.

Diagnosis. This typically relies on cross-sectional imaging using ultrasound, CT or MRI scanning. Transcutaneous ultrasonography is particularly useful in jaundiced patients, detects larger liver metastases and is relatively inexpensive. However, its resolution is relatively low (tumours smaller than 2 cm in diameter are often difficult to detect) and the pancreas may be obscured by overlying bowel gas. The use of endoscopic ultrasound is being evaluated, although its accuracy is currently only around 70%.

CT scanning is perhaps the most widely used imaging technique and has a diagnostic accuracy of 90–5%. However, small tumours may lead to subtle changes in attenuation that can mimic those of pancreatitis or necrosis. Contrast enhancement helps to demonstrate invasion of vascular structures, enlarged lymph nodes and distant liver

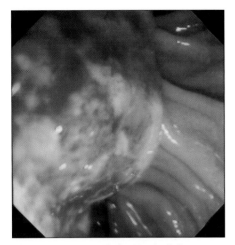

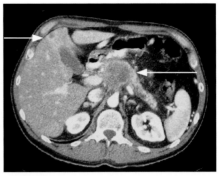

Fig. 5.14 *Advanced pancreatic cancer. Intravenous contrast-enhanced CT scan of the abdomen, demonstrating an adenocarcinoma arising from the neck of the pancreas (right arrow) that is invading the coeliac axis and splenoportal confluence. Metastasis to the liver has already occurred (left arrow). A CT scan of pancreatic cancer arising from the tail is shown in Fig. 4.30.*

Fig. 5.13 *Cancer of the head of the pancreas. Endoscopic view, showing pancreatic cancer invading the second part of the duodenum.*

metastases, avoiding unnecessary laparotomy for inoperable cases (**Fig. 5.14**). Spiral CT scanning increases the likelihood of detecting smaller tumours.

ERCP is especially useful in jaundiced patients and the signs of pancreatic cancer include the 'double duct' appearance, pooling of contrast in necrotic areas and stenosis or displacement of the ducts. Biopsies or cytology brushings can be taken and palliative therapeutic manoeuvres such as stent insertion can be performed.

Laparoscopy, with or without laparoscopic ultrasound, may be used to stage the disease if 'curative' surgery is being considered.

Blood tests are generally of little diagnostic use in suspected cases of pancreatic cancer. Serum levels of the epithelial mucins CA 19–9 or CAM 17–1 can be used as 'tumour markers', although their specificity is much reduced in jaundiced patients as levels may be raised by non-neoplastic pancreaticobiliary disease. That said, a CA 19–9 level that is persistently raised above 40 iu/l has a specificity and sensitivity for pancreatic cancer of around 80 and 90% respectively. As levels climb into the hundreds, the raised serum CA 19–9 becomes even more specific, but the sensitivity falls. Other tumour markers under investigation include SPAN-1, DUPAN-2, CA 242 and islet amyloid polypeptide (IAPP), though they have yet to prove useful in clinical practice.

Confirming the diagnosis of pancreatic cancer with histological biopsy is clearly desirable in theory, but may be of little practical benefit for many patients. This is a controversial area but patients with pancreatic cancer can roughly be divided into three groups:

1. Those with unresectable advanced disease or who are otherwise unfit for surgery
2. Those with obstruction (either biliary or duodenal) and a mass lesion
3. Those without obstruction and who have a potentially resectable lesion

Patients in the first group are likely to be referred for palliative therapy only or perhaps included in trials of non-surgical treatments such as chemotherapy. Confirmation of the diagnosis by histology is therefore important and may occasionally discover an alternative condition (such as lymphoma) that is treatable by other means. Percutaneous guided biopsy does carry some risks (such as peritoneal seeding or haemorrhage) but these are rare in practice.

The remaining two groups of patients are potential candidates for surgery, either palliative (in the case of group 2) or possibly curative in some of the remainder. In these circumstances, percutaneous biopsy is unlikely to alter the management algorithm and is usually unnecessary, although it may be useful in cases where a small asymptomatic mass is detected in the pancreatic tail of a patient with chronic pancreatitis, for example.

In most cases of pancreatic cancer, the diagnosis is made on the radiological appearance and confirmed by brush cytology. Histological biopsy may be used in different circumstances depending on the preference of the local surgical team. Recently, researchers have explored the diagnostic use of detecting mutant oncogenes (such as K-ras) in the blood, stools or pancreatic juice of patients with pancreatic cancer. These tests are currently undergoing further evaluation.

Management and prognosis. Pancreatic cancer has a very poor prognosis, with the overall 5-year survival rate being less than 5%. At the time of presentation, 80% of cases will have detectable spread of tumour to the regional lymph nodes, adjacent structures or distant organs and micrometastases will already be present in a proportion of the remainder. For the minority of patients whose cancer is still confined to the pancreas, a Whipple's pancreaticoduodenectomy is the only hope of cure. Even then, up to half of cases thought to be operable radiologically are found to be inoperable at the time of laparotomy; in any event, surgical resection only raises the 5-year survival rate to around 20% of its recipients.

Adjuvant treatment with radiation and/or chemotherapy may give a modest improvement in survival to a few selected patients but usually at the expense of significant toxicity.

Despite these statements, it is important not to be nihilistic about the treatment of pancreatic cancer. Recent years have seen improved results with palliative approaches, reflecting advances in surgical technique and more appropriate selection of patients for surgery. There have been a number of studies that suggest patient outcomes (and particularly perioperative complication rates) are much improved in specialist centres managing larger numbers of cases as opposed to general hospital units that perform relatively few pancreatic resections.

Resection rates for 'palliative' purposes differ between centres; some surgeons operate on up to 40% of their patients, while the average for most pancreatic surgeons is probably nearer to 15%. As well as tumour resection, surgical bypass can be created to relieve biliary or duodenal obstruction and permit a reasonable quality of life. Similarly, endoscopic stenting may be useful, particularly in the very elderly and those unfit for surgery.

Achieving adequate pain relief is a key aspect of palliative care and may require strong opioids by oral or parenteral routes, with nerve block procedures (such as epidural anaesthesia or coeliac plexus block) sometimes being necessary.

Given the generally poor response to 'conventional' cancer treatments, pancreatic cancer therapy is currently the subject of much research. For example, clinical trials of immunotherapy using vaccines derived from modified tumour cells are under way and other scientists are investigating approaches based on cytoreductive gene therapy. These techniques remain some way from the clinical arena, but may one day give rise to the therapeutic breakthrough needed.

Hormone-secreting neuroendocrine tumours of the pancreas

Tumour type*	Main hormone secreted	Other hormones often produced	Clinical manifestations
Insulinoma	Insulin	PP, glucagon	Fasting hypoglycaemia
Gastrinoma	Gastrin	PP, glucagon, insulin	Zollinger–Ellison syndrome, hyperacidity, severe peptic ulceration, diarrhoea
VIPoma	VIP	PP, calcitonin, glucagon, PHI	Severe watery diarrhoea, achlorhydria, hypokalaemia
Glucagonoma	Glucagon	PP, insulin, somatostatin	Diabetes mellitus, necrolytic migratory erythema
Somatostatinoma	Somatostatin	PP, gastrin, insulin	Steatorrhoea, diabetes mellitus, achlorhydria

*Shown in order of decreasing frequency. Insulinomas and gastrinomas between them account for around 80% of cases. The remainder are very rare. PP = pancreatic polypeptide, VIP = vasoactive intestinal polypeptide, PHI = peptide histidine isoleucine.

Fig. 5.15 *Hormone-secreting neuroendocrine tumours of the pancreas.*

Neuroendocrine tumours of the pancreas

Neoplasms derived from the pancreatic islet cells are rare. The tumours themselves are usually relatively small in size, but may become clinically apparent due to the secretion of one or more peptide hormones (**Fig. 5.15**), although around 50% are thought to be non-functional. Mixed patterns of hormone secretion do occur and PP is produced by around half of the tumours.

They are typically slow-growing and the histological distinction between benign and malignant is often blurred, with the detection of invasion or metastasis being the only reliable indicator of malignancy. Some pancreatic neuroendocrine tumours occur as part of the multiple endocrine neoplasia syndrome type I (MEN-I).

Diagnosis relies on the detection of high levels of secreted hormones (if present) and the identification of tumour masses. Most lesions are visible on CT scanning, but smaller tumours may require endoscopic or laparoscopic ultrasound, selective venous sampling or octreotide scintigraphy (see **Fig. 4.44**) to be identifiable.

Treatment involves the medical control of symptoms (such as diazoxide to reduce insulin secretion or high-dose proton pump inhibitors to block uncontrolled gastric acid output), surgical resection or debulking and the use of somatostatin analogues to inhibit hormone release.

chapter 6

Systemic Manifestations of Digestive Tract Diseases

It is not unusual for gastrointestinal diseases to lead to complications elsewhere in the body. The most obvious examples are those due to malnutrition and vitamin deficiencies, but many digestive conditions are associated with systemic disorders that may have a shared aetiology such as immunological or infective processes. In many cases, the basis for the association is unknown.

SKIN CONDITIONS

Inflammatory bowel disease (IBD)

Direct but relatively rare consequences of Crohn's disease are swollen lips (orofacial granulomatosis) and perineal involvement. Occasionally there may be skin involvement elsewhere, with granulomatous lesions in the umbilicus, for example.

Pyoderma gangrenosum (**Fig. 6.1**) is more common in patients with ulcerative colitis (UC) than in those Crohn's disease. It is characterised by pustular-looking lesions, usually on the legs, which go on to ulcerate. Treatment is with oral steroids, but sometimes the lesions do not improve until patients have had a colectomy.

Conversely, *erythema nodosum* (**Fig. 6.2**) occurs more frequently in Crohn's disease than UC and is often associated with other extra-intestinal features, such as arthritis and iritis. It can also occur as an adverse reaction to sulphasalazine therapy. The condition usually responds to treatment of the underlying disease, although systemic steroids are sometimes necessary for erythema nodosum alone.

Small vessel leucocytoclastic vasculitis (**Fig. 6.3**) is rare, but generally patients respond to immunosuppressive regimes with steroids and, if necessary, cyclophosphamide.

Aphthous ulceration of the buccal mucosa is relatively common in IBD and usually correlates with the severity of the intestinal inflammation. Local steroid mouthwashes can be helpful.

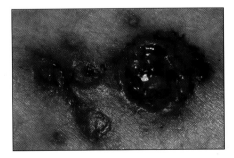

Fig. 6.1 *Pyoderma gangrenosum. Close-up view of ulcerated pyoderma gangrenosum in a patient with inflammatory bowel disease.*

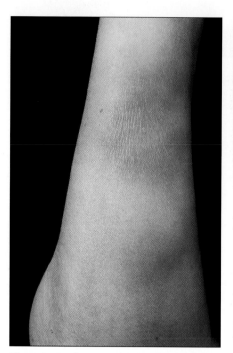

Fig. 6.2 *Erythema nodosum. The typical appearance of erythema nodosum, with painful, tender red nodules usually found on the anterior aspect of the shins.*

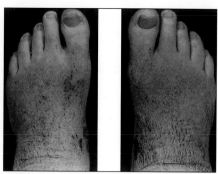

Fig. 6.3 *Cutaneous vasculitis in ulcerative colitis. Histological analysis of skin biopsies from this patient confirmed a leucocytoclastic vasculitis.*

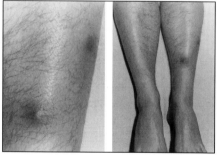

Fig. 6.4 *Panniculitis in a patient with chronic pancreatitis.*

Pancreatitis

Patients with acute haemorrhagic pancreatitis may develop Grey Turner's or Cullen's signs, skin discolouration due to tracking of blood into fascial planes under the flanks or umbilicus respectively.

In chronic pancreatitis, panniculitis may develop, resulting in painful skin nodules similar to erythema nodosum (**Fig. 6.4**).

Cutaneous signs of gastrointestinal malignancy

Skin metastases from gastric, pancreatic and, more rarely, colonic carcinomas usually occur on the abdominal wall and may be single or multiple. They generally have a nodular appearance; isolated lesions in the umbilicus have been termed 'Sister Mary Joseph's nodule'.

Paraneoplastic cutaneous disorders

Acanthosis nigricans (**Fig. 6.5**) is a velvety-looking pigmented rash involving the axillae, hands and joint flexures. It can occur in association with non-malignant conditions such as insulin resistance but may also be found in patients with adenocarcinomas, particularly those of the stomach, pancreas, colon and breast.

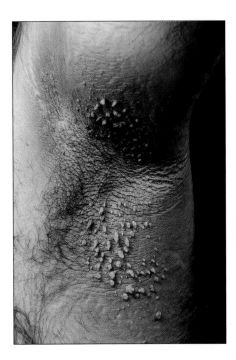

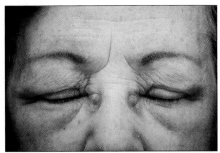

Fig. 6.5 *Acanthosis nigricans. The typical velvety pigmented appearance of acanthosis nigricans, affecting the axilla.*

Fig. 6.6 *Dermatomyositis. Violaceous 'heliotrope' rash affecting the eyelids of a patient with dermatomyositis.*

Dermatomyositis (**Fig. 6.6**) is associated with underlying malignancy in up to 40% of cases, colorectal and stomach tumours being the most common gastrointestinal associations. A violaceous (heliotrope) rash affecting the hands and the eyelids is accompanied by elevated creatine kinase levels and limb girdle weakness.

Much rarer skin conditions include hyperkeratosis of the hands and feet associated with the autosomal dominant oesophageal carcinoma syndrome, tylosis.

Hereditary polyposes

Perioral freckling is part of the Peutz–Jeghers syndrome (an autosomal dominant inherited condition with small intestinal hamartomas and an increased risk of malignancy, not only in the gut but at distant sites too). These dark melanin flecks can occur on the fingers, toes and also on the perianal skin.

Cowden's syndrome is characterised by multiple hamartomas of the skin, mucous membranes, thyroid and breast, associated with hamartomatous polyps of the gastrointestinal and urinary tracts. The condition is autosomal dominant in its inheritance and has a strong association with the development of breast, thyroid and colonic carcinoma.

FINGER CLUBBING

As well as being found in a number of cardiac and respiratory conditions, digital clubbing (**Fig. 6.7**) may occur in patients with chronic liver disease, malabsorption (including coeliac disease) and sometimes IBD.

JOINT AND CONNECTIVE TISSUE DISORDERS (IBD)

Up to 20% of patients with Crohn's disease and UC have joint problems. Any joint can be affected, but the most commonly involved are the knees and ankles in an asymmetrical

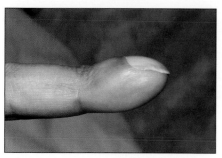

Fig. 6.7 Clubbing. Classical finger clubbing in a patient with cryptogenic liver cirrhosis and the hepatopulmonary syndrome. Note the complete loss of the normal angle between the proximal end of the nail and the nail-fold. This is accompanied by an increased curvature of the fingernail in all planes and expansion of the tissues of the fingertip.

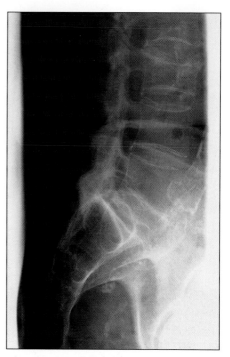

Fig. 6.8 Spondylitis in ulcerative colitis. Lateral radiograph of the lumbar spine, from the same patient shown in Fig. 6.9. Here there are early changes similar to ankylosing spondylitis, with loss of the normal lumbar lordosis and early formation of bridging calcification across the intervertebral discs. This condition occurs in about 1–2% of patients with UC and the majority of those affected are HLA-B27-positive.

pattern. However, patients may present with small joint arthritis, sacroiliitis (**Fig. 6.8**) and a spondylitis similar to idiopathic ankylosing spondylitis (**Fig. 6.9**).

Treatment of most IBD-associated arthropathies usually concentrates on the underlying bowel disease. Sulphasalazine was first introduced as an anti-inflammatory agent for rheumatoid arthritis and is effective for both the gut and joint problems in IBD, but often only standard analgesics and sometimes intra-articular injection of steroids are required for the arthritis.

In ankylosing spondylitis associated with IBD, the condition may develop at any stage and its activity or progression can be unrelated to that of the underlying bowel disorder. Indeed, ankylosing spondylitis can occur before colitis has even developed and is unaffected by proctocolectomy. It is usually treated with physiotherapy and non-steroidal anti-inflammatory drugs (NSAIDs).

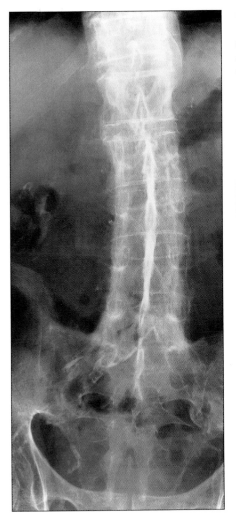

Fig. 6.9 *Sacroiliitis in ulcerative colitis. Typical radiographic appearance of sacroiliitis, with marked loss of the normal joint space between the sacrum and ilium. Up to 15% of patients with UC will develop sacroiliitis at some stage.*

Non-rheumatological features of post-enteric reactive arthritis	
Eyes	Conjunctivitis Anterior uveitis
Oral ulceration	

Skin	Erythema nodosum
	Keratoderma
	  blenorrhagicum
	  (pustular lesions
	  on the soles of
	  the feet)
	Circinate balanitis
	Nail dystrophy

Urethritis	(Usually sterile)

Cardiovascular	Aortitis
	Aortic incompetence
	Carditis with
	  conduction
	  abnormalities

Myositis	

Neurological	Peripheral and
	  cranial
	  neuropathies

Fig. 6.10 *Non-rheumatological features of post-enteric reactive arthritis*

Reactive arthritis

A Reiter's-type syndrome with arthritis and ocular and skin involvement can develop after episodes of diarrhoea (**Fig. 6.10**). Classically, in individuals who are HLA-B27-positive, infections with *Salmonella enteritidis*, *Yersinia enterocolitica*, *Campylobacter jejuni* and *Shigella flexneri* can provoke a post-enteric reactive arthritis (PERA). Unlike the sexually acquired syndrome which predominantly affects young men, females acquire PERA in similar numbers to males.

The arthritis is usually asymmetrical, involving the knees, ankles and the small joints of the feet. Spondylitis and sacroiliitis are common and enthesiopathies, particularly involving the insertion of the Achilles' tendon, are typical. The syndrome is usually self-limiting over a period of a few months and symptomatic treatment with NSAIDs is generally all that is required.

Coeliac disease

Metabolic bone disease (osteomalacia and osteoporosis) is common in coeliac disease. Some patients have muscle weakness and a seronegative arthritis which involves the hips, knees and shoulders in an asymmetric pattern. Adherence to a gluten-free diet usually improves these symptoms.

Other joint abnormalities

Autoimmune chronic active hepatitis can cause a non-destructive migratory polyarthritis. Arthralgia is a common feature of viral hepatitis, while primary biliary cirrhosis is associated with a Sjögren's syndrome (dry eyes, dry mouth and arthralgia) as well as a small-joint arthropathy (Fig. 6.11).

Chondrocalcinosis, osteochondritis and osteomalacia patellae occur in Wilson's disease, and patients with haemochromatosis may develop an arthropathy with joint space narrowing and chondrocalcinosis. The respective underlying conditions should be treated appropriately, but treatment of the rheumatological sequelae is essentially symptomatic.

OCULAR MANIFESTATIONS (IBD)

Anterior uveitis (iritis and episcleritis) are commoner in UC than Crohn's disease. Blurred vision, ocular pain and photophobia are the presenting symptoms of an iritis, which in patients with IBD is often bilateral. Posterior synechiae may be seen, where the iris sticks down to the lens behind. Episcleritis is a differential diagnosis of a painful red eye; a painful red nodule appears on the sclera. Both conditions may resolve spontaneously or with treatment of the underlying IBD, but specific ophthalmological advice should be sought. Pupillary dilatation with atropine and topical steroids are effective measures.

Other conditions

Patients with PERA may have conjunctivitis or anterior uveitis (iritis). Primary biliary cirrhosis is associated with a sicca syndrome with dry eyes, while the Kayser–Fleischer ring caused by copper deposition at the limbus of the cornea is the classical ocular finding in patients with Wilson's disease. This abnormality should not be confused with arcus senilis and has a greenish-yellow appearance (see Fig. 4.76). Mild cases can be demonstrated using a slit-lamp examination.

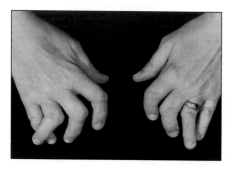

Fig. 6.11 *Small joint arthropathy in primary biliary cirrhosis. This patient with PBC has a severe, deforming, psoriatic-type arthropathy affecting the small joints of the hands.*

NEUROLOGICAL MANIFESTATIONS

Wilson's disease

This is also known as hepatolenticular degeneration. There is copper deposition, especially in the globus pallidus and the putamen. The cerebral cortex and other basal ganglia structures may also be damaged. Patients display personality changes, tremor, dysarthria, drooling, extrapyramidal signs (chorea, dystonia, akinesia, rigidity) and ultimately dementia. Provided the disease is recognised early enough, the neurological symptoms can be completely controlled with copper chelation by D-penicillamine, but if left untreated for too long, the neurological abnormalities are usually irreversible.

Paraneoplastic syndromes

The commonest cause of neurological problems in patients with gastrointestinal malignancy is metastatic spread, but paraneoplastic syndromes (presumably as a result of cytokine production or immune responses) can occur. Dementia, cerebellar degeneration, optic neuritis and amyotrophic lateral sclerosis (lower motor neurone weakness combined with spasticity and fasciculation) may occur. Colorectal carcinoma may cause these syndromes, but oesophageal carcinoma can provoke a paraneoplastic peripheral neuropathy.

Neurocysticercosis

The larval stages of the pork tapeworm, *Taenia solium*, can encyst in the muscle and the central nervous system (CNS). The neurological manifestations are protean, depending on the number and the localisation of the cysts. Epilepsy is the predominant symptom, but hydrocephalus may occur.

Botulism

This is an acute, symmetrical, descending paralysis of the autonomic and cranial nerves produced by the potent, heat-labile protein neurotoxin of *Clostridium botulinum*. It is mercifully rare, but usually results from the ingestion of poorly produced canned foods which contain *C. botulinum* spores. It is destroyed by the normal cooking process. The toxin primarily affects the cranial nerves and blocks cholinergic transmission at the neuromuscular junction, autonomic ganglia and parasympathetic nerve terminals. Presenting symptoms include nausea, vomiting, dry mouth, dizziness and blurred vision. It is often mistaken for a simple gastrointestinal upset, but difficulty in swallowing, generalised muscular weakness and respiratory depression ensue. An antitoxin should be administered, because it may shorten the course of the illness. However, most patients require extended respiratory support until neurological recovery takes place.

RENAL MANIFESTATIONS

IBD

Crohn's disease is associated with renal stones (uric acid and also calcium oxalate stones in hyperoxaluric patients with ileal Crohn's disease), with renal amyloid deposition and by direct extension with the formation of enterovesical fistulae. UC is also associated with nephrolithiasis and amyloid deposition (this may present as a nephrotic syndrome). There is also an increased incidence of pyelonephritis in these patients, but the mechanism is unknown.

PULMONARY MANIFESTATIONS

Oesophageal disease

Patients with hiatus hernias, oesophageal atresia and pharyngeal pouches, depending on the nature of the underlying condition, are prone to aspiration of oesophageal or gastric contents. This may present as recurrent chest infections, a cough or wheezing. Associated pathology includes pneumonia, bronchiectasis, chronic airway obstruction and lung abscesses. Patients need to be treated symptomatically and the underlying condition needs to be corrected.

Pancreatitis

Pleural effusions, atelectasis, pneumonitis and the acute respiratory distress syndrome (ARDS) are common associations of acute pancreatitis.

IBD

Pulmonary fibrosis is a rare association of UC. An idiosyncratic sulphasalazine-induced alveolitis is also well recognised with cough, fever, dyspnoea, eosinophilia and patchy shadowing on plain chest radiography. The syndrome usually responds to withdrawal of the drug.

CARDIAC ABNORMALITIES

IBD

Patients with joint involvement may develop aortic regurgitation, but this is probably associated with HLA-B27 tissue type. There are rare associations with myocarditis, pericarditis and dilated cardiomyopathy.

INFECTIONS

Typhoid

Enteric or typhoid fever is caused by *Salmonella typhi*, but the syndrome (see chapter 2) may also be caused by other *Salmonella* species such as *S. enteritidis*. The illness has a number of distinct phases. Patients often present with a fever, but with a characteristic relative bradycardia. A typical truncal 'rose spot' rash appears towards the end of the first week. After ingestion, the organisms multiply in the duodenum, before a septicaemic phase ensues. Pneumonia, lung abscesses, pericarditis, myocarditis, osteomyelitis, joint involvement, meningitis, peripheral neuropathy and orchitis may develop in addition to gastrointestinal manifestations such as cholecystitis, hepatitis, pancreatitis and severe ulceration of the small intestine. Treatment is discussed in chapter 2.

MULTISYSTEM DISORDERS

Whipple's disease

This rare malabsorptive condition is caused by the organism, *Tropheryma whippelii* (see chapter 2). It has protean systemic manifestations including skin pigmentation, lymphadenopathy and a seronegative arthritis which affects both large and small joints. A classical sacroiliitis and spondylitis are less common than involvement of the knees, wrists and the small joints of the hands. Finger clubbing can occur. The organism may cause endocarditis and valvular thickening, while pulmonary infiltrates, pleurisy and a chronic cough are common. Rarely, there may be involvement of the CNS with cranial nerve lesions, myoclonus, meningitis and an encephalopathy. However, the manifestations of CNS involvement are usually non-specific, with depression, dizziness, apathy, epilepsy, behavioural disturbances and memory loss prominent features. The organism may be seen in the cerebrospinal fluid on lumbar puncture. Although systemic Whipple's disease responds to antibiotic treatment, this is not usually the case with the neurological sequelae.

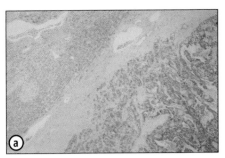 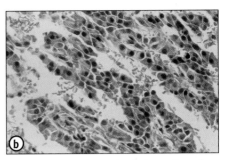

Fig. 6.12 *Carcinoid tumour in the liver. Haematokylin and eosin-stained views show the typical histological appearance of carcinoid tumour deposits, with aggregates of small, uniform cells and prominent, basophilic, rounded nuclei. Similar appearances may be seen with other tumours of neuroendocrine origin, although immunohistochemistry techniques can be used to identify specific secretory granules. (a) Low-power view. (b) High-power view.*

Carcinoid tumours and the carcinoid syndrome

Pathogenesis. Carcinoid tumours are neoplasms arising from neuroendocrine cells (**Fig. 6.12**) that either secrete or contain serotonin (otherwise known as 5-hydroxytryptamine or 5-HT). They can occur anywhere in the gut, particularly in the appendix, small intestine, stomach and rectum. Carcinoids account for around 1–2% of all gastrointestinal tumours and are frequently an incidental finding at autopsy or in a resected appendix. In most cases, they are benign and grow in a slow and indolent fashion, but in some instances they develop a more malignant phenotype and produce liver metastases. Extra-intestinal tumours may arise in the pancreas, and more rarely, the bile ducts, bronchus, ovary and testis.

The main significance of the tumour site concerns its ability to drain into the systemic circulation. Carcinoid cells produce a wide range of vasoactive amines and hormones, including serotonin, histamine, substance P, bradykinin, prostaglandins, neuropeptide Y, gastrin and adrenocorticotrophic hormone (ACTH). The liver would normally metabolise such substances originating from the portal venous territory before they can exert systemic effects, but if liver metastases have developed (or if the tumours drain directly into the systemic veins, such as with ovarian, bronchial or retroperitoneal carcinoids) then the carcinoid syndrome may occur.

Clinical features. Overall, the carcinoid syndrome is present in probably only 3–4% of all cases of carcinoid tumours. The range of substances secreted by the tumours can lead to quite striking clinical manifestations, most notably the various combinations of flushing, diarrhoea and bronchospasm:

- Flushing
- Diarrhoea
- Dyspnoea/wheezing
- Abdominal discomfort
- Palpable abdominal mass or hepatomegaly

- Cardiac valvular lesions
- Fatigue/lethargy
- Morphoea
- Pellagra

Facial flushing occurs in around 80% of cases and may be transient, lasting only seconds, or more prolonged and lasting several hours. The flushing is often not restricted to the face, and the neck and upper thorax are frequently affected. Gastric carcinoids tend to produce more histamine, which may lead to weal formation along with the flushing. Around 30% of carcinoid patients eventually develop widespread telangiectasia and a permanently plethoric facies.

319

Causes of diarrhoea in the carcinoid syndrome are as follows:
- Secretion of amines and hormones – e.g. serotonin may cause secretory diarrhoea by direct stimulation of epithelial cells or indirectly by activating enteric neurones: motility is also usually increased
- Bowel resection – e.g. terminal ileum, leading to bile malabsorption or bacterial overgrowth
- Octreotide-induced exocrine pancreatic hypofunction

The primary tumour may cause intestinal obstruction, while hepatic metastases are a cause of right upper quadrant pain and may reach such a size that there may not be much normal functioning hepatic tissue left.

Pellagra may occur because of increased production of serotonin and demands on its precursors (the amino acid tryptophan is diverted into excessive synthesis of 5-hydroxytryptamine at the expense of its other use as the precursor of nicotinamide). Other skin abnormalities include thickened areas of morphoea which can be confused with scleroderma.

Cardiac abnormalities are common and occur as a result of endomyocardial fibrosis with valve thickening. Cardiac lesions can be found at echocardiography in approximately 25–40% of all patients with the carcinoid syndrome. The lesions are usually right-sided, unless there is bronchial carcinoid or an atrial septal defect. The relative frequencies of the valvular abnormalities are shown here, based on a survey of patients at the Hammersmith Hospital, London:
- Tricuspid regurgitation   (83%)
- Pulmonary stenosis   (39%)
- Pulmonary regurgitation   (22%)
- Tricuspid stenosis   (17%)
- Mitral stenosis   (5%)

Diagnosis. The diagnosis of carcinoid syndrome is confirmed by demonstrating excessive urinary levels (on 24-hour collection) of the serotonin metabolite, 5-hydroxyindole acetic acid (5-HIAA). A raised urinary 5-HIAA level is present in nearly 100% of cases, although false positives may occasionally be seen with excessive consumption of serotonin-rich foods such as bananas or tomatoes, as well as with some drugs such as phenothiazines and reserpine.

The liver metastases will usually be readily apparent on cross-sectional imaging (Fig. 6.13) and if necessary this can be confirmed histologically (see **Fig. 6.12**). Extensive searching for the primary tumour is unlikely to alter the initial management, as most small bowel primaries are not resected unless an obstruction develops. In any event, a primary

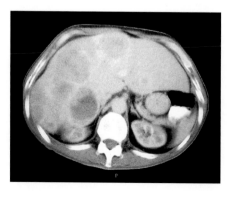

Fig. 6.13 *Extensive liver metastases in the carcinoid syndrome. Abdominal CT scan showing multiple large carcinoid tumour deposits throughout the liver.*

source can only be identified in 50–70% of cases of carcinoid syndrome. In addition to CT scanning, the extent of the tumour may be staged using radiolabelled octreotide scintigraphy, as most carcinoid tumours express somatostatin receptors (see **Fig. 4.40**).
Management. For the vast majority of patients with carcinoid syndrome, the management approach is palliative. However, carcinoid tumours in general are slower-growing than other gastrointestinal cancers and it is not unusual for patients to survive 10–20 years after liver metastases have developed.

There are a number of different treatment options available, the primary aim being symptom control:
- Symptomatic relief – e.g. codeine or loperamide for mild diarrhoea
- Nicotinamide supplementation
- Inhibition of secretion of amines and hormones using somatostatin analogues
- Oral serotonin antagonists – e.g. cyproheptadine.
- Reduction of tumour bulk
    Surgical resection
    Chemotherapy – e.g. streptozotocin and 5-fluorouracil
    Percutaneous alcohol injection
    Selective hepatic arterial embolisation
    Targeted radiotherapy using labelled somatostatin analogues e.g. [111]indium octreotide
Orally active serotonin antagonists, such as cyproheptadine, may offer partial benefit but usually only in controlling diarrhoea with little effect on vasomotor symptoms. Instead, the most widely used therapy is to give injections of somatostatin analogues to reduce secretion from the carcinoid tumour cells. Octreotide is the most widely used and is administered by subcutaneous injection, usually two or three times a day. Recently, two longer-acting analogues have been developed: lanreotide (given by intramuscular injection every 2 weeks) and sandostatin-LAR (long-acting octreotide acetate, injected intramuscularly once every 4 weeks).

For many patients, a reduction in tumour bulk is necessary, either to reduce the carcinoid-related symptoms or to relieve the discomfort from large abdominal tumour masses. Partial hepatectomy has attendant risks, but can be useful if there is a reasonable margin of normally functioning liver.

Hepatic deposits can also be targeted by percutaneous alcohol injection to induce necrosis. However, one of the most effective debulking treatments is selective arterial embolisation at angiography (**Fig. 6.14**). This technique is generally safe in experienced hands, but a full 'blocking' regime (including octreotide infusion, prophylactic antibiotics, nicotinamide and steroids) is usually instituted to guard against the 'carcinoid crisis' that can arise due to massive release of hormones from necrotic tumours.

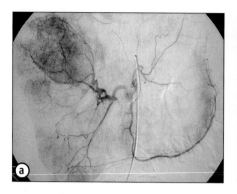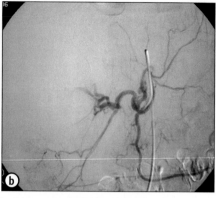

Fig. 6.14 *Hepatic artery embolisation of carcinoid tumour deposits. Hepatic arteriograms from the same patient as in Fig. 6.13. (a) There are several areas of abnormal circulation, known as tumour 'blushes', particularly in the upper and outer aspects of the right lobe. (b) Embolisation coils are inserted via the angiography catheter and the arterial supply to the carcinoid deposits is occluded.*

SYSTEMIC MANIFESTATIONS OF LIVER DISEASE

STIGMATA OF CHRONIC LIVER DISEASE

Patients may be icteric, pigmented and occasionally even cyanosed (due to pulmonary venous shunts). Digital clubbing (see **Fig. 6.7**), leuconychia, palmar erythema (see **Fig. 4.20**), Dupuytren's contracture and a flapping tremor (asterixis) may be present in the hands. Scratch marks from pruritus and purpura are often widespread, while spider naevi (see **Fig. 4.19**) are distributed in the territory of the superior vena cava. There is usually a paucity of body hair; men may have gynaecomastia (**Fig. 6.15**) and testicular atrophy, while women have breast atrophy. Patients with primary biliary cirrhosis may have xanthelasmata. Patients with haemochromatosis often have a slate-grey pigmentation ('bronze diabetes').

HEPATORENAL SYNDROME (HRS)

HRS is a syndrome of progressive acute renal failure that occurs in patients with advanced liver disorders who have no identifiable cause of intrinsic renal disease:

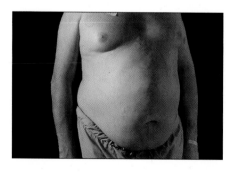

Fig. 6.15 *Signs of chronic liver disease. This patient with liver cirrhosis demonstrates gynaecomastia, loss of body hair, distended abdominal wall veins (caput medusae) and ascites.*

Major criteria

- Acute or chronic liver disease with synthetic liver failure and/or portal hypertension
- Absence of hypovolaemic shock, active sepsis or treatment with nephrotoxic drugs
- Low glomerular filtration rate (creatinine clearance < 40 ml/min)
- Failure to improve renal function after fluid challenge with 1.5 litres of normal saline i.v.
- Proteinuria < 0.5 g/day with no evidence of renal tract disease on ultrasound

Minor criteria

- Urinary sodium excretion < 10 mmol/day
- Urine volume < 500 ml per day
- Urinary osmolality < plasma osmolality
- Serum sodium level < 130 mmol/l
- Urinary red cell count < 50 cells per high-power field

This is an important distinction, as the commonest causes of renal failure in patients with liver disease are hypovolaemia (due to recent gastrointestinal bleeding or post-paracentesis circulatory disturbance, for example) and nephrotoxic drugs, including the overzealous use of diuretics. Additionally, some liver disorders are associated with specific renal lesions such as glomerulonephritis (chronic viral hepatitis, autoimmune hepatitis, α_1-antitrypsin deficiency), the Fanconi syndrome (Wilson's disease) or polyarteritis nodosa (hepatitis B).

Evidence that HRS has a functional rather than structural basis is suggested by the following facts: renal function returns to normal after liver transplantation, while kidneys from donors with chronic liver disease work normally if given to renal transplant recipients.

Pathophysiology. The main feature of HRS is one of paradoxical renal vasoconstriction in the face of systemic vasodilatation. Most investigators agree that this is the result of imbalances between competing pressor and vasodilator influences in cirrhosis. Features of the systemic 'hyperdynamic circulation' in cirrhosis are:

- Peripheral vasodilatation
- Diminished *systemic* response to vasoconstrictor agents
- Increased cardiac output
- Increased heart rate
- Bounding pulse
- Warm peripheries

Splanchnic vasodilatation occurs early in portal hypertension, mainly as a result of sheer stress and the release of local vasodilators such as nitric oxide. Many of these vasodilators escape into the systemic circulation and cause a diminished systemic response to the normal endogenous vasoconstrictors such as angiotensin that are produced in response to the hyperdynamic circulation. In contrast, the renal blood vessels remain highly sensitive to these pressor agents and consequently blood flow through the kidneys is restricted. This theory is known as the 'peripheral vasodilatation hypothesis'.

It is likely that other factors are involved. Not least, portal hypertension itself is clearly important for the development of HRS and this may be mediated partly by autonomic neural reflexes restricting splanchnic blood flow. Conjugated hyperbilirubinaemia also appears to increase the renal vascular responsiveness to vasoconstrictors.

The net result is that urine output falls as the serum creatinine rises. Urine sodium is usually low or non-existent, but the urine is concentrated with a high urine/plasma creatinine ratio and urine/plasma osmolality. In severe cases, urine osmolality may begin to fall as renal failure progresses.

Clinical features. The probability of developing HRS after the onset of ascites is about 20% at 1 year and 40% at 5 years. The syndrome typically develops in patients with frank hepatic decompensation, and clinical features include ascites, hypotension, oliguria and jaundice.

Some authors have classified HRS into two distinct clinical patterns. Type 1 is said to describe those patients with a relatively acute clinical course (usually < 2 weeks), generally in the setting of a precipitating event such as a variceal bleed or bacterial peritonitis. The more chronic type 2 HRS usually represents those patients with refractory ascites whose renal function has steadily deteriorated over a period of several weeks or months.

Management. Acutely ill patients with HRS should ideally be managed in an intensive care setting, with invasive monitoring to optimise fluid balance and intravascular volumes. Management involves excluding other causes of renal failure, establishing adequate circulatory volume and restricting sodium and water intake. Nephrotoxic agents must be avoided and consideration given to haemodialysis. While having little beneficial effect on most cases of HRS, haemodialysis may be useful as a temporary holding measure in patients awaiting urgent liver transplantation. The suitability of all patients for liver transplantation needs to be actively considered because most will be dead within 2 months of the onset of HRS.

Otherwise there are few specific therapies. Some recent success has been reported with the use of vasopressin analogues that selectively constrict the splanchnic circulation while preserving renal blood flow, such as ornipressin. This agent has been shown to cause a temporary improvement in renal function (sustainable for up to 14 days) and may prove useful as a holding agent prior to transplantation.

HEPATOPULMONARY SYNDROME (HPS)

The hepatopulmonary syndrome is a triad of:
- Liver disease
- Increased alveolar-arterial oxygen gradient when breathing room air
- Evidence of intrapulmonary vascular dilatations or shunts

Many patients with cirrhosis have pulmonary disease. Indeed, it has been estimated that abnormal arterial oxygenation can be found in up to 50% of patients referred for liver transplantation. Often this is due to comorbidity from cigarette smoking and the development of chronic obstructive airways disease, but there are other important disease associations. Examples include portopulmonary hypertension, α_1-antitrypsin deficiency, recurrent or persistent respiratory infections (including tuberculosis) and HPS.

HPS is increasingly being recognised as a cause of hypoxaemia in patients with cirrhosis and/or portal hypertension. Its hallmark is the intrapulmonary right-to-left shunting of blood due to the presence of microvascular shunts. Importantly, hypoxia due to HPS was previously considered to be a contraindication to liver transplantation, but we now know that the condition itself can be corrected by the procedure and may be the main indication for receiving a liver graft in some cases.

Pathophysiology. The exact cause of the microvascular shunting is still unknown, but many clues have now been gathered. Typically, the condition occurs in patients with chronic liver disease of any aetiology (but most commonly alcoholic cirrhosis, cryptogenic cirrhosis, chronic active hepatitis and primary biliary cirrhosis). It has been described in acute liver failure, but such reports are very rare. However, as HPS is well documented in non-cirrhotic portal hypertension it appears that the raised portal pressure itself is an important factor.

The main pulmonary findings at autopsy studies are the presence of multiple precapillary vascular dilatations, giving rise to gross dilatation of the alveolar capillaries themselves (**Fig. 6.16**). The consequence of this has been termed a diffusion-perfusion defect – the blood flows too quickly through dilated capillaries that are themselves too wide to allow adequate diffusion of oxygen to all the erythrocytes.

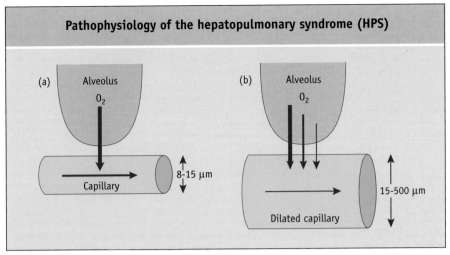

Fig. 6.16 *Pathophysiology of the hepatopulmonary syndrome (HPS). (a) Under normal circumstances, alveolar oxygen easily diffuses into the 8–15 μm diameter pulmonary capillaries. (b) In HPS, the precapillary arteriolar vasodilatation leads to the formation of much wider capillaries, with high flow rates. Consequently, the oxygen is unable to diffuse adequately into the centre of the vessels and oxygenate enough red cells.*

However, the cause of the precapillary vasodilatation itself is still unknown. Investigators have described abnormalities in the same vasoactive mediators involved elsewhere in the hyperdynamic circulation of cirrhosis, such as nitric oxide, prostaglandins and endothelins.

Clinical features. Most patients with HPS present with the usual symptoms and signs of liver disease, their respiratory problem being discovered only later. However, dyspnoea is the presenting symptom in about 20% of cases, the liver disease being found coincidentally. The severity of HPS does not always correlate with that of the liver disease and may progress to respiratory failure even while liver function remains stable.

On examination, patients usually have marked finger clubbing (see **Fig. 6.7**) and may have multiple spider naevi. HPS itself has been referred to as 'spider naevi of the lung'. Patients with severe right-to-left shunting may be cyanosed. Examination of the respiratory system usually reveals no further signs.

Most patients (around 90%) demonstrate *orthodeoxia* whereby, in contrast to most other cardiorespiratory diseases, the arterial oxygenation falls on changing from the supine position to standing up. This is the result of the microvascular dilatations being most severe in the lower lobes of the lungs, which are preferentially perfused in the upright position. Some of these patients may complain of *platypnoea*, breathlessness relieved by lying down.

Investigations. The chest radiograph is usually normal, although there may occasionally be some fine interstitial shadowing due to larger microvascular dilatations in the lower lobes. Similarly, routine pulmonary function testing usually shows normal spirometry (although HPS can coexist with other lung diseases).

The presence of intrapulmonary microvascular 'shunting' is confirmed by imaging techniques. The two most commonly used tests are ^{99}Tc MAA scanning and contrast-enhanced echocardiography.

325

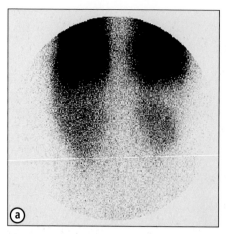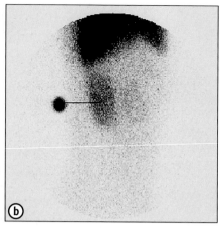

(a)   (b)

Fig. 6.17 *⁹⁹Tc MAA scanning in the hepatopulmonary syndrome. Gamma camera images of the lower chest and abdomen from a patient with HPS. Normally, the injected albumin macroaggregates are exclusively taken up by the lungs (darker shadows on these images), but here we can see that there is also considerable impaction of the tracer in the kidneys. The cobalt 57 marker is present as an internal control. The relative densities of the pulmonary and renal shadows are used to calculate the percentage right-to-left shunt. (a) Posterior view. (b) Right lateral view.*

⁹⁹Tc MAA scanning involves injecting radiolabelled macro-aggregates of albumin into a peripheral vein. Normally, these aggregates would be almost entirely filtered out of the circulation by impacting in the pulmonary capillaries. In HPS, however, the tracer is able to pass through the lungs and can be detected by scintigraphy in other organs (**Fig. 6.17**). A mathematical formula can be used to calculate the proportion of ⁹⁹Tc MAA that has been shunted and so grade the severity of the condition.

Right-to-left shunting can also be demonstrated using two-dimensional echocardiography. Injected microbubbles are usually filtered out by an intact pulmonary capillary bed, but when injected intravenously into patients with HPS they can be observed arriving back into the left side of the heart on echocardiography. By measuring the time taken for the bubbles to arrive, intrapulmonary shunts can be distinguished from intracardiac right-to-left shunts. Unlike ⁹⁹Tc MAA scanning, it is not possible to quantify the percentage shunt using echocardiography.

Pulmonary angiography is usually performed in patients with HPS, principally to ascertain the presence of macroscopic arteriovenous malformations (AVMs). Based on angiography, HPS can be classified into two distinct forms – types 1 and 2 (**Fig. 6.18**). *Management.* The natural history of HPS is variable, although a steady degree of deterioration in arterial oxygenation is seen in most cases. Many patients will succumb to other complications of their chronic liver disease (such as variceal haemorrhage) before the HPS is life-threatening, but the condition may worsen rapidly in some individuals even if their liver function remains stable. Spontaneous resolution of HPS is well recognised although uncommon.

Supplemental oxygen should be supplied and most patients respond at least initially. A variety of drug therapies have been tried, mostly with vasoactive properties, including prostaglandin inhibitors, somatostatin analogues, corticosteroids, sympathomimetics and inhibitors of nitric oxide synthesis, with little convincing efficacy.

Classification of the hepatopulmonary syndrome based on angiography and clinical differences

Type	Angiographic appearance	Clinical features
Type 1 HPS	Usually normal angiogram or very fine, diffuse spider-like branching of small vessels	Most common type Favourable response to breathing 100% oxygen (i.e. 'functional' R→L shunt) Usually reversible after liver transplantation
Type 2 HPS	Focal, discrete abnormalities similar to other causes of arteriovenous malformations	Less common May have only limited improvement with 100% oxygen (i.e. 'true' R→L shunt) Tends to be less responsive to liver transplantation Focal lesions can be blocked by coil embolisation

Fig. 6.18 *Classification of the hepatopulmonary syndrome based on angiography and clinical differences.*

Interventional radiology offers hope for some patients. Relief of portal hypertension using TIPSS (see chapter 4) has been associated with reversal of HPS. Focal pulmonary AVMs in those with type 2 HPS can also be blocked at angiography using coil embolisation.

However, liver transplantation remains an effective therapy for many patients with HPS. There is some evidence that the larger AVMs seen in type 2 HPS may not respond to transplantation, but the majority of patients with the more common type 1 HPS will see some improvement if not full resolution. On this basis, severe progressive HPS in the presence of stable liver disease may itself become the indication for hepatic transplantation. Careful patient selection is clearly important.

HEPATIC ENCEPHALOPATHY, ASCITES AND SPONTANEOUS BACTERIAL PERITONITIS

These complications of liver disease are discussed in chapter 4.

LIVER DISORDERS WITH MULTISYSTEM MANIFESTATIONS

Haemochromatosis

The hepatic manifestations of this autosomal recessive disorder are detailed in chapter 4. Iron overload can occur throughout the body. Diabetes and a bronze or metallic grey skin pigmentation (so-called 'bronze diabetes') are frequent accompaniments to primary haemochromatosis. The skin colour is due to melanin and iron deposition. Arthralgia is common and involves the small joints in the hand, wrist, hips and knees. Some patients develop chondrocalcinosis. Cardiac involvement includes ventricular muscular hypertrophy which behaves like a dilated cardiomyopathy in its later stages, conduction abnormalities and, rarely, a constrictive cardiomyopathy. Regular venesection may improve or arrest these cardiac manifestations.

Primary biliary cirrhosis

Features are skin pigmentation, excoriation, xanthelasmata around the eyes and in the palmar creases and, more rarely, tuberous xanthomas on extensor surfaces including the knees, elbows, wrists and ankles. Primary biliary cirrhosis is also associated with other autoimmune conditions including scleroderma, the CREST syndrome (calcinosis, Raynaud's syndrome, oesophageal dysmotility, sclerodactyly and telangiectasia), Sjögren's syndrome, autoimmune thyroiditis, renal tubular acidosis and myasthenia gravis. Pulmonary fibrosis, seronegative and seropositive arthritis and coeliac disease are also disease associations.

NUTRITION

MALNUTRITION

Severe malnutrition in children can be divided into three syndromes: marasmus, kwashiorkor and nutritional dwarfism (**Fig. 6.19**), while the easiest assessment of malnutrition in adults is the body mass index (BMI). This is defined as weight (in kilograms) divided by the square of the height (in metres). The values for defining grades of malnutrition are as follows:
- BMI > 20: Normal
- 18.5–20: Marginal
- 17–18.5: Mild malnutrition
- 16–17: Moderate malnutrition
- < 16: Severe malnutrition

The mid upper arm circumference is another useful measure.

Childhood malnutrition

Malnutrition and starvation, particularly in the developing world, can give rise to specific clinical patterns. It is often possible to make a distinction between protein-energy malnutrition, resulting in *kwashiorkor*, and the total malnutrition seen in *marasmus*. However, the boundaries are often blurred by an accompanying reduction in total calorific intake in patients with kwashiorkor and the occurrence of other causes of protein loss such as diarrhoeal illnesses.

Features of protein-energy malnutrition include:
- Weight loss >10%
- Growth failure
- Anorexia, lethargy, apathy
- Diarrhoea
- Muscle wasting
- Oedema
- Hair thinning
- Stomatitis
- Signs of specific vitamin deficiencies
- Triceps skinfold thickness < 10 mm (males). < 13 mm (females)
- Serum albumin < 35 g/l
- Serum transferrin < 1.5 g/l
- Blood lymphocyte count < 1.5 × 10⁹
- Impaired cell-mediated immunity (negative *Candida* skin test)

In kwashiorkor, oedema is the salient feature, with fullness of the cheeks (**Fig. 6.20**), abdominal swelling, polyserositis, skin rashes, alopecia, hepatomegaly, general apathy, osteomalacia and signs of specific nutrient deficiencies. The glomerular filtration rate and sodium excretion are reduced and urinary tract infections are common. Body temperature is often low and patients frequently develop secondary opportunistic infections.

In classical marasmus (**Fig. 6.21**), there is no oedema, while some children with nutritional dwarfism may look normal apart from being small for their age.

Wellcome classification of the clinical types of malnutrition in children		
Weight for age*	No oedema	With oedema
60–80%	Undernutrition	Kwashiorkor
Less than 60%	Marasmus	Marasmic kwashiorkor

* Percentage of the median US National Center for Health Statistics standard.

Fig. 6.19 *Wellcome classification of the clinical types of malnutrition in children.*

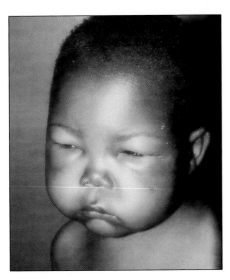

Fig. 6.20 *Childhood malnutrition. Facial swelling due to oedema in a child with kwashiorkor. (Courtesy of AVS Department, Imperial College School of Medicine at St Mary's Hospital).*

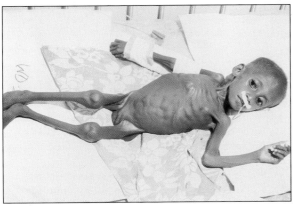

Fig. 6.21 *Marasmus. Severe childhood malnutrition due to starvation. (Courtesy of AVS Department, Imperial College School of Medicine at St Mary's Hospital).*

Adult malnutrition

This may be due to famine in developing nations or secondary to chronic malabsorption, such as coeliac disease. The marasmic features of starvation are similar to those seen in anorexia nervosa in countries with fully developed economies. There is gross loss of muscle mass, particularly from the limb girdles, and almost no subcutaneous fat. The skin is usually thin and atrophic. Patients with malabsorption may have features more akin to kwashiorkor with oedema secondary to hypoproteinaemia.

329

Vitamin deficiency syndromes	
Vitamin A	Night blindness, dry eyes, keratomalacia, corneal ulceration, follicular hyperkeratosis
Thiamin (B$_1$)	Wet beri-beri: muscle weakness, congestive cardiac failure Dry beri-beri: peripheral neuropathy, Wernicke's encephalopathy, Korsakoff's syndrome
Riboflavin (B$_2$)	Angulostomatitis, cheilosis, magenta tongue, red mucous membranes, seborrhoeic dermatitis
Niacin (B$_3$)	Photosensitive dermatitis, diarrhoea, mental disturbance (confusion, disorientation, loss of memory)
Pyridoxine (B$_6$)	Nasolabial seborrhoea, glossitis, peripheral neuropathy, kidney stones
B$_{12}$	Pallor, mild icterus, anorexia, diarrhoea, paraesthesia, ataxia, optic neuritis, mental disturbance
Vitamin C	Scurvy
Vitamin D	Osteomalacia
Vitamin E	Anaemia, peripheral neuropathy, spinocerebellar degeneration
Vitamin K	Bleeding disorders
Biotin	Fatigue, depression, nausea, dermatitis, muscular pains
Pantothenic acid	Fatigue, sleep disturbances, impaired coordination, nausea
Folic acid	Pallor, glossitis, stomatitis, diarrhoea, anaemia

Fig. 6.22 *Vitamin deficiency syndromes.*

Specific nutrient deficiencies

Vitamin deficiencies are listed in **Fig. 6.22**.

Thiamin (vitamin B$_1$). Alcoholics are prone to thiamin deficiency, but clinical features of deficiency only develop in a small proportion of patients. Occasionally, deficiency is seen in other patients with poor diet or in the intractable vomiting of hyperemesis gravidarum. In the developing nations, deficiency typically occurs in populations where the staple diet consists mainly of polished rice. The cardiovascular and nervous systems are classically affected by thiamin deficiency.

'Wet beri-beri' comprises left and right ventricular failure, peripheral vasodilatation with high-output cardiac failure and marked peripheral oedema (**Fig. 6.23**). Neurological manifestations comprise peripheral neuropathy, Wernicke's encephalopathy (cerebral beri-beri) and the Korsakoff syndrome. Patients may have vomiting, nystagmus, ophthalmoplegia, ataxia, confusion, retrograde amnesia and confabulation. It is vital to treat all patients prophylactically where thiamin deficiency is considered to be a risk, because ensuing neurological damage may be irreversible. All alcoholic patients admitted to hospital should have intravenous or oral thiamin supplementation.

'Dry beri-beri' typically presents insidiously with a symmetrical mixed polyneuropathy. Wernicke's encephalopathy or the Korsakoff syndrome may also occur.

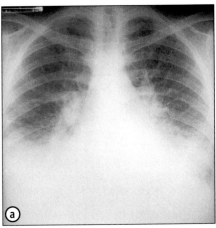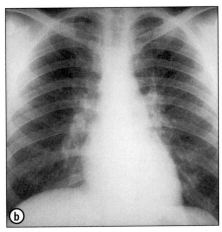

Fig. 6.23 *Wet beri-beri. (a) Chest X-ray taken before treatment. (b) After thiamin treatment, showing resolution of cardiac failure. (Courtesy of AVS Department, Imperial College School of Medicine at St Mary's Hospital).*

Nicotinic acid (vitamin B$_3$). Deficiency of niacin (nicotinic acid) causes pellagra (**Fig. 6.24**), but the full triad of dermatitis, dementia and diarrhoea is rare. Niacin is derived from the amino acid tryptophan, which is also used for 5-hydroxytryptamine synthesis, and therefore deficiency may occur in the carcinoid syndrome. It is usually alcoholics with a poor diet who develop pellagra, but the condition may also be seen if there is a pyridoxine deficiency (or if the patient is taking a pyridoxine antagonist such as isoniazid), as this vitamin is required for the biosynthetic pathway of niacin. The symptoms of pellagra usually improve with replacement therapy, which routinely includes pyridoxine.

Vitamin B$_{12}$ and folate. Deficiency of either may cause a megaloblastic anaemia (**Fig. 6.25**). Neurological complications may occur with B$_{12}$ deficiency, including peripheral neuropathy and subacute combined degeneration of the spinal cord. Response to treatment with hydroxocobalamin is usually very good.

Vitamin C. Deficiency of ascorbic acid leads to impaired collagen synthesis and the features of scurvy, such as poor wound healing, capillary fragility – purpura, easy bruising, splinter haemorrhages, haemarthroses, perifollicular haemorrhages, and gum swelling, friability and bleeding (**Fig. 6.26**). This is rare in the developed world, but can occur in alcoholics and socially disadvantaged people living on convenience foods.

Zinc. Acrodermatitis enteropathica is a pustular eruption on the body extremities and around the mouth, nose and perineum. It may be associated with a congenital zinc malabsorption in children, but is acquired in adults. Zinc deficiency may occur with jejunal pathology such as Crohn's disease and in alcoholic patients.

EATING DISORDERS

Anorexia nervosa

This is largely a disease of adolescent girls in the developed world, where self-induced starvation leads to severe weight loss and clinical features similar to marasmus. It is estimated to affect around 4% of the female population at some time, with the female to male ratio being approximately 15:1. Around 1 in 20 of those affected will die because of the condition.

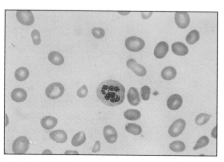

Fig. 6.25 *Vitamin B$_{12}$ deficiency. Blood film from a patient with severe pernicious anaemia, including a hypersegmented neutrophil. Similar blood film appearances may occur with folic acid deficiency.*

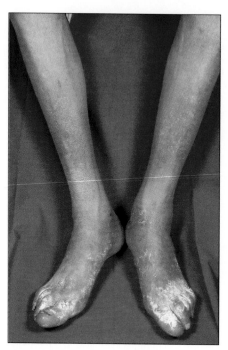

Fig. 6.24 *Pellagra. Symmetrical dermatitis affecting the lower limbs in a patient with pellagra. Other typical sites include sun-exposed areas such as the hands and face, as well as the perianal skin and vulva. (Courtesy of AVS Department, Imperial College School of Medicine at St Mary's Hospital).*

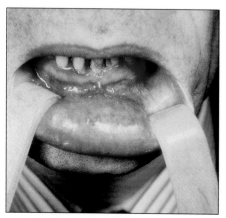

Fig. 6.26 *Vitamin C deficiency. Gingivostomatitis due to scurvy. (Courtesy of AVS Department, Imperial College School of Medicine at St Mary's Hospital).*

There is an associated distortion of body image, where affected individuals perceive themselves as being overweight, sometimes because of a history of previous obesity and associated unhappiness with it. Laxative and/or diuretic abuse is common and there is some overlap with bulimia, discussed below.

The typical clinical features are:

- Onset in female under the age of 25 years
- Absence of body fat
- Loss of > 25% of ideal body weight
- Secondary amenorrhoea
- Peripheral oedema
- Lanugo hair on the body
- Parotid enlargement
- Relative hypotension and bradycardia
- Restlessness, lack of energy
- Normocytic normochromic anaemia
- Hypercholesterolaemia
- Low luteinising hormone and follicle stimulating hormone levels
- Osteopenia, osteoporosis
- Reversible 'pseudoatrophy' of the brain with widened sulci and prominent ventricles (seen on MRI or CT)
- Cardiomyopathy, conduction defects

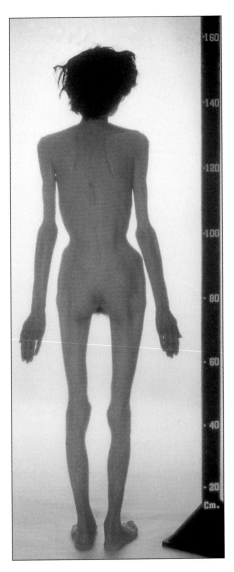

Fig. 6.27 *Anorexia nervosa. Severe wasting in a patient with the eating disorder anorexia nervosa. (Courtesy of AVS Department, Imperial College School of Medicine at St Mary's Hospital).*

Severe wasting may be particularly obvious on examination (**Fig. 6.27**). Investigations may reveal anaemia, a low serum albumin, reduced thyroxine and gonadotrophic hormone secretion. Treatment must be supportive and generally involves a combined nutritional and psychotherapeutic approach.

Bulimia nervosa

Binge eating and subsequent self-induced vomiting, a condition termed *bulimia nervosa*, is related to anorexia nervosa and often affects a slightly older age group. In addition to dietary deficiencies, patients may suffer the metabolic consequences of chronic vomiting and develop local complications such as dental caries. Sufferers tend to have greater insight into their illness than those with anorexia nervosa and so the prognosis is somewhat better. Behavioural therapy is the most effective approach.

Neurological sequelae of alcoholism	
Alcohol intoxication	Drunkenness, coma, blackouts
Withdrawal syndrome	Tremulousness, hallucinosis, delirium tremens
Nutritional diseases	Wernicke–Korsakoff syndrome, peripheral neuropathy, optic neuropathy, pellagra
Direct associations	Cerebellar degeneration Marchiafava–Bignami syndrome (degeneration of the corpus callosum) Cerebral atrophy
Hepatic encephalopathy	

Fig. 6.28 *Neurological sequelae of alcoholism.*

ALCOHOLISM

Alcohol abuse has widespread manifestations apart from alcoholic liver disease, pancreatitis and gastritis. Abnormalities may be found in just about every organ system in the body. Apart from specific vitamin deficiencies, chronic alcohol abuse has a variety of neurological sequelae (Fig. 6.28). Although not directly attributable to alcohol, there is an increased incidence of traumatic lesions such as intracranial haemorrhage (see Fig. 4.107). Bone marrow suppression with anaemia and thrombocytopenia is common in such patients. It is difficult to distinguish the direct effect of alcohol from the effects of thiamin deficiency in alcoholic myopathy and cardiomyopathy. Hyperlipidaemia may be secondary to chronic alcohol ingestion. Abstinence (with the psychosocial support that this entails) and correction of vitamin deficiencies are the salient points of treatment.

chapter 7

Digestive Tract Manifestations of Systemic Disease

The normal activities of the alimentary tract can easily be affected by disease elsewhere. Its complex physiology depends on the integrity of an adequate blood supply, autonomic nervous system, smooth muscle motility, neuroendocrine functions and a constant turnover of epithelial cells. Any of these aspects may be influenced by pathological processes originating from other parts of the body. Furthermore, the daily exposure of the gastrointestinal mucosa to foreign antigens and infective agents means that an appropriately regulated gut immune system is vital.

VASCULAR DISORDERS

HEREDITARY HAEMORRHAGIC TELANGIECTASIA (HHT)
This condition, also known as Osler–Weber–Rendu disease, is probably a group of related disorders that can lead to multiple telangiectasia and arteriovenous malformations (AVMs) in the respiratory and gastrointestinal systems. Pathologically, it is characterised by a microvascular dilatation of capillaries and venules.

Genetics
HHT has long been recognised as a familial disease and two Anglo-American groups working independently have isolated the faulty gene to the long arm of chromosome 9. It is inherited in a Mendelian, autosomal dominant fashion, with a 97% penetrance.

Clinical features
The usual clinical presentation is of recurrent epistaxes in childhood (96% of cases), followed by the development of mucocutaneous telangiectasia and AVMs (**Fig. 7.1**). In the majority of cases, the epistaxes develop before the age of 25 years, but the gastrointestinal manifestations are more likely to develop with increasing age. HHT may present as a cause

Clinincal manifestations of hereditary haemorrhagic telangiectasia	
Feature	Frequency (% of cases)
Recurrent epistaxis	96%
Mucocutaneous telangiectasia	75%
Gastrointestinal lesions	25%
Pulmonary arteriovenous malformations	15%
Cerebral arteriovenous malformations	4%

Fig. 7.1 *Clinical manifestations of hereditary haemorrhagic telangiectasia.*

of occult gastrointestinal bleeding, with iron deficiency, or (less commonly) as obvious overt haemorrhage from any part of the gastrointestinal tract.

On examination, patients may display the classic telangiectatic lesions (**Fig. 7.2**) on their nasal or oral mucosa, lips and perioral skin. There may be clinical signs of iron deficiency, such as koilonychia or glossitis, and there may be evidence of a hyperdynamic circulation due to AVMs. Patients with pulmonary shunts may be cyanotic and the abdomen should be auscultated for bruits associated with hepatic lesions (**Fig. 7.3**).

Diagnosis and management

The diagnosis of HHT may be a clinical one based on the above features and usually backed up by a positive family history. Telangiectatic lesions may be visualised at endoscopy in the stomach (**Fig. 7.4** and also see **Fig. 1.15**), small bowel or colon. Angiography may also demonstrate abnormal vascular communications (see **Fig. 7.3**) and Doppler ultrasound examination of the liver may be revealing in severe cases. Screening for pulmonary AVMs can be achieved with pulse oximetry, chest radiography and ^{99}Tc MAA scanning (as used in the hepatopulmonary syndrome, see chapter 6).

Medical treatment may help to reduce the frequency of gastrointestinal bleeding in some patients. There is evidence that oestrogen and progesterone therapy can diminish the

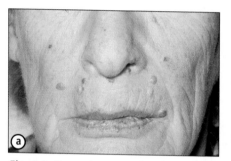

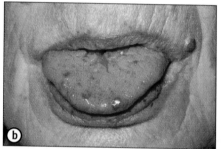

Fig. 7.2 *Mucocutaneous telangiectasia. This 65-year-old female patient had a history of recurrent nose bleeds, lethargy and iron deficiency. (a) There are multiple large telangiectatic lesions visible on her lips and nostrils. (b) Lesions of the tongue in the same patient.*

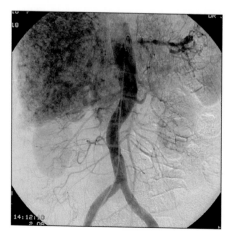

Fig. 7.3 *Severe hepatic involvement with HHT. Digital subtraction visceral angiography from the patient shown in Fig. 7.2. There are multiple large arteriovenous malformations in the liver, affecting all areas, with direct shunting of blood. Arterial blood flow through the liver is abnormally high, as represented by the attenuation of the infrahepatic aorta. Additionally, there are abnormal communications between the portal and systemic venous circulations. The patient developed high-output cardiac failure.*

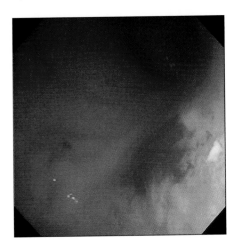

Fig. 7.4 *Gastric telangiectasia. Endoscopic view showing a large telangiectatic lesion in a patient with iron-deficiency anaemia.*

transfusion requirement, presumably by a direct action on the HHT lesions, which are known to worsen in oestrogen-deficient states (such as after the menopause).

Gastrointestinal lesions within reach of the endoscope can be ablated using a heater probe, argon beamer or Nd YAG laser, but frequently recur. Coil embolisation at arteriography can be useful, particularly for large, actively bleeding AVMs or those difficult to reach endoscopically. This technique can also be employed for hepatic or pulmonary AVMs, the latter being particularly important in view of the potential for paradoxical cerebral embolism to occur if left untreated.

Affected patients should receive appropriate genetic counselling and their family members will need screening for the manifestations of HHT.

ATHEROSCLEROSIS, ISCHAEMIA AND CARDIAC FAILURE

It is not uncommon for cardiovascular disease to lead to involvement of the gastrointestinal tract in some form. Obvious examples are where atheromatous disease involves the mesenteric arteries, leading to chronic ischaemia of the small or large bowel (discussed in chapters 2 and 3, respectively) or where an intracardiac thrombus may embolise to the gut, causing an acute infarction.

Atheroma of the abdominal aorta may lead to aneurysm formation. Massive gastrointestinal bleeding results if an aortic aneurysm fistulates into the gut, the most common site being the duodenum. Primary aorto-enteric fistulae are less common than secondary forms, which may occur 3–5 years after reconstructive graft surgery for abdominal aortic aneurysms.

In patients with right ventricular failure (most commonly congestive cardiac failure, cor pulmonale or constrictive pericarditis), chronic venous congestion can cause a protein-losing enteropathy. Drug absorption may also be affected, an example being the reduced bioavailability of frusemide as compared to bumetanide in congestive heart failure.

Right ventricular failure can lead to hepatomegaly (which may be pulsatile, particularly if there is significant tricuspid valvular regurgitation) and ascites. The reduced hepatic perfusion that occurs in patients with heart failure leads to hepatocyte damage, particularly around the centrilobular region, and serum transaminases may become elevated. In the longer term, atrophic changes, sinusoidal distension and fibrosis may occur, ultimately giving rise to what has been termed 'cardiac cirrhosis' in some cases.

CARDIAC VALVULAR LESIONS AND GASTROINTESTINAL BLEEDING

Over the last 30 years there have been a number of reports linking cardiac valvular lesions to chronic gastrointestinal bleeding. This association has been questioned by many and may reflect coexisting factors such as chronic intestinal ischaemia, anticoagulant therapy or just coincidence in an ageing population.

The majority of published reports have described patients with aortic valve stenosis as having an increased incidence of bleeding from angiodysplasia, particularly on the right side of the colon. One hypothesis has suggested that chronic intestinal hypoperfusion may lead to the development of angiodysplastic lesions, with an increased likelihood of haemorrhage if the patient is subsequently anticoagulated for a prosthetic valve graft.

VASCULITIS

The systemic vasculitides are characterised by the presence of fibrinoid necrosis and inflammation of blood vessel walls. These conditions can be classified as either primary or secondary processes or, alternatively, according to the predominant size of the vessels involved.

Involvement of the mesenteric circulation may occur with many of these diseases (**Fig. 7.5**), together with subsequent complications such as mucosal ulceration, inflammation, ischaemia, haemorrhage or chronic fibrosis.

The management of these conditions is best undertaken in collaboration with a rheumatologist and usually involves immunosuppressive therapy.

Vasculitic disorders affecting the gastrointestinal tract	
Systemic lupus erythematosus (SLE)	Mesenteric vasculitis in 2% of SLE cases High mortality (about 50%) May cause pancreatitis, ileocolitis, protein-losing enteropathy, gastritis Treat with high-dose steroids and/or cyclophosphamide
Polyarteritis nodosa (PAN)	Mesenteric involvement in 80% of PAN cases Frequently leads to ischaemia, haemorrhage, perforation, infarction Angiography may show multiple aneurysms
Churg–Strauss syndrome	40–50% of patients have GI symptoms Usually abdominal pain, bloody diarrhoea Diffuse ulceration – stomach, small bowel, colon Eosinophilic infiltration
Wegener's granulomatosis	Mesenteric vasculitis in 5% Infarction, ileocolitis, pancreatitis, appendicitis
Henoch–Schönlein purpura	Usually children, but can affect any age Abdominal pain in 65% GI bleeding in 40% May cause intussusception, appendicitis, cholecystitis, atypical ulceration of mucosae

Fig. 7.5 *Vasculitic disorders affecting the gastrointestinal tract.*

Special mention should be given to the variant of polyarteritis nodosa (PAN) that occurs in some patients with hepatitis B infection. Although this is clinically indistinguishable from 'classical' PAN, treatment should include some form of antiviral agent as well as immunosuppression. One such regimen utilises interferon-α and prednisolone (1 mg/kg), the latter drug being tapered over a few weeks with concomitant plasma exchange. Cyclophosphamide is more commonly used in 'classical' PAN patients who do not have viral hepatitis.

A number of rheumatological conditions that are associated with vasculitis may affect the gastrointestinal tract in other ways (see p. 342).

ENDOCRINE DISEASES

THYROID DISEASE

Gastrointestinal symptoms are common in patients with abnormal thyroid function and this should always be kept in mind when patients present with changes in bowel habit or body weight.

Thyrotoxicosis can cause a rapid gastrointestinal transit time and increased mucosal secretions, leading to diarrhoea and occasionally steatorrhoea. Mild abnormalities in liver function tests may be found, particularly raised transaminases, hyperbilirubinaemia and an elevated alkaline phosphatase (although this latter enzyme is usually of bony origin in these patients). In some cases a true histological hepatitis may develop. Importantly, antithyroid drug treatments may cause abnormal liver function tests themselves, particularly propylthiouracil.

Not surprisingly, *hypothyroidism* has the opposite effect on gut motility. It can lead to constipation, megacolon and intestinal pseudo-obstruction and may also impair the gastro-oesophageal sphincter mechanism so that reflux is more common. Weight gain and obesity are further complications. Liver function tests are also abnormal in about half of patients with hypothyroidism, although histologically the liver appears unchanged. Myxoedema is a well-recognised cause of exudative ascites as well as pleural effusions.

DIABETES MELLITUS

Given that diabetes mellitus affects virtually all organ systems, with particular effects on the microvasculature and innervation, it is not surprising that gastrointestinal complications commonly occur (**Fig. 7.6**).

Diabetic gastroparesis

Gastric motility is frequently affected in diabetes mellitus, with almost 60% of patients developing a form of gastroparesis. Normal gastric emptying may be retained for liquids, but is usually abnormal for solids (**Fig. 7.7**). The syndrome results from varying combinations of unusually high pyloric pressures, reduced gastroduodenal pressure gradients and absent or diminished migratory motor complexes.

The reasons for the development of diabetic gastroparesis are not fully understood, but there are demonstrable abnormalities of both neuronal and humoral mechanisms. Acute hyperglycaemia itself can also lead to a short-term inhibition of gastric emptying in both diabetic patients and healthy subjects.

The most common symptoms include early satiety, abdominal bloating, nausea and vomiting. Their severity does not always correlate with the degree of measurable gastroparesis. An accurate drug history should always be taken, as many drugs with anticholinergic or opioid actions may reduce gastric motility.

Gastrointestinal manifestations of diabetes mellitus

Clinical syndrome	Pathophysiology
Nausea, early satiety, bloating	Slow gastric emptying (gastroparesis)
Heartburn, dysphagia, odynophagia	Oesophageal dysmotility Oesophageal candidiasis
Diarrhoea, steatorrhoea	Small bowel dysmotility Bacterial overgrowth Impaired luminal fluid absorption
Mesenteric 'angina'	Intestinal ischaemia Atherosclerosis
Constipation	Large bowel dysmotility
Unexplained abdominal pain	Diabetic radiculopathy Pancreatitis
Abnormal liver function tests	Hepatic steatosis Gallstones and their complications Sclerosing cholangitis Hepatobiliary sepsis

Fig. 7.6 *Gastrointestinal manifestations of diabetes mellitus.*

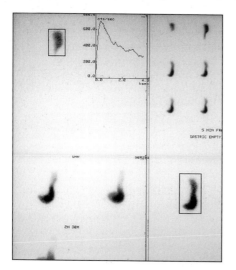

Fig. 7.7 *Diabetic gastroparesis. These scintigraphic images demonstrate the rate of gastric emptying in a patient with longstanding diabetes mellitus. The patient consumes a meal of ^{99}Tc-labelled baked beans and mashed potato before the gamma camera images are recorded. In this case, there is no visible gastric emptying in the first hour (normally 30–45 minutes) and food does not even begin to appear in the small bowel until 2 hours have elapsed.*

Patients should initially be investigated with a barium meal or gastroscopy, in order to exclude anatomical lesions such as pyloric stenosis. Impaired gastric emptying may occasionally be seen on the barium study but, as gastroparesis is significantly worse for solids than liquids, scintigraphic techniques using solid-phase meals (as in **Fig. 7.7**) are usually necessary. A number of other conditions may also cause a similar gastroparesis (**Fig. 7.8**).

Treatment of diabetic gastroparesis is often difficult. Simply improving diabetic control can sometimes be beneficial, but some form of promotility drug is usually required. Success

Causes of impaired gastric motor function

Central nervous system disorders	Multiple sclerosis Parkinsonism Brainstem vascular disease or neoplasia Psychiatric illness Acute psychological stress
Spinal cord lesions	Trauma Tumours Vascular disease
Autonomic neuropathies	Diabetes mellitus Amyloidosis Paraneoplastic Primary autonomic neuropathy
Metabolic disturbance	Acute hyperglycaemia Hypokalaemia Hypothyroidism Porphyria
Drugs	Opioids Anticholinergics Nicotine Levodopa β-adrenergic stimulants
Infiltrative conditions	Systemic sclerosis Amyloidosis
Miscellaneous	Post-vagotomy Postoperative ileus Radiation-induced Idiopathic pseudo-obstruction Myotonic dystrophy

Fig. 7.8 *Causes of impaired gastric motor function.*

has been reported with the dopamine agonists metoclopramide and domperidone, both of which have the added effect of increasing locally released acetylcholine at the myenteric plexus. Side-effects and the development of tachyphylaxis may limit their use.

The macrolide antibiotic, erythromycin, has agonist effects at motilin receptors (which partly explains the diarrhoea that often accompanies its use in infectious illnesses). Randomised studies have shown that oral erythromycin gives similar results to cisapride in improving gastric emptying. Recent animal studies have explored the possibility of transdermal delivery of erythromycin, with some success. The main long-term difficulty with erythromycin, as with other agonist drugs, is a degree of receptor down-regulation leading to tachyphylaxis.

Finally, a number of researchers in Europe and North America are exploring the possibility of implanting electrical 'gastric pacemakers' to stimulate motility in patients with gastroparesis, with promising results to date.

Diabetic diarrhoea

Diarrhoea is a common symptom in diabetes mellitus, occurring in about 20% of patients, particularly those with evidence of autonomic neuropathy. Its pathogenesis results from a combination of disordered motility, small bowel bacterial overgrowth (in some patients) and impaired reabsorption of fluids, the latter possibly being the result of a functional sympathetic denervation.

A complete drug history is important. In patients with type II (so-called 'non-insulin-dependent') diabetes mellitus, diarrhoea may be induced by antidiabetic drugs, such as metformin, acarbose and occasionally by sulphonylureas.

True diabetic diarrhoea seems to affect men more than women. Nocturnal diarrhoea is particularly common and about a third of patients will have episodes of faecal incontinence.

As with diabetic gastroparesis, improving glycaemic control may cause some improvement in symptoms. Antidiarrhoeal drugs are commonly required and many patients achieve symptomatic relief with loperamide or codeine phosphate.

Some therapeutic regimens have tried to correct the relative sympathetic deficiency and clinical benefit has been reported with the adrenergic agonist clonidine, with an improvement in luminal salt and water reabsorption.

The somatostatin analogue octreotide may also be helpful, by reducing intestinal secretions, although pancreatic insufficiency may be a side-effect as the drug also inhibits the production of digestive enzymes by the exocrine pancreas. If this complication develops, the patient may need to take oral pancreatic enzyme supplementation at meal times.

ACROMEGALY

Individuals with acromegaly, even if successfully treated, have an increased risk of developing colonic adenomatous polyps and colorectal cancer. Patients should ideally undergo a screening examination of the colon (barium enema or colonoscopy) and follow-up studies have been recommended, although their necessity and frequency have yet to be firmly established.

RHEUMATOLOGICAL DISORDERS

SCLERODERMA (SYSTEMIC SCLEROSIS)

Although these two terms are often used interchangeably, 'systemic sclerosis' best describes those scleroderma patients who have visceral involvement. The condition is characterised by tissue fibrosis, vascular damage and immunological activation. Histologically, there is an increased extracellular deposition of matrix proteins, vascular luminal narrowing, and an excess of fibroblasts, macrophages and activated CD4 lymphocytes, often in a perivascular distribution.

The gastrointestinal tract is commonly affected (**Fig. 7.9**). For example, over 90% of patients with either limited or diffuse systemic sclerosis have evidence of oesophageal dysmotility. A wide range of abnormal motility patterns can be demonstrated, including poorly coordinated contractions, complete paralysis and, in some cases, achalasia-like spasms. Gastro-oesophageal reflux is common (often exacerbated by a coexisting gastroparesis) and may lead to complications such as oesophageal ulcers, strictures and Barrett's metaplasia.

Therapeutic benefit may be seen with the usual remedies for reflux disease, such as proton pump inhibitors and promotility agents including metoclopramide. Non-steroidal

Gastrointestinal complications of systemic sclerosis	
Site	**Problem**
Mouth	Microstomia Sicca syndrome Increased dental caries Gingival atrophy
Oesophagus	Hypomotility Dysphagia Reflux symptoms Strictures Barrett's oesophagus
Stomach	Delayed gastric emptying NSAID-induced ulceration
Pancreas	Exocrine hypofunction Calcific pancreatitis Vasculitic pancreatic necrosis
Liver	Increased incidence of primary biliary cirrhosis Nodular hyperplasia Calcification
Small intestine	Fibrosis Dysmotility Intussusception Pseudo-obstruction Bacterial overgrowth *Pneumatosis intestinalis* Arteritis
Colon	Dysmotility Constipation Pseudodiverticula Pseudo-obstruction Anal sphincter dysfunction

Fig. 7.9 *Gastrointestinal complications of systemic sclerosis.*

anti-inflammatory drugs (NSAIDs) and drugs which relax the lower oesophageal sphincter, such as nifedipine, should be avoided if possible.

Small intestinal involvement may be the result of a number of different pathological processes (see **Fig. 7.9**) and treatment should be directed at the underlying mechanism. Small bowel stasis frequently leads to bacterial overgrowth and steatorrhoea is reported to occur in about a third of patients with systemic sclerosis. In some cases, malabsorption may be the direct result of excessive collagen deposition within the bowel wall. Patients with neuropathic pseudo-obstruction may derive benefit from treatment with erythromycin or cisapride, although efficacy may be lost later in the disease as smooth muscle damage progresses.

Colonic dysmotility usually presents as constipation. Patients can develop large pseudodiverticula, particularly in the left hemicolon. Anal sphincter dysfunction, with or without rectal prolapse, may cause faecal incontinence.

SYSTEMIC LUPUS ERYTHEMATOSUS (SLE)

Mesenteric vasculitis is the most serious complication of this multisystem disorder, but it is fortunately uncommon, occurring in about 2% of patients. Gastrointestinal symptoms have a high prevalence rate in individuals affected by SLE, with foregut symptoms being particularly prominent. Anorexia, nausea, heartburn and dysphagia may occur and oesophageal motility is often abnormal.

Protein-losing enteropathy, malabsorption, lupus peritonitis and *pneumatosis cystoides intestinalis* are all recognised complications. SLE patients may develop ascites for a number of reasons, including nephrotic syndrome, cardiac failure, polyserositis or peritoneal vasculitis.

RHEUMATOID DISEASE

The most common gastrointestinal abnormalities seen in this condition relate to the drugs used to treat it. NSAID-induced erosions or ulcers are endoscopically detectable in about a third of rheumatoid patients taking these drugs.

Rheumatoid arthritis may affect the temporomandibular joint, leading to difficulty in mastication. As with the rheumatic disorders already mentioned, oesophageal dysmotility is common.

Rheumatoid disease may be complicated by amyloidosis or mesenteric vasculitis. Some patients develop Felty's syndrome, with leucopenia and hypersplenism, which may be further exacerbated by portal hypertension.

BEHÇET'S SYNDROME

This chronic multisystem disorder is characterised by the development of oral and genital ulceration, uveitis and inflammatory lesions affecting nerves, skin, joints, blood vessels and viscera (**Fig. 7.10**). As well as the oral mucosa, ulceration may affect the oesophagus, small bowel and colon, where the appearance may mimic Crohn's disease.

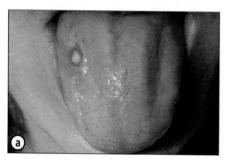

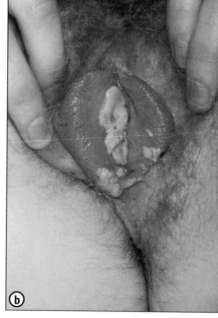

Fig. 7.10 *Behçet's syndrome. (a) Ulceration of the tongue in a patient with Behçet's syndrome. (b) Vaginal ulceration. (Courtesy of AVS Department, Imperial College School of Medicine at St Mary's Hospital).*

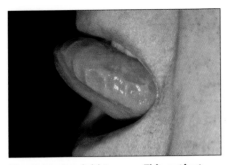

Fig. 7.11 *Amyloid tongue. This patient has macroglossia due to amyloidosis. The degree of enlargement can be judged by the teethmarks on the side of the tongue. (Courtesy of Dr Janice Main, St Mary's Hospital).*

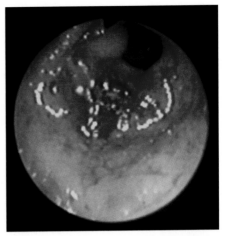

Fig. 7.12 *Haemorrhagic amyloidosis. This patient developed multiple gastric antral amyloid deposits. The gastroscopic view shows active haemorrhage from these lesions.*

AMYLOIDOSIS

Gut involvement in systemic amyloidosis is sufficiently common for a rectal biopsy to be part of the routine diagnostic work-up. Amyloid fibrils become deposited in blood vessel walls, which may cause ischaemia and infarction or, in some cases, encourage haemorrhage by losing vascular reactivity. Deposits within the intestinal mucosa may impair absorption of nutrients and muscular involvement leads to dysmotility syndromes.

Clinical manifestations of these effects include

- Macroglossia (**Fig. 7.11**)
- Oral haemorrhagic bullae
- Temporomandibular arthritis
- Achalasia
- Gastrointestinal bleeding (**Fig. 7.12**)
- Gastric outlet obstruction (functional or mechanical)
- Intestinal pseudo-obstruction
- Malabsorption (from bacterial overgrowth, pancreatic insufficiency, mucosal ischaemia or physical effects of amyloid protein deposition in enteric mucosa)
- Protein-losing enteropathy
- Constipation
- Hepatosplenomegaly
- Ascites

The diagnosis of amyloidosis rests upon the demonstration of birefringent apple-green and gold extracellular protein deposits on Congo red-staining of histological biopsies (**Fig. 7.13, 7.14**). Immunohistochemical techniques may allow specific typing of the amyloid fibrils.

Recently, the technique of 'SAP scanning' (**Fig. 7.14**) has been developed, using radiolabelled serum amyloid P component (SAP) to image amyloid deposits. Contrary to traditional teaching, research using SAP scans has recently demonstrated that amyloid deposits are not irreversible and can begin to regress if the supply of the precursor protein can be eliminated.

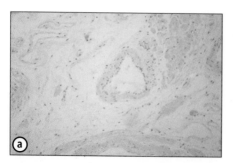

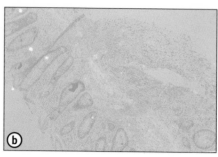

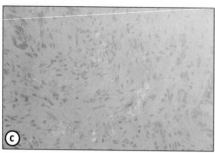

Fig. 7.13 *Histological appearances of amyloid protein deposition. (a) Haematoxylin and eosin-stained colonic biopsy, demonstrating pink-staining amyloid protein around a blood vessel. (b) Specific staining of biopsies using the Congo red technique can be used to reveal the gold colour and apple-green birefringence of amyloid fibrils under plane-polarised light. Low-power view. (c) High-power view.*

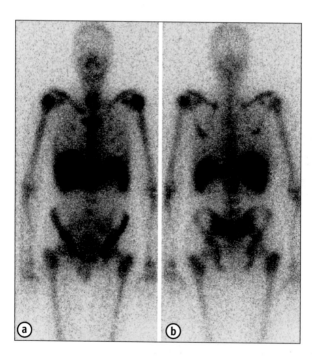

Fig. 7.14 *Serum amyloid protein (SAP) scintigraphy in a 60-year-old man with Waldenstrom's macroglobulinaemia complicated by systemic amyloid light (AL) amyloidosis. These images were recorded 24 hours after an injection of ^123I-labelled SAP and show amyloid deposits in the liver, spleen and bones. Follow-up scans taken after successful treatment of the Waldenstrom's macroglobulinaemia with fludaribine demonstrated gradual regression of the amyloid deposits. (a) Anterior view. (b) Posterior view. (Courtesy of Professor P Hawkins, Royal Free Hospital).*

FOOD ALLERGY AND FOOD INTOLERANCE

Patients often focus on dietary elements as the cause of chronic gastrointestinal symptoms. Care must be taken to establish a firm diagnosis, as a spurious label of 'food allergy' may lead to unnecessary exclusion diets and even nutritional deficiency. The term should only be applied in those situations where an immunological basis can be demonstrated. In most cases, the allergic mechanism is via immunoglobulin E (IgE) or type I hypersensitivity, although in a few instances it may be a type IV delayed hypersensitivity reaction. The allergic response usually occurs quickly after consuming only a small quantity of food.

Where patients develop food-induced symptoms without an immunological mechanism, the term 'food intolerance' should be used. One example is the lack of enzymes leading to cows' milk (or lactose) intolerance. As a general rule, intolerant reactions tend to occur more slowly than allergies and a larger 'dose' of food is required. Some of the differences between food allergy and food intolerance are highlighted in **Fig. 7.15**.

FOOD ALLERGY

The true prevalence of food allergies is actually quite low. One study has suggested that while 20% of individuals attributed their symptoms to food allergy, the condition could only be demonstrated in about 1%.

Patients who have a genuine IgE-mediated allergy to a dietary component tend to develop a rapid immunological response when challenged with the relevant agent. Characteristically, the patient develops oral symptoms, including itching and mucosal oedema in the mouth and pharynx which may be followed by more generalised manifestations affecting the lungs, gastrointestinal tract and skin. In some instances, life-threatening anaphylaxis, laryngeal oedema or severe bronchospasm may occur. Typical examples of such allergic reactions are seen in hypersensitivities to peanuts, fish (particularly shellfish), hens' eggs, some citrus fruits and certain food additives.

The diagnosis rests largely on an accurate history of typical symptoms and an identifiable precipitant. Some degree of dietary manipulation is often necessary to confirm suspicion of an allergy, including the use of short-term elimination diets. The help of a dietician in devising these diets can be invaluable.

Specific allergy testing can be carried out, using skin prick tests (although there has been some difficulty with standardisation of food extracts). Ideally, the food challenge is

Differences between food allergy and food intolerance	
Food allergy	**Food intolerance**
Mediated by IgE	Not immunologically mediated
Can occur after ingestion of only minute amounts of relevant food	Usually requires large amount of food to exert effect
Usually rapid onset	Symptoms often delayed
May cause anaphylaxis, acute bronchospasm, diarrhoea, abdominal pain, skin rashes	Usually chronic vague symptoms – bloating, flatulence, discomfort, fatigue
IgE levels may be raised	IgE levels normal
Skin prick, radioallergosorbent (RAST) testing useful	Skin prick, RAST testing unhelpful

Fig. 7.15 *Differences between food allergy and food intolerance.*

carried out in a double-blind, placebo-controlled manner. Radioallergosorbent (RAST) tests may identify allergen-specific IgE in the patient's serum.

The clinching of the diagnosis should come from the disappearance of symptoms during treatment with an elimination diet. Re-challenge with allergen confirms the diagnosis, but should obviously be avoided if the allergic reactions have been severe. If an oral food challenge is made, it should again be in a double – blind manner by masking the suspected ingredient in other foods, for example. Facilities for resuscitation (in the event of anaphylaxis) should be available.

Recently, the technique of colonoscopic allergen provocation (COLAP) has been described. This involves the submucosal injection of suspected food allergens directly into the caecum. Weal and flare reactions may be observed locally to allergens which failed to invoke positive skin tests. More than 80% of their patients achieved symptomatic improvement after avoiding food allergens identified in this way. This technique remains experimental, but may be useful where the usual tests have failed to identify a specific allergen.

Individuals with true food allergies require careful counselling about foods to be avoided. This is not always easy, as peanut extracts, for example, are found in a wide range of foodstuffs, often with little obvious identification. Patients' diets should be formulated with the help of a dietician.

In some cases, patients will 'grow out' of their allergies. This is true for about 90% of infants with cows' milk allergy and for about 50% of those allergic to eggs. Allergic reactions to peanuts, however, tend to persist.

A preloaded injection syringe of adrenaline, along with appropriate training in its use, should be issued to patients with severe allergies. Prompt administration could be life-saving in the event of an anaphylactic reaction.

FOOD INTOLERANCE

This term covers a wide range of non-allergic adverse reactions to foods. A variety of different mechanisms may be involved. For example, pharmacologically active substances such as caffeine may give rise to adverse effects if consumed in excess. Another example would be the consumption of tyramine-containing foods (such as yeast extracts or certain cheeses) in patients taking monoamine-oxidase inhibitors. In some instances, abnormal fermentation of foodstuffs by intestinal bacteria may give rise to toxic substances. Post-infectious malabsorption (secondary lactase deficiency) is another cause of food intolerance.

There seems to be a paucity of reliable data regarding the true prevalence of food intolerance. It has been estimated that symptoms caused by food intolerance may be found in up to 50% of those patients thought to have the irritable bowel syndrome. These symptoms tend to be chronic, vague and often difficult to explain. There may be lethargy, headaches, diarrhoea, abdominal pain, bloating and flatulence.

Given the degree of symptomatic overlap with other conditions, the diagnostic work-up should exclude other significant gastrointestinal disorders. Patients with diarrhoea should have stool sent for microscopy and culture, a sigmoidoscopy should be performed and, depending on age and comorbidity, a barium enema or colonoscopy obtained. Routine blood tests should be taken, including a full blood count, thyroid function and inflammatory markers. Serum anti-endomyseal antibodies should be measured as a screen for coeliac disease. Skin-prick and/or RAST testing can be used in cases where a true food allergy is suspected.

For diagnostic purposes, a short-term (2-week) exclusion diet, under close supervision, is usually necessary. The most common causative foods are wheat, cows' milk, cheeses, caffeine, oats, maize and certain artificial food additives. Foods can be carefully reintroduced to the diet to see if symptoms are induced. Again, the involvement of a dietician should be obtained to minimise the risk of nutritional deficiency.

GASTROINTESTINAL DISORDERS ASSOCIATED WITH PREGNANCY

Pregnant women may be under the care of a gastroenterologist in a number of different circumstances. Firstly, the physiological changes that occur during pregnancy predispose to certain gastrointestinal conditions and may alter the presenting features of others. Secondly, there are certain specific and unique pregnancy-related diseases (such as acute fatty liver) and, thirdly, patients with some chronic gastrointestinal disorders (ulcerative colitis, for example) may become pregnant and require closer attention.

GASTROINTESTINAL ANATOMY AND PHYSIOLOGY DURING PREGNANCY

Pregnancy has both anatomical and functional effects on the gastrointestinal tract. Most obviously, as gestation progresses, the gravid uterus displaces many intra-abdominal organs, particularly the stomach, small bowel and the mobile areas of the colon, including the appendix. As a result, abdominal pain may be less easily localised to its usual site. For instance, appendicitis may cause pain in the right upper quadrant rather than the right iliac fossa. Clinical diagnosis of intra-abdominal pathology is made more difficult by the presence of the enlarged uterus on palpation, and the risks to the fetus from irradiation mean that many of the common imaging techniques cannot be used.

Pregnancy has diffuse effects on the motility of the stomach, intestines and biliary tract. Most of these are hormonally mediated (**Fig. 7.16**).

Gastrointestinal effects of pregnancy	
Clinical problem	**Pathophysiology**
Gastro-oesophageal reflux	Reduced lower oesophageal sphincter pressure (progressively weakens throughout pregnancy) Raised intra-abdominal pressure
Nausea and vomiting	May be due to abnormal motility Exclude urinary tract infection, cholecystitis, gastroenteritis, etc *Hyperemesis gravidarum* (rare)
Constipation	Altered motility (progesterone-induced) Changes in diet, physical activity
Haemorrhoids	Raised intra-abdominal pressure Constipation
Cholelithiasis	Oestrogens reduce bile salt production* Progesterone inhibits gall bladder motility* (Cholecystitis risk *not* increased)

*May predispose to gallstones.

Fig. 7.16 *Gastrointestinal effects of pregnancy.*

CLINICAL PROBLEMS

Although the most serious gastrointestinal complications of pregnancy are those affecting the liver (discussed in chapter 4), symptoms originating from elsewhere in the gastrointestinal tract are much more common.

Nausea and vomiting ('morning sickness')

These occur in about 50% of pregnant women. Symptoms are worst in the first trimester, beginning as early as 4 weeks after conception. The nausea may worsen between 5 and 10 weeks, but usually resolves by the 15-week stage. Emesis is often worse during twin pregnancies. It is important to exclude secondary causes of vomiting, such as urinary sepsis, biliary disease or gastroenteritis.

Most cases are managed by eating small, frequent meals, but anti-emetics may be necessary in some individuals. The usual cautions regarding prescribing in pregnancy should be observed; suitable anti-emetics that are considered 'safe' include doxylamine, cyclizine and diphenhydramine. Metoclopramide is probably safe in the third trimester.

Hyperemesis gravidarum

This is a rare condition (affecting about 1 in 1000 pregnancies) characterised by persistently severe nausea and vomiting, together with weight loss of more than 5% and depletion of fluids, electrolytes and some B vitamins. Complications include hypovolaemia, renal failure and Mallory–Weiss tears. Patients should be admitted to hospital and resuscitated with intravenous fluids. Anti-emetic therapy and B vitamins are given as appropriate. An ultrasound scan should be performed to exclude multiple pregnancy or a hydatidiform mole.

Gastro-oesophageal reflux disease

This is also very common in pregnancy. It tends to progress, being worst in the second and third trimesters. Management involves introducing the lifestyle measures described in chapter 1, including stopping smoking, eating small frequent meals, raising the head of the bed and reducing intake of caffeine, chocolate and cheese. If drug therapy is necessary, then simple antacids should be used, such as magnesium hydroxide, calcium carbonate or aluminium hydroxide. Ranitidine seems safe during pregnancy, but there is presently insufficient safety data to support the use of proton pump inhibitors.

Constipation

Constipation in pregnancy is best combatted by taking an adequate intake of fluids and dietary fibre. Non-absorbable stool softeners (such as lactulose, sorbitol or magnesium hydroxide) may be effective, but stimulants are best avoided as they may increase uterine activity in some patients.

INFLAMMATORY BOWEL DISEASE IN PREGNANCY

Given that inflammatory bowel disease (IBD) tends to affect people most during the 'reproductive' years of life, pregnancy is not an uncommon event.

Ulcerative colitis itself does not appear to cause reduced fertility, although this may occur in some patients with Crohn's disease. A number of mechanisms may be implicated, such as direct inflammatory involvement of pelvic structures, dyspareunia, reduced libido, poor nutrition or the systemic effects of chronic disease.

The natural history of IBD is most often unaffected by pregnancy, although there have been some reports of active disease being suddenly brought under control and, conversely, quiescent IBD becoming more severe. The aim of managing the pregnant IBD patient is to

Safety of drugs used to treat inflammatory bowel disease during pregnancy

Medication	Clinical aspects
5-aminosalicylates	Generally safe Sulphasalazine may cause folate malabsorption (supplements necessary)
Corticosteroids	Generally safe Fetal morbidity and mortality unchanged
Azathioprine	Organ transplant studies suggest increased risk of prematurity Appears safe in data on IBD pregnancies Avoid during lactation
Cyclosporin	Little data on use in IBD pregnancies Not teratogenic in animals Slightly increased incidence of prematurity and growth retardation reported in pregnancies after renal transplantation
Methotrexate	Contraindicated in pregnancy Dose-related fetal toxicity Craniofacial abnormalities, growth retardation, prematurity Avoid pregnancy for several months after drug stopped
Metronidazole	Should be avoided during pregnancy Possible teratogenicity, particularly with high doses in first trimester

Fig. 7.17 *Safety of drugs used to treat inflammatory bowel disease during pregnancy.*

ensure a successful outcome for mother and fetus, which is aided by achieving a low level of IBD activity during the pregnancy.

There is a large body of evidence showing that patients with poorly controlled, pre-pregnancy IBD are at higher risk of pre-term delivery. Reassuringly, there appears to be no increase in the incidence of stillbirths or congenital abnormalities.

Careful consideration is given to the risk:benefit ratio for the drugs used to treat IBD in pregnancy (**Fig. 7.17**). In general, treatment that has successfully maintained the mother in remission before conception should be continued during the pregnancy, as withdrawal may expose both mother and fetus to the risks of uncontrolled IBD.

For the newer immunomodulatory drugs, such as cyclosporin and azathioprine, women of childbearing age should be aware of the possible risks before starting treatment, as teratogenesis may potentially occur in the first trimester even before the patient is aware of the pregnancy. In the cases of those women who conceive whilst taking azathioprine or cyclosporin, the teratogenic risks are not thought to be sufficiently high, however, to justify elective termination.

HAEMATOLOGICAL DISEASES

Digestive disorders can certainly lead to haematological complications. Examples include pernicious anaemia, iron deficiency and both hypersplenism and splenic atrophy. However, certain blood diseases may also lead to profound effects on the gastrointestinal tract.

LYMPHOMA

Lymphomas that occur in the gut may have their primary origin there or may have spread from elsewhere. Indeed, the gastrointestinal tract is the commonest extranodal site of spread for lymphomas. Any part of the gut may be affected, although the most common sites are the stomach, small bowel, caecum and colon. The vast majority are of B cell origin (**Fig. 7.18**), although there are certain variants.

For example, some low-grade gastric lymphomas have the morphological appearance of mucosa-associated lymphoid tissue (MALT). These 'MALTomas' have been closely linked to *Helicobacter pylori* infection and there have been a number of reports of lymphoma regression after successful *Helicobacter* eradication therapy.

Approximately 10% of patients with coeliac disease will develop a small intestinal lymphoma, known as enteropathy-associated T-cell lymphoma (EATL), which seems to originate from intra-epithelial T8 lymphocytes. An example is shown in **Fig. 2.23**.

The clinical features of gastrointestinal lymphomas depend to a large extent on the site involved. In many cases, general malaise and so-called 'B symptoms' (fevers, night sweats, loss of more than 10% body weight) are found.

Treatment methods also depend on the grade, stage and site of the lymphoma but will usually involve surgery, chemotherapy or radiotherapy. Surgery can be particularly important in debulking or resecting small bowel lymphomas, as successful radiotherapy or chemotherapy may cause perforation or bleeding as the lymphoma becomes necrotic.

LEUKAEMIAS

Gastrointestinal complications frequently occur in patients with leukaemia. These can relate to the disease process itself, the development of immunodeficiency and the adverse effects of chemotherapy, radiotherapy and bone marrow transplantation.

Direct leukaemic invasion of the gut may occur and lead to ulceration, polypoid lesions, intussusception and bleeding, the latter made much worse by the frequent coexistence of thrombocytopenia or coagulopathy.

Leukaemic patients are at risk of opportunistic infections and further immunosuppression occurs with the neutropenic states induced by chemotherapy and the pre-engraftment phase of bone marrow transplantation (**Fig. 7.19**).

Patients who undergo an allogeneic bone marrow transplant (BMT) can develop many possible gastrointestinal complications, which range from the almost ubiquitous oral

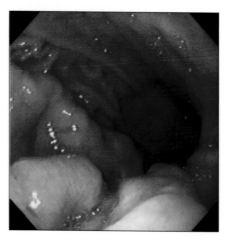

Fig. 7.18 Gastric lymphoma. This 72-year-old man presented with anaemia and weight loss. The gastroscopic view demonstrates grossly enlarged mucosal folds with a 2 cm ulcer visible in the foreground. Biopsy specimens revealed a high-grade B-cell lymphoma.

Gastrointestinal complications of allogeneic bone marrow transplantation

Complications related to pre-transplant conditioning (chemotherapy and total body irradiation)	Nausea and vomiting Abdominal pain Diarrhoea Brush-border enzyme deficiencies Abnormal liver function tests Hepatic veno-occlusive disease Pancreatitis Radiation enteritis
Neutropenia and immunosuppression	Early (first month): bacteria, fungi Later (second month): viruses Mucositis Gram-negative sepsis Bacteraemias post-endoscopy Candidal oesophagitis, hepatitis Antibiotic-associated diarrhoeas Antiviral drug reactions Cytomegalovirus (CMV) oesophagitis, hepatitis, colitis *Herpes simplex* virus (HSV) oesophagitis, hepatitis, colitis Disseminated varicella zoster
Graft versus host disease (GvHD)	Acute cholestasis Diarrhoea Mucositis Gastrointestinal bleeding Chronic ductopenic cholestasis Intestinal strictures Chronic malabsorption
Late complications	Chronic GvHD Gastrointestinal B-cell lymphomas

Fig. 7.19 *Gastrointestinal complications of allogeneic bone marrow transplantation.*

mucositis (painful and distressing stomatitis) to life-threatening conditions such as hepatic veno-occlusive disease (VOD). Mucositis is managed with analgesia, topical anaesthetics, antifungals and mouthwashes.

Hepatic VOD is thought to be related to pre-transplant conditioning with high-dose chemotherapy and total body irradiation. It tends to develop in the first 100 days post-transplant and is often fatal. Patients may present with hepatomegaly, portal hypertension, ascites, jaundice and abnormal liver function tests. The differential diagnosis can be wide, as post-BMT hepatic disorders may occur with graft versus host disease, viral hepatitis, drug reactions and critical illness-related ductopenia. Hepatic venography with wedged portal venous pressure measurement may be diagnostic and also allows an opportunity for transjugular liver biopsy.

Graft versus host disease (GvHD) occurs in two distinct forms: an early (1–3 months post-transplant) acute form and a later (beginning 3–12 months post-BMT) chronic disease. Once the newly transplanted marrow engrafts, an immune response may be mounted against the host's own tissues.

Acute GvHD is characterised by a triad of effects on the skin, liver and gastrointestinal tract. There is often inflammation, ulceration and sloughing of intestinal mucosa which leads to diarrhoea and sometimes severe gastrointestinal bleeding. Histological biopsies taken at gastroscopy or sigmoidoscopy may be diagnostic. Treatment is by manipulation of the immunosuppressive therapy. One recent study has suggested that prophylactic administration of ursodeoxycholic acid may reduce the incidence of hepatic GvHD.

Chronic GvHD has a more insidious course and in many ways resembles systemic sclerosis. Complications include fibrotic intestinal strictures, malabsorption and a chronic ductopenic cholestasis.

HYPERCOAGULABLE STATES

Thrombosis of the hepatic, portal and mesenteric veins may be the result of myeloproliferative disorders such as polycythemia rubra vera, chronic myeloid leukaemia, myelofibrosis and essential thrombocythaemia. Such diseases are the commonest cause of the Budd–Chiari syndrome in adults.

DRUGS, ALCOHOL AND THE GUT

Adverse reactions to therapeutic drugs are a common source of gastrointestinal complaints. 'Recreational' drug use may also have gastrointestinal consequences, particularly in the case of alcohol abuse. The hepatic manifestations of alcoholism are discussed in chapter 4. Many of the common gastrointestinal problems induced by drugs are shown in **Fig. 7.20**

Drug-induced gastrointestinal problems		
Clinical Manifestation	**Associated Drugs**	**Mechanisms**
Nausea and vomiting	Many examples: Metronidazole Erythromycin Iron preparations Potassium supplements NSAIDs Theophyllines Alcohol Digoxin Opiates L-Dopa Cytotoxic drugs	Gastric irritation Chemoreceptor trigger zone
Heartburn and oesophagitis	Alcohol Anticholinergics Phenothiazines Calcium antagonists NSAIDs Potassium chloride Tetracyclines	Relax lower oesophageal sphincter Mucosal injury

Fig. 7.20 *Drug-induced gastrointestinal problems.*

Drug-induced gastrointestinal problems

Clinical manifestation	Associated drugs	Mechanisms
Dyspepsia, gastritis and peptic ulceration	NSAIDs Alcohol Cytotoxic drugs Oral gold	Direct mucosal injury Diminished mucosal protection
Pancreatitis	Alcohol Corticosteroids Azathioprine Thiazide diuretics Didanosine Pentamidine Oestrogens Sulphonamides Many others	
Diarrhoea	Numerous antibiotics Erythromycin H$_2$ antagonists, proton pump inhibitors Magnesium salts Sorbitol Acarbose	*Clostridium difficile* infection Stimulation of motilin receptors Increased enteric infections Osmotic diarrhoea
	Alcohol Beta-blockers Misoprostol Salicylates Bile acids Colchicine Constipating drugs (see below)	Altered bowel motility Increased bacterial colonisation Elevated faecal bile acids Direct mucosal toxicity Increased motility Increased motility Increased intestinal secretions Increased intestinal secretions Colonic irritation Villous atrophy Fat malabsorption Overflow diarrhoea
Constipation	Opioids Anticholinergics Tricyclic antidepressants Gonadorelin analogues Mebeverine Sucralfate Iron Chronic laxative abuse Vinca alkaloids	Reduced motility Enteric neurotoxicity
Colitis	NSAIDs Antibiotics Penicillamine Oral gold	Mucosal injury Pseudomembranous colitis
Colonic strictures	Pancreatin (high potency)	Fibrosing colonopathy

Fig. 7.20 *(Cont).*

NSAIDS AND ULCERATION

The first NSAID, aspirin, became widely available in 1898. The drug proved hugely successful, but within a few years reports began to appear of an association with gastric toxicity, leading to erosions, ulcers and bleeding. Pharmaceutical manufacturers have since searched for less toxic drugs and from the 1960s onwards there have been numerous new NSAID drugs brought to the market. Gastrointestinal toxicity has not been avoided, however, and these drugs remain a source of considerable morbidity, not least in the elderly.

The scale of the problem

In the UK, there are currently over 20 different non-aspirin NSAIDs on the market. They provide symptomatic benefit for a great many patients and are among the most commonly prescribed agents in medical practice. However, adverse effects are common and may affect the gastrointestinal tract, skin, kidneys, bone marrow, bronchial smooth muscle and central nervous system. Indeed, NSAIDs have provided the UK's Committee on the Safety of Medicines (CSM) with more 'yellow card' adverse event reports than any other class of drug.

The consumption of NSAIDs, both prescribed and sold over-the-counter, has risen steadily since the 1970s, particularly amongst women and the elderly. In the USA, each year, approximately 1 in 7 adults will receive treatment with an NSAID. About 30% of the elderly will receive either aspirin or another NSAID in a given 12-month period.

NSAIDs may cause inflammation and ulceration in almost any part of the gastrointestinal tract, from the oesophagus to the colon. Small intestinal ulceration and bleeding, for example, is well recognised and the drugs may exacerbate cases of ulcerative colitis. However, the most significant problems have been with NSAID-induced gastric and duodenal ulceration and their complications.

Mechanisms of toxicity and clinical consequences

Nobel prize-winning studies by John Vane demonstrated that the inhibition of prostaglandin synthesis by the enzyme cyclo-oxygenase (COX) formed the basis of NSAID-induced analgesia, as well as the adverse effects on the gut and kidney. Mucosal prostaglandins have a key role in protecting the gastric mucosa against damage from acidity, alcohol, bile, hypertonic solutes and heat. Prostaglandins (mainly E_2, I_2 and $F_{2\alpha}$) encourage the secretion of protective mucus and bicarbonate, increase mucosal blood flow and help stabilise membrane phospholipids.

Endoscopic studies have shown that gastric erosions can develop within 90 minutes of a single 75 mg oral dose of aspirin. Theoretically, such erosions may develop into ulcers with sustained NSAID administration and lead to haemorrhage or perforation, both of which are 3–4 times more common in NSAID users than control populations.

About one-third of patients taking an NSAID will develop dyspeptic symptoms. Gastric or duodenal ulcers can be found endoscopically in 20–30% of all NSAID users, many of whom are asymptomatic (**Fig. 7.21**).

Epidemiologically, NSAID-related ulceration is a major problem, reflecting their widespread use. For the individual patient, however, the absolute risks seem less dramatic. NSAID users can expect to be hospitalised due to a gastrointestinal complication once every 40–50 patient-years. It is possible to identify certain risk factors, related to characteristics of the patient and their individual drug therapy (**Fig. 7.22**).

Certain risk factors, such as a dose-response relationship, are well established. Recently, a number of large case-control studies and epidemiological data have identified marked differences between individual NSAIDs. The incidence of serious gastrointestinal complications in patients taking azapropazone is over ten times that seen with ibuprofen.

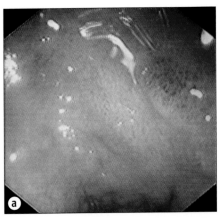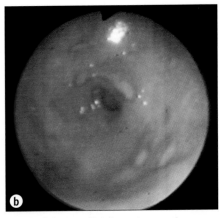

Fig. 7.21 *Gastroduodenal pathology in NSAID users. (a) Superficial erosions and mucosal inflammation are common findings in patients taking NSAID therapy, as shown here in the duodenum. (b) Multiple pre-pyloric gastric ulcers in a patient taking diclofenac to relieve arthritic symptoms.*

Risk factors for NSAID-related gastroduodenal ulcers and their complications	
Patient age	Absolute risk increases with age
Past medical history	Previous peptic ulcer disease Bleeding diathesis
Other medication	Corticosteroids increase ulceration risk Bleeding more likely with warfarin use

Type of NSAID prescribed	Highest risk
	  Azapropazone
	High risk
	  Piroxicam
	  Ketoprofen
	Medium risk
	  Diclofenac
	  Indomethacin
	  Naproxen
	Low risk
	  Ibuprofen

NSAID dosage	Risk increases with dose Possibility of increased risk in first 3 months of therapy

Fig. 7.22 *Risk factors for NSAID-related gastroduodenal ulcers and their complications.*

Some risk factors remain controversial. Approximately half of all NSAID-related acute upper gastrointestinal haemorrhages occur in the first 3 months after initiating therapy. This presumably reflects some 'unmasking' of previously silent peptic ulceration. The significance of concomitant infection with *H. pylori* in patients taking NSAIDs is also in dispute. The data have often been contradictory as to whether or not *H. pylori* increases the risk of bleeding in NSAID users, but in general it appears that NSAIDs and *H. pylori* act independently (rather than additionally) as ulcerogenic agents. Interestingly, a number of studies have shown that *Helicobacter*-positive NSAID users achieve better protection with acid-suppressing drugs than uninfected individuals. Possible mechanisms for a protective effect of *H. pylori* include a stimulation of mucosal prostaglandin secretion by the bacterium and the higher intragastric pH seen in infected patients. This area remains the subject of intense study.

MINIMISING NSAID TOXICITY

A knowledge of the risks of NSAID-associated complications should lead to more rational usage of these drugs and certain steps can be taken to reduce the incidence of adverse events (**Fig. 7.23**).

Recent studies have demonstrated that there are two forms of cyclo-oxygenase in the body: COX-1, which is constitutively expressed in gastric mucosal protection, and COX-2, which is induced elsewhere at sites of inflammation. This finding has prompted a search for selective COX-2 inhibitors, which could reduce pain and inflammation without significantly damaging the gastrointestinal tract. One such drug, meloxicam, has recently been marketed and early reports suggest fewer gastroduodenal side-effects than with similar NSAIDs such as piroxicam. However, COX-2 can be induced in the gastrointestinal tract at sites of inflammation such as colitis or at the edge of established ulcers, and this may be of significance in the longer term.

Enteric coating of NSAID has been tried in an attempt to reduce gastric injury. With the possible exception of aspirin (and even here the benefit is disputed), this does not confer any reduction in NSAID-related gastroduodenal side-effects. The pathogenic mechanism is related more to the systemic absorption and distribution of NSAIDs than any local irritant effect.

Co-prescription of certain 'gastroprotective' drugs may offer some prophylaxis against NSAID-induced ulceration (see **Fig. 7.23**). The gastroprotective agent, sucralfate, however, seems to have no efficacy as prophylaxis against NSAID injuries, which draws further attention to the fact that the proven prophylactic agents have antisecretory activity.

Suppression of acid secretion is an important factor in reducing NSAID injury. Interestingly, raising the intragastric pH may reduce the bioavailability of NSAIDs, as they are predominantly weak acids themselves and so are best absorbed (in a non-polar form) at low pH values.

When patients develop an ulcer on an NSAID, the drug should ideally be stopped as, even with antisecretory treatment, healing rates are slower if the NSAID is continued. At present, the data from clinical trials suggest that omeprazole is the most efficacious and best-tolerated treatment for NSAID ulceration. Whether this can be generalised to other proton pump inhibitors is currently unknown.

ALCOHOL AND THE GUT

Excessive alcohol consumption can cause significant injury to the liver and pancreas (see chapters 4 and 5). However, there are also numerous effects on the rest of the gastrointestinal tract (**Fig. 7.24**).

The morbidity of chronic alcoholism is often complicated by a combination of factors including poor diet, low general health and an increased risk of non-gastrointestinal illnesses such as hypertension, trauma, cardiomyopathy, neuropathy and tuberculosis.

Malnutrition is relatively common in alcoholics. Although ethanol has a high calorific content (7 kcal/g) and may contribute to obesity in some individuals, it has no real nutritional value. The poor dietary intake of many alcoholics may be due to adverse social circumstances, self-neglect, anorexia or persistent nausea. The postprandial pain of chronic pancreatitis sometimes acts as a deterrent to eating.

Reducing the risk of NSAID-associated gastroduodenal complications

NSAID prescribing habits	Use other analgesics 'Disease-modifying' drugs in rheumatological diseases Preferential use of ibuprofen Minimise dosage
Misoprostol	Prostaglandin analogue Reduces incidence of gastric and duodenal ulceration May be more effective for healing erosions than ulcers Shown to reduce hospitalisation rates (in one study, by 40–50% over 6 months) Dose-related side-effects, particularly diarrhoea May exacerbate colitis
Omeprazole	Recently shown to be better at preventing and healing NSAID ulcers than ranitidine At least equal to misoprostol 20 mg daily dose is as good as 40 mg Better tolerated than misoprostol
Ranitidine	Licensed for prophylaxis of duodenal ulcers only (not gastric) Healing rates worse than omeprazole
Nizatidine	Some reduction in gastric and duodenal ulcers, if previous history of ulceration or patient aged over 65 years
Famotidine	Standard dose protects only against duodenal ulcers High-dose regimen protects against gastric and duodenal ulcers
Modified NSAID therapies: **Cox-2 inhibitors**	Reduced rate of GI adverse events Do not affect platelets – may reduce severity of bleeding episodes
Nitro-ester NSAIDs	Animal studies suggest nitro moiety reduces toxicity Clinical studies awaited
Zwitterionic NSAIDs	NSAID preformed with phospholipids Increases mucosal protection

Fig. 7.23 *Reducing the risk of NSAID-associated gastroduodenal complications.*

A degree of malabsorption may be present, due to the direct toxicity of alcohol on small bowel villous architecture and active transport mechanisms. Exocrine pancreatic insufficiency and abnormal bile salt metabolism may also contribute.

Patients with alcoholic liver disease often have abnormal amino acid metabolism and decreased storage of certain vitamins and minerals. Certain specific vitamin deficiencies are common in alcoholics. Examples include vitamin A, thiamin (because of inadequate dietary intake and impaired hepatic storage and conversion to its active metabolite), pyridoxine, folic acid, vitamin C and vitamin D.

The serum levels of vitamin B_{12} are sometimes elevated, as a result of increased hepatic release and high levels of the specific vitamin-binding protein, transcobalamin.

Gastrointestinal effects of alcohol abuse	
Non-specific	Nausea Retching Anorexia Altered bowel habit
Mouth and pharynx	Increased risk of pharyngeal cancer Parotitis Signs of nutritional deficiencies

Oesophagus	Increased gastro-oesophageal
	  reflux
	Increased risk of oesophageal
	  cancer
	Mallory – Weiss mucosal tears
	Oesophageal rupture (Boerhaave
	syndrome)
	Oesophageal varices

Stomach	Gastritis Erosions Increased risk of NSAID injury Slow ulcer healing
Small intestine	Diarrhoea Dysmotility Abnormal villous architecture
Colon	Irritable bowel syndrome Increased risk of rectal cancer
Pancreas	Acute pancreatitis Chronic calcific pancreatitis

Fig. 7.24 *Gastrointestinal effects of alcohol abuse.*

GASTROINTESTINAL MANIFESTATIONS OF THE ACQUIRED IMMUNODEFICIENCY SYNDROME (AIDS)

Gastrointestinal problems are common in individuals with AIDS and affect almost all patients with the condition at some stage (**Fig. 7.25**). Indeed, certain gastrointestinal complications can be AIDS-defining events, such as Kaposi's sarcoma, chronic cryptosporidiosis or disseminated *Mycobacterium avium* infection. Diarrhoea and wasting are frequent developments in AIDS patients, as are oesophagitis and oesophageal ulceration (discussed in chapter 1). Less commonly, patients may develop hepatobiliary (**Fig. 7.26**) or anorectal disease (**Fig. 7.27**).

To some extent, the likely pathogens causing a given problem may be predictable, based on the patient's degree of immunosuppression. For example, infections with cytomegalovirus (CMV) or *Mycobacterium avium* complex (MAC) are more likely with lower CD4 counts (particularly below 100). A glance at the infectious agents listed in **Figs 7.25–7.27** will confirm that these organisms are often disseminated, affecting numerous sites in the gut and elsewhere (**Fig. 7.28**). The physician should always be alert to the possibility of unusual and atypical infections. One example, only recently described, is that of bacillary angiomatosis (**Fig. 7.29**), which may cause granulomatous lesions in the skin, liver, bones, brain or

Gastrointestinal problems in patients with AIDS

Diarrhoea	May be due to pathogens in **Fig. 7.31**
	Often non-specific, multifactorial (see text)
Weight loss	Reduced oral intake
	Malabsorption
	Hypercatabolic metabolism
Oesophagitis/oesophageal ulceration	*Candida albicans*
	Cytomegalovirus (CMV)
	Idiopathic oesophageal ulcer (IOU)
	Herpes simplex virus (HSV)
	Reflux oesophagitis
	Drug-induced (e.g. zidovudine)
	Mycobacterium avium complex (MAC)
	Histoplasma capsulatum
	Oesophageal neoplasia
Gastric ulceration	CMV
	Cryptosporidium spp.
Small bowel enteritis or focal ulceration	CMV
	MAC
	Cryptosporidium spp.
Colitis	CMV
	HSV
	Salmonella, Shigella
Gastrointestinal mass lesions	Lymphoma
	Kaposi's sarcoma

Fig. 7.25 *Gastrointestinal problems in patients with AIDS.*

intestines. The clinical picture of AIDS is often complicated by simultaneous infections with more than one pathogen and recurrences after courses of treatment are common.

These issues mean that patients are best managed with a symptom-based approach. The three commonest presentations to the gastroenterologist are oesophageal symptoms, weight loss and diarrhoea.

WEIGHT LOSS AND WASTING IN AIDS

Losing more than 10% of ideal body weight without an obvious cause is one of the primary diagnostic criteria for AIDS. The wasting that occurs seems to be the result of a combination of factors (**Fig. 7.30**), with preferential loss of body fat. Numerous studies have linked poor nutritional status to adverse clinical outcome.

Management of the patient with weight loss requires an evaluation of the most likely underlying cause. For example, in patients with chronic diarrhoea, a potentially treatable malabsorptive process may be identified. Continued weight loss is often associated with specific pathogens such as protozoal gut infections.

Dietary advice, enteral nutrition and (occasionally) parenteral nutrition may be of benefit in reducing weight loss. Some clinicians use anabolic steroids or testosterone as appetite stimulants and synthetic human growth hormone has also been shown to increase lean body mass in some cases.

Hepatobiliary complications of AIDS	
Hepatomegaly	Common finding (50–80%) Often non-specific, but may result from conditions below
Hepatic parenchymal infections	*Mycobacterium avium* complex Cytomegalovirus (CMV) Coinfection with hepatitis B, C or D *Microsporidium* spp. *Pneumocystis carinii* *Mycobacterium tuberculosis* *Cryptococcus* spp. Pyogenic abscess Histoplasmosis
Hepatic drug reactions	Sulphonamides (including cotrimoxazole) Zidovudine Didanosine Zalcitabine Protease inhibitors Nevirapine
Focal liver lesions	Lymphoma Kaposi's sarcoma Candidal abscess Tuberculous abscess Pyogenic abscess
Acalculous cholecystitis	CMV *Salmonella* spp. *Campylobacter* spp. *Microsporidium* spp. *Cryptosporidium* spp. *Isospora belli*
Sclerosing cholangitis	'AIDS cholangiopathy' CMV *Cryptosporidia* *Microsporidia*
Pancreatitis	Drug-induced (pentamidine, didanosine) CMV *Herpes simplex* virus *Mycobacteria* *Cryptococcus*

Fig. 7.26 *Hepatobiliary complications of AIDS.*

DIARRHOEA IN AIDS

Diarrhoeal illnesses are very common in patients with AIDS and have a significant bearing on their quality of life. There is a wide spectrum of severity, varying with the stage of the patient's illness and the relevant enteric pathogens (see **Fig. 7.25**). As well as being vulnerable to the same infectious agents as the immunocompetent individual, patients with AIDS are at risk of infections (often multiple and concurrent) with a range of opportunistic organisms. Importantly, finding a single pathogen should not necessarily halt the diagnostic process, as other occult organisms may underlie the current illness.

Fig. 7.27 *Anorectal complications of AIDS.*

Anorectal complications of AIDS*

Anorectal infections	*Chlamydia trachomatis* *Neisseria gonorrhoea* CMV *Herpes simplex* *Entamoeba histolytica* *Candida albicans*
Perianal abscesses **Perianal fistulae** **Idiopathic ulceration or proctitis** **Anorectal neoplasia**	Lymphoma Kaposi's sarcoma Squamous cell carcinoma Condyloma acuminatum

* These disorders are generally more common in male homosexuals than other patients. Anorectal carcinoma, for example, does not appear to be purely related to immunosuppression and may reflect sexually transmitted papillomavirus infection.

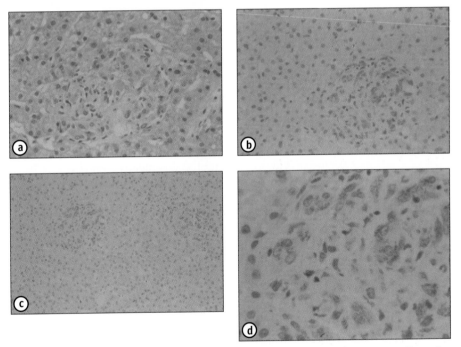

Fig. 7.28 *Hepatic infection with atypical mycobacteria in AIDS. (a) Haematoxylin and eosin stained liver biopsy also showing the formation of a granuloma. (b and c) Ziehl–Neelsen staining under low power. (d) High-power view.*

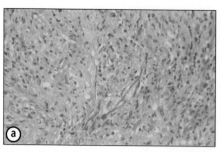
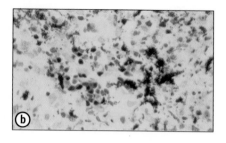

Fig. 7.29 *Bacillary angiomatosis in AIDS. Rectal biopsy specimens. (a) H&E stain. Histologically, the lesion is characterised by an inflammatory myxoid stroma. (b) Bacilli and eosinophilic granular clumps on Warthin–Starry staining.*

Causes of weight loss in AIDS	
Poor intake of food*	Anorexia Depression Neurological disease Odynophagia
Malabsorption	Small bowel cryptosporidiosis Intestinal MAC infection Secondary lactose intolerance Exocrine pancreatic insufficiency Bacterial overgrowth Villous atrophy
Increased catabolism	Acute-phase responses Circulating cytokines Increased metabolic rate Adrenal insufficiency

* Reduced oral intake in the single commonest cause.

Fig. 7.30 *Causes of weight loss in AIDS.*

There are numerous pathogenic mechanisms in AIDS-related diarrhoeas. Intracellular pathogens may lead to a loss of epithelia and consequently a reduced surface area for absorption. Villous atrophy and crypt hyperplasia are often found in the small bowel. Terminal ileal dysfunction, often the result of protozoal or bacterial infection, may lead to bile salt malabsorption or B_{12} deficiency. There may be alterations in gut motility and changes in the balance between mucosal secretion and absorption caused by inflammatory cytokines.

Localised enteric infection with human immunodeficiency virus (HIV) itself may also lead to diarrhoea. The mechanism seems to be a combination of local inflammation, antiproliferative effects of the virus and direct stimulation of vasoactive intestinal polypeptide (VIP) receptors by gp120.

Investigation of diarrhoea in AIDS

The diagnostic work-up for diarrhoeal illnesses in these patients is summarised as follows:
Clinical assessment
- Description of diarrhoea, stool frequency
- Stage of immune deficiency
- Previous gastrointestinal disease

- Medication history
- Dietary habits
- Signs of weight loss, dehydration, fever, anaemia
- Usual routine blood tests
  Examination of stools (at least three)
- Samples for microscopy and culture
- Screen for ova, cysts and parasites
- Specific mention of *giardia* spp., *cryptosporidia* spp., *isospora* spp., amoeba and *microsporidia* spp.
- Check for common pathogens including *salmonella* spp., *campylobacter* spp., *shigella* spp. and *Clostridium difficile*
- Send stool for AFB culture if CD4 count <100

Colonoscopy or flexible sigmoidoscopy, with biopsies*

- If no pathogen identified
  or
- No response to treatment
  or
- If evidence of malabsorption
- Upper GI endoscopy with small-bowel biopsies**

* Large bowel biopsies should be sent for microbiological culture, as well as histopathology, in order to increase the yield of bacterial pathogens.

** Small-bowel biopsies should additionally be sent for electron microscopy to aid detection of viruses or *Microsporidium* spp.

As the diarrhoea is usually related to infection, radiological investigations are seldom helpful. The most useful tests are the serial examination of stools (at least 3–6) for microscopy and culture, together with sigmoidoscopy and mucosal biopsy. In some patients, more invasive tests such as duodenal aspiration, duodenal biopsy or colonoscopic terminal ileal biopsy may be necessary if the above measures fail. Performing routine duodenal biopsies in all patients, however, seems unnecessary, altering management in less than 20% of cases.

The common opportunistic pathogens causing diarrhoea in AIDS are summarised in **Fig. 7.31**. The diagnosis of CMV or adenovirus infection requires mucosal biopsy (**Fig. 7.32**), which also detects a protozoal cause in the 10% of infected patients who have negative stool examination. In some patients, investigations fail to find a specific pathogen. This is more common in patients with relatively little immunosuppression, a low-volume diarrhoea and little or no weight loss. Most cases eventually resolve spontaneously and severe long-term pathogen-negative diarrhoea only occurs in about 1% of cases.

Treatment of AIDS-related diarrhoea

As with all diarrhoeal illnesses, resuscitation is required for patients who are dehydrated or have electrolyte imbalances. Where a specific pathogen is isolated, then antimicrobial therapy as listed in **Fig. 7.31** should be given. If the initial investigations have failed to isolate a cause, empirical antibiotic therapy (with a quinolone or metronidazole) can be efficacious in some circumstances, although there is a high rate of spontaneous resolution (up to 38%) of acute cases of diarrhoea.

Symptomatic treatment for chronic AIDS-related diarrhoea is often required and can be achieved with a number of different agents. Opioids such as codeine or loperamide may slow bowel actions and increase anal sphincter tone. Cholestyramine is helpful in patients with terminal ileal dysfunction.

Enteric pathogens in AIDS-related diarrhoea

Pathogen	Diagnosis	Treatment
Viruses		
Cytomegalovirus	Mucosal biopsy	Ganciclovir or foscarnet
Herpes simplex	Mucosal biopsy Viral culture	Aciclovir or valaciclovir or famciclovir
Adenovirus	Mucosal biopsy	Symptomatic treatment only
Bacteria		
Campylobacter spp.	Stool cultures	Ciprofloxacin or erythromycin
Salmonella spp.	Stool cultures	Ciprofloxacin or amoxycillin or cotrimoxazole
Shigella spp.	Stool cultures	Ciprofloxacin or cotrimoxazole or amoxycillin
Mycobacterium tuberculosis	Mucosal biopsy Culture	Rifampicin, isoniazid, ethambutol and pyridoxine for 9 months
Mycobacterium avium	Mucosal biopsy	Clarithromycin or azithromycin
Parasites		
Cryptosporidium spp.	Stool analysis (modified Ziehl–Neelsen stain) or mucosal biopsy	Paromomycin or nitazoxidine or azithromycin
Microsporidium spp.	Stool microscopy (trichrome stain) or electron microscopy of duodenal biopsy	Albendazole or metronidazole for *Encephalitozoon* or *Septata* spp. *Enterocytozoon bienusi* usually resistant
Isospora belli	Mucosal biopsy	Cotrimoxazole Pyrimethamine and folinic acid
Entamoeba histolytica	Stool microscopy	Metronidazole Paromomycin
Giardia lamblia	Stool microscopy Duodenal biopsy	Metronidazole or tinidazole or mepacrine
Cyclospora spp.	Stool microscopy	Cotrimoxazole

Fig. 7.31 *Enteric pathogens in AIDS-related diarrhoea.*

The somatostatin analogue, octreotide, may be beneficial by reducing intestinal secretions, slowing motility and inhibiting release of enteric peptides from neuroendocrine cells.

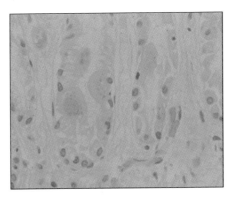

Fig. 7.32 *Cytomegalovirus infection.* *Rectal biopsy demonstrating intraepithelial CMV inclusions.*

Exocrine pancreatic secretions are also reduced, however, and this may worsen malabsorption in some patients. A reduction in diarrhoeal volume has also, somewhat surprisingly, been found with administration of NSAIDs.

Phenothiazines have some antimotility and antisecretory actions and can be useful in some cases of severe cryptosporidial diarrhoea. Bulking agents, such as ispaghula or methylcellulose, may help in certain cases by absorbing luminal water.

SEXUALLY TRANSMITTED GASTROINTESTINAL DISEASE

The gastrointestinal tract can be a portal of entry for sexually transmitted diseases (STDs) in heterosexuals and homosexuals, where there is orogenital, oro-anal or peno-anal contact:

Oropharyngeal route*
- *Neisseria gonorrhoeae*
- *Treponema pallidum*
- *Chlamydia trachomatis*
- *Herpes simplex* virus 1 and 2
- Hepatitis A
- Cytomegalovirus
- *Salmonella* spp.
- *Shigella* spp.
- *Campylobacter* spp.
- Giardiasis
- *Entamoeba histolytica*
- *Strongyloides stercoralis*

Anorectal route
- *Neisseria gonorrhoeae*
- *Treponema pallidum*
- *Chlamydia trachomatis*
- *Herpes simplex* virus 1 and 2
- Hepatitis B
- Cytomegalovirus
- HIV
- Human papillomavirus
- *Haemophilus ducreyi*
- *Calymmatobacterium granulomatis*
- Human herpes virus 8

* May be the result of orogenital or oro-anal contact.

If a gastrointestinal STD is suspected, a carefully taken sexual history should be documented. Particular care should be taken to establish the dates when the 'at risk' sexual activity occurred and enquiry made about travel to tropical regions or sexual contact with returning travellers. This may be especially relevant when investigating diarrhoeal symptoms. Specific enquiry should be made about activities such as oral sex or anal intercourse and whether there is any previous history of syphilis, viral hepatitis, herpes simplex or gonorrhoea.

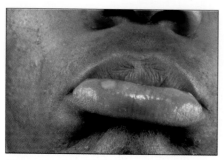

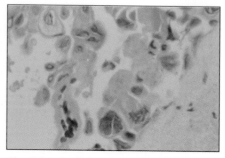

Fig. 7.33 *Mucosal lesions due to* Herpes simplex *virus infection.*

Fig. 7.34 *Anal* Herpes simplex *infection. High-power view of the anal mucosa, showing viral inclusions due to Herpes simplex.*

ORAL AND PHARYNGEAL LESIONS

Oral ulceration may be the result of syphilis or herpes simplex (1 or 2); the latter may also cause vesicular lesions on the lips or tongue (**Fig. 7.33**). Pharyngeal gonorrhoea is usually asymptomatic and should be sought by taking a swab from the tonsils and adjacent fossae. Patients with HIV infection may develop oral manifestations such as hairy leucoplakia, erosive gingivitis, Kaposi's sarcoma or candidiasis.

ANORECTAL DISORDERS

Pruritus ani is a common, non-specific symptom in anally receptive, sexually active individuals. It may be due to a combination of anal discharge, chronic anal fissures, fungal infections or hypersensitivity to lubricants.

Ulceration of the anal canal is a common manifestation of certain STDs. Primary syphilis may cause a single painless ulcer, but multiple lesions (which are usually very painful) are seen with anal *Herpes simplex* (**Fig. 7.34**). There is often an associated inguinal lymphadenopathy and a fever with the first attack of anal herpes, but subsequent attacks are usually less 'toxic'.

Anal and perianal warts may be the result of a human papillomavirus infection and need to be differentiated from the *condylomata lata* of secondary syphilis.

PROCTITIS AND COLITIS

Patients with STDs affecting the rectum and distal colon present with the usual proctitic symptoms of tenesmus, lower abdominal discomfort, bloody motions or a mucopurulent discharge. Colonic infection (such as with *Campylobacter* spp. acquired by the oral route) may present with bloody diarrhoea as described in chapter 3, and stools should be sent for culture. Proctoscopy and sigmoidoscopy should be performed. As mentioned above, lone ulceration is often a feature of syphilis or a chlamydial lymphogranuloma, whereas multiple painful ulcers are seen with *Herpes simplex* infection. Chronic diarrhoea in the absence of local colorectal symptoms should prompt consideration of giardiasis, which may be diagnosed by stool microscopy or on small bowel biopsy.

SEXUAL TRANSMISSION OF VIRAL HEPATITIS

Both CMV and the Epstein–Barr virus may be acquired by sexual activity. Of the major hepatotropic viruses, hepatitis A and B can be sexually transmitted. Hepatitis C infection can be transmitted in this way, although infection rates are relatively low (about 5% of patients' spouses are seropositive).

Index

scintigraphy (*contd*)
  diabetic gastroparesis, 340
  hepatopancreaticobiliary
    disease, 188–9
  hepatopulmonary syndrome,
    325–6
  hindgut, 108
  inflammatory bowel disease,
    108
  Meckel's diverticulum, 66, 86
  pancreatic neuroendocrine
    tumours, 309
  ulcerative colitis, 125
scleroderma (systemic sclerosis),
  342–3
  oesophageal dysmotility, 19
  primary biliary cirrhosis, 242,
    328
secretin, 168
SeHCAT (selenium homocholic
  acid taurine) test, 72
Sengstaken–Blakemore tube,
  260
sentinel piles, 102
serotonin
  (5-hydroxytryptamine),
    319–21
serum amyloid protein (SAP)
  scanning, 345
sexually transmitted diseases,
  217, 367–8
Shigella spp., 77, 315
shock, hypotensive, 10
short gut syndrome, 88, 122
sicca syndrome, 316
sigmoid colon
  colorectal cancers, 142
  diverticulosis, 134
  volvulus, 103
sigmoidoscopy, 110
  acute colitis, 113
  colorectal cancer screening,
    110, 152
  diverticulosis, 134
  ischaemic colitis, 121
  ulcerative colitis, 124–5
Sister Mary Joseph's nodule,
  312
Sjögren's syndrome, 241, 316,
  328
skin disorders, 311–13
skin prick tests, 347, 348
small bowel enema, 66, 84
small intestine
  absorption, 55
  adenocarcinomas, 88
  adenomas, 87
  anatomy, 53–4
  atresia, 53
  bacterial overgrowth, 69–70
  biopsies, 68–9
  carcinoma, 74, 88
  Crohn's disease, 84–5
  cryptosporidiosis, 81

cytomegalovirus infection, 82
  diarrhoea, 100
  digestion, 56
  duplication, 53
  embryology, 53
  endoscopy, 68–9
  haemorrhage, 64, 67
  Herpes simplex virus, 82
  hormones, 58
  immunology, 58–61
  intussusception, 67, 88
  investigations, 65–72
  leiomyomas, 88
  leiomyosarcomas, 88
  lymphomas, 74, 88
  microsporidiosis, 82
  motility studies, 72
  mucosa-associated lymphoid
    tissue (MALT), 58–61
  nuclear medicine, 66
  obstruction
    abdominal pain, 64
    neonatal, 53
    radiation enteropathy, 90
    ultrasound, 107
  parasitic infections, 82–4
  physical signs of disease, 65
  physiology, 55–62
  symptoms and signs, 62–5
  tumour blush, 67
  tumours, 86–8
  ulceration, 85, 356–8
smoking
  bezoars, 43
  Crohn's disease, 122, 130
  duodenal ulceration, 44
  gastric cancer, 40
  gastric ulceration, 38
  inflammatory bowel disease,
    122
  oesophageal cancer, 24
  pancreatic cancer, 305
  ulcerative colitis, 122, 130
sodium benzoate, 270
sodium picosulphate, 111
sodium valproate, 228
somatostatin, 299
somatostatin analogues, 260,
  309, 321
somatostatinomas, 309
Sonde-type enteroscope, 68–9
sorbitol, 155, 350
space of Disse (perisinusoidal
  space), 163
sphincter of Oddi
  dysmotility, 156, 288
  manometry, 184, 288
  motility, 168
sphincteroplasty, balloon, 288
sphincterotomy, endoscopic
  biliary dysmotility, 288
  chronic pancreatitis, 304
  gallstone pancreatitis, 297
  idiopathic pancreatitis, 294

spider naevi, 174, 227
  autoimmune hepatitis, 240
  chronic liver disease, 322
  hepatopulmonary syndrome,
    325
  primary biliary cirrhosis, 242
spiramycin, 81
spironolactone, 264
splanchnicectomy, thorascopic,
  304
spleen
  coeliac disease, 73
  portal hypertension, 176
  varices, 182
sprue
  non-tropical *see* coeliac disease
  tropical, 71, 74–5
Staphylococcus aureus, 78
steatohepatitis, 227–8
steatorrhoea, 62–3, 71, 173
  chronic pancreatitis, 302,
    304
  coeliac disease, 71, 73
  scleroderma, 343
  tropical sprue, 75
steatosis (fatty liver)
  acute fatty liver of pregnancy,
    228, 250–52
  alcoholic, 224–6
  microvesicular, 228
  non-alcoholic (NASH
    syndrome), 227–8
stents
  biliary tree, 185, 283
  chronic pancreatitis, 304
  oesophageal strictures, 25
  pancreatic cancer, 185, 308
stercobilinogen, 167
steroids *see* corticosteroids
stomach
  see also gastric entries
  anatomy, 1–2
  cancer, 9, 35, 40–42
  carcinoid tumours, 43
  digestion, 56
  diseases, 32–43
  embryology, 1–2
  heterotopic pancreatic rests,
    43
  infection, 35–7
  innervation, 1
  leiomyomas, 43
  leiomyosarcomas, 43
  lymphomas, 43, 352
  physiology, 6
  telangiectasia, 12, 335–7
  tumours, 40–43
  watermelon, 37
stomatitis, angular, 18
streptomycin, 80
streptozotocin, 321
string test, 79, 80
Strongyloides spp., 69, 75, 80
substance P, 255